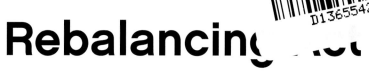

Rebalancing Act

Updating U.S. Food and Farm Policies

2012 Hunger Report

22nd Annual Report on the
State of World Hunger

Published with the generous support of
Margaret Wallhagen and Bill Strawbridge

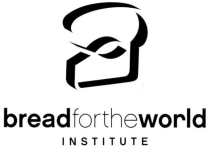

breadfortheworld
INSTITUTE

425 3rd Street SW, Suite 1200
Washington, DC 20024 USA
www.bread.org/institute

Bread for the World Institute provides policy analysis on hunger and strategies to end it. The Institute educates its network, opinion leaders, policy makers, and the public about hunger in the United States and abroad.

© 2011 by Bread for the World Institute
425 3rd St. SW, Suite 1200
Washington, DC 20024
Telephone (202) 639-9400
Fax (202) 639-9401
Email: institute@bread.org
www.bread.org/institute

Printer: HBP, Hagerstown, MD. Printed on recycled paper.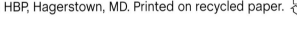

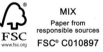

MIX
Paper from
responsible sources
FSC
www.fsc.org   FSC® C010897

Cover photo: Laura Elizabeth Pohl

Manufactured in the United States of America
First Edition Published in November 2011
978-0-9843249-2-7

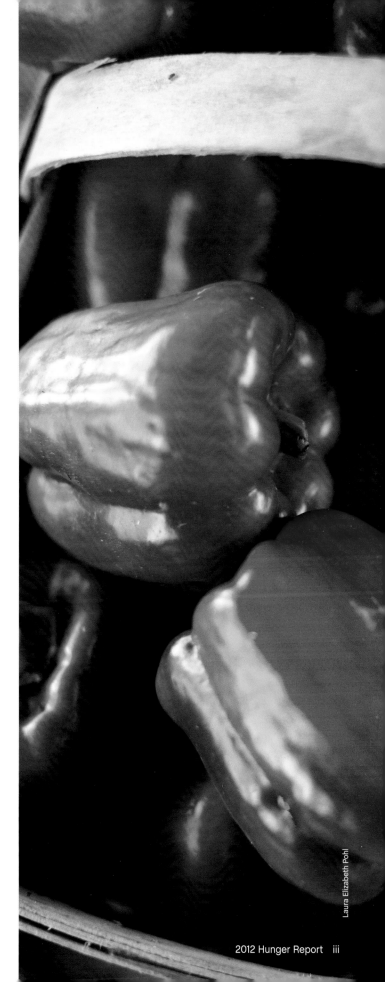

Laura Elizabeth Pohl

CONTENTS

CONTENTS

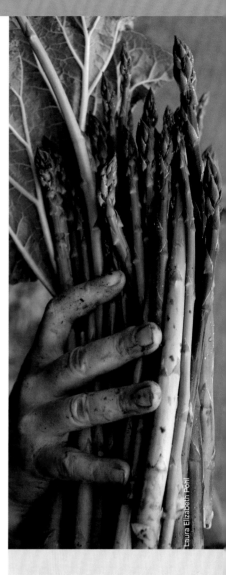

Laura Elizabeth Pohl

On the Web

For interactive maps and graphs, additional content, data tables, and other material from Bread for the World Institute, visit the Hunger Report website:

www.bread.org/go/hunger2012

CONTENTS

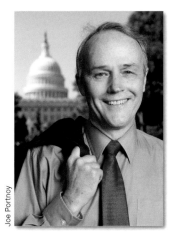

Joe Portnoy

Congress is starting work on a new farm bill at a time of increased hunger. One in five U.S. children now lives in a household that runs out of food sometimes. The number of hungry people in the world declined gradually for several decades, but has now surged to nearly one billion. This is also a moment of intense political pressure to reduce U.S. federal spending. Congress and the president have bound themselves by law to make deep cuts in the federal budget deficit.

A relatively small group of farmers, mostly large landowners, have long dominated U.S. farm policy. But budget pressures may finally help to achieve long overdue reforms that would make our nation's farm policies work better for farmers and, at the same time, save money for taxpayers. Bread for the World and Bread for the World Institute are focused on hunger and poverty, so we want farm policies that will help farm and rural families who really need help, protect the environment, and contribute to a nutritious food supply. We also want farm policies that will promote the expansion of food production globally, especially in low-income developing countries, in order to help reduce world hunger.

The farm bill includes SNAP (formerly called food stamps) and other food programs that help hungry people in this country. It's important to protect SNAP, which has been a lifeline for millions of struggling families, and the new farm bill could help to get more nutritious food into the school meals of low-income children. The farm bill also includes international food aid, which is a matter of life and death in famine situations such as the Horn of Africa today. This report explains how to use food aid dollars more efficiently and provide more nutritious food to hungry people around the world.

During the current battles over the federal budget, Bread for the World is working to form a Circle of Protection around funding for hungry and poor people. All the programs focused on poor people in the United States amount to 19 percent of federal spending. All the U.S. programs focused on reducing poverty in developing countries amount to an additional 0.6 percent of federal spending. Yet when the House of Representatives first formally proposed deep cuts in government spending in April 2011, it voted to take two-thirds of the cuts from SNAP and other programs for hungry and poor people. In the House's agricultural appropriations bill for 2012, it voted to take away nutrition assistance from 600,000 young children and their mothers who now participate in the WIC program and to eliminate food aid rations for 14 million of the most desperate people in the world.

It is possible to reduce the federal deficit without making poor people hungrier. Bread for the World members are campaigning to protect funding for hungry and poor people. The farm bill debate will present a clear choice between wasteful payments to large landowners and desperately needed help for hungry people.

The 2012 Hunger Report explores opportunities to rebalance U.S. farm policies. It stresses the need for a healthier diet—for all of us and, especially, for people who sometimes have to go without food. It recommends replacing the current patchwork of farm policies with a new system that would cost less, provide better help to U.S. farmers, and be better in other respects as well. It explores the continuing plight of U.S. farm workers and suggests a way forward that would be good for farm workers and their employers. It also documents the importance of food assistance in this country and food aid internationally and proposes reforms to make both more nutritious.

The government publishes annual statistics on hunger and food insecurity in the United States, and the data for 2009 and 2010 tell an encouraging story. Hunger surged during the financial crisis of 2008, but did not increase in 2009 and 2010, even though unemployment and poverty continued to rise.

The U.S. poverty measure does not include the income that poor people receive from government programs, while the hunger measure focuses simply on whether people are eating. So the hunger statistics for 2009 and 2010 show that anti-poverty programs are working. Notably, SNAP and the other national nutrition programs are now reaching 60 percent of food-insecure households.

SNAP and several other federal anti-poverty programs expand automatically when need increases and then shrink when the economy picks up. Congress and the president strengthened SNAP and other anti-poverty programs in 2009 and 2010. Groups like Bread for the World played a crucial advocacy role. Our grassroots efforts have helped to keep hunger at bay in a time of severe need.

There are lots of reasons to feel discouraged nowadays. The economy remains dour, and our nation is deeply divided by partisan differences. At times like this, we need to reach more deeply within ourselves for inspiration. I have been struck by reports showing that people who experience God as a loving presence in their lives are more likely to support government programs that help hungry and poor people.

I'm a Christian preacher, so it's my job to remind people that God loves you and me and everybody, including single moms who have trouble feeding their kids—and Somali moms who have trouble keeping their kids from dying of hunger.

Rev. David Beckmann
President
Bread for the World and Bread for the World Institute

ACKNOWLEDGMENTS

Bread for the World Institute wishes to thank the following people individually for their contribution to this report. Several people contributed articles to the report: Ken Cook, Environmental Working Group; Vicki Escarra, Feeding America; Matt Newell-Ching, Bread for the World; Jeannie Economos, Farm Worker Association of Florida; Ivone Guillen, Sojourners (formerly an Institute Immigration Policy Fellow); Philip Martin, University of California, Davis; Stephanie Hanson, One Acre Fund; Rebecca Vander Meulen, Anglican Diocese of Niassa (Mozambique).

Others who shared their insights: Robin Robbins, Appalachian Sustainable Development; Arlyn Schipper, Foods Resource Bank; Jennifer Fike, Michigan Department of Agriculture; Paul Green, North American Millers Association; Tianna Gaines-Turner, Mariana Chilton, and Jenny Rabinowich, Witnesses to Hunger; Thomas Melito, Phil Thomas, and Joy Labez, U.S. Government Accountability Office; Stuart Clark, Canadian Foodgrains Bank; Kathleen Kurz, DAI; Mary Minette, Evangelical Lutheran Church in America; David DeGennarro, Environmental Working Group; Adrienne DeVartanian, Miriam Strauss, and Victoria Kornick with Farm Worker Justice; Sophie Milam, Feeding America; Christopher Goldthwait and Mary Chambliss, food aid consultants; Jennifer N'gandu, National Council of La Raza; Jasmine N. Hall Ratliff and Arielle Traub, Robert Wood Johnson Foundation; Heather Hanson, Mercy Corps; Gabrielle Serra, Meridian Institute; Judit Ruis, Médecins Sans Frontières (Doctors Without Borders); Laura Demmel, National Farmers Union; Kendell Keith, National Feed and Grain Association; Eric Muñoz, Oxfam America; Elizabeth Kucinich, Physicians Committee for Responsible Medicine; Rick Swartz, Strategic Solutions; Charles Uphaus, U.S. Agency for International Development; Jay Hirschman, Lindy Haffey, Kelly Kennison, Jessica Shahin, Julie Brewer, Loren LaCorte, Tom Hertz, Cynthia Reeves Tuttle, Isabel Walls, and Christina Conell, U.S. Department of Agriculture; Daniel Carroll, U.S. Department of Labor; Allan Jury, World Food Program; Gabriel Laizer and Daniel Gustafson, Food and Agriculture Organization of the United Nations; Margaret Ziegler, Congressional Hunger Center; Marie Brill, ActionAid; Teresa Hendricks, Migrant Legal Aid; Beatriz Maya, Farm Labor Organizing Committee; Rubén Martinez and William Knudson, Michigan State University; Diego Reyes, Farm Labor Organizing Committee; Nancy Foster, U.S. Apple Association; Jerry Gonzalez, Georgia Association of Latino Elected Officials; Bryan Tolar, Georgia Agribusiness Council; Janine Duron and Chuck Barrett, CITA/Amanecer; Bert Perry and Lariza Garzón, National Farm Worker Ministry, Florida; Rob Williams, Florida Legal Services; Jeannie Economos and Elva Rincón, Farm Worker Association of Florida; Manuel Cunha, Nisei Farmers League; Dawson Morton, Georgia Legal Services; Greg Schell, Migrant Farmworker Justice Project; Lynnette Asselin and Mary DeLorey, Catholic Relief Services; Dennis Harding and Dave Miller, Iowa Farm Bureau; Chris Peterson, Iowa Farmers Union; Michael Duffy and Chad Hart, Iowa State University; Donald Coe, Michigan Department of Agriculture; Renne DeWindt, Food Services Director, Benzie County (MI); Doug Davis, Food Services Director, Burlington (VT); Lee LaVanway, Benton Harbor Fruit Market; Carey Miller, Iowa Food Bank; Kathy Mulvey, Community Food Security Coalition; Dianne Conners, Michigan Land Institute; and a number of farmers and farm workers from around the United States.

For helping us think through the Comprehensive Risk Management proposal, we wish to thank Bruce Babcock, Iowa State University; Dan Sumner, University of California, Davis; David Orden, International Food Policy Research Institute; Charlotte Hebebrand, International Food and Trade Policy Council; David Blandford, Penn State; Douglas Hedley, former Deputy Minister of Agriculture for Canada; and special thanks to Robert L. Thompson, Johns Hopkins University, and Stephanie Mercier, former Chief Economist for the Senate Agricultural Committee.

Finally, we wish to thank all of our colleagues at Bread for the World and the Alliance to End Hunger. Some of these deserve special notice: Tammy Walhof, Nancy Neal, Carter Echols, and Zachary Schmidt of Organizing and Church Relations for their work on the Christian Study Guide; Laura Elizabeth Pohl, Molly Marsh, Hans Friedhoff, Doug Puller, Kristen Youngblood, Racine Tucker-Hamilton, Jeannie Choi, and Adlai Amor for help with text, images and technology; Mannik Sakayan, Christine Melendez-Ashley, and Monica Mills of Government Relations.

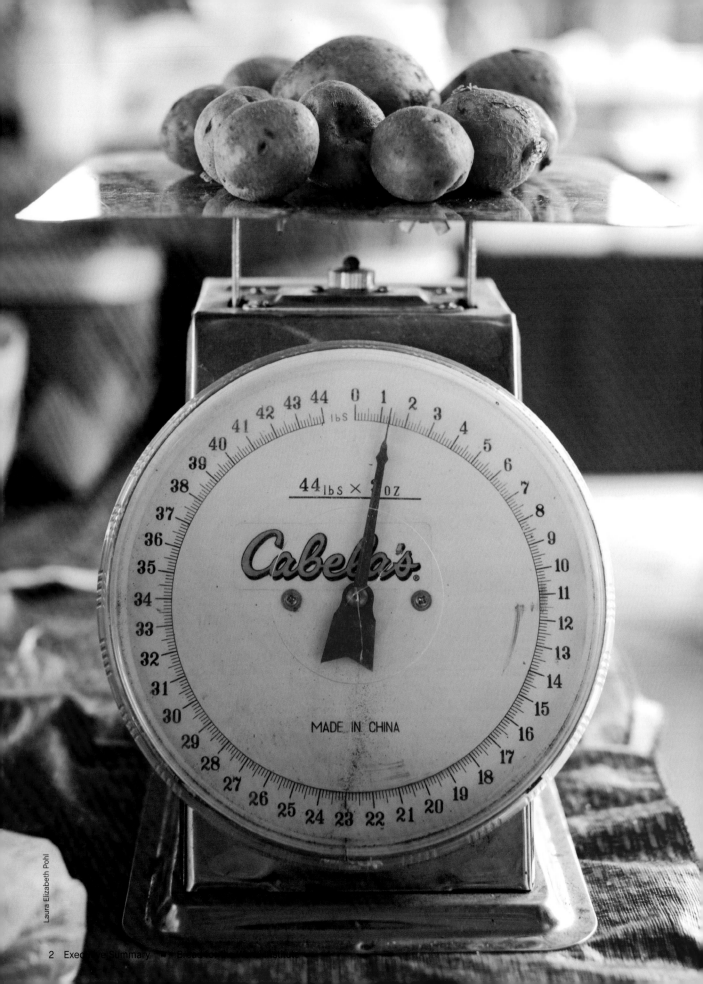

Rebalancing Act
Updating U.S. Food and Farm Policies

Scan the QR code below or visit www.bread.org/go/hunger2012 for updates throughout 2012.

On the eve of 2012, Congress is negotiating dramatic cuts in the federal budget. Cuts to programs designed to overcome the effects of poverty are in neither the short- nor the long-term interests of the nation. The recommendations in the 2012 Hunger Report are all the more relevant because the budget decisions are so urgent.

People may disagree about what items in the federal budget are necessary for the public good, but we take for granted that it's in everyone's interest for the government to fight hunger. In fact, there should be zero tolerance for hunger— no matter what the size, ideology, or other responsibilities of the government may be, it must do what is necessary to keep people from going hungry.

The 2012 Hunger Report recommends ways for the federal government to better respond to the agriculture and nutrition challenges of today and tomorrow. Normally, change in food and farm policy occurs incrementally. The 2012 Hunger Report calls for bolder, more determined thinking about how U.S. food and farm policies can meet the global and domestic challenges of the 21st century.

With one in four Americans participating in a federal nutrition program, the nation's nutrition and farm policies absolutely need to be aligned. Farm policies should significantly increase production of healthy foods. But farm policies alone can't automatically improve access to nutritious foods for low-income families. Strengthening the nutrition safety net is also critical. Nutrition programs need to do more than provide food for hungry people; they must ensure that healthy food is available to all.

The 2012 Hunger Report recommends ways for U.S. development assistance and food aid programs to work together more efficiently. Food aid programs should follow the lead of Feed the Future—the new U.S. Global Hunger and Food Security Initiative—by focusing more deliberately on improving nutrition outcomes for the most vulnerable people, especially pregnant and lactating women and children under the age of 2. This will help achieve the strongest possible nutrition and development outcomes with the limited resources available.

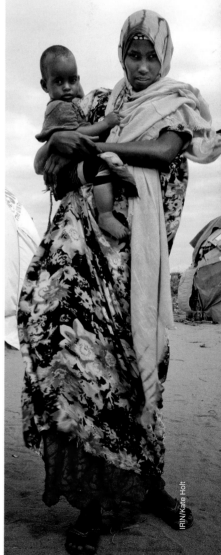

IRIN/Kate Holt

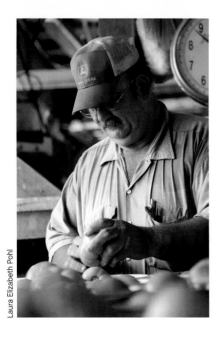

Laura Elizabeth Pohl

Chapter 1:
Farm Policies for Today and Tomorrow

America's farmers and the federal government are natural allies in the fight against domestic hunger and malnutrition—and this alliance is enshrined in the nation's farm policies. The U.S. public needs farm policies to ensure a safe and affordable food supply, to protect the sustainability of vital natural resources that agricultural production depends on, and to produce well-balanced, nutritious foods.

A cursory look at the U.S. food system reveals the latter—producing well-balanced, nutritious foods—as badly in need of attention. Rising healthcare costs associated with chronic diet-related diseases should lead policymakers to reassess the balance of farm policies. Current policies favor production of calories, not nutrients. Today, the United States does not even produce enough fruits and vegetables for Americans to meet the recommended daily allowances (RDAs) of vitamins and minerals. Thus, farm policies should lean more towards the production of healthy foods.

A rapidly growing segment of the U.S. population is demanding healthy, sustainably produced foods. Small and medium-size producers, the farmers best suited to meet this demand, receive virtually no support from U.S. farm policy. The largest, wealthiest producers of a limited number of crops are the biggest beneficiaries of government support in good times and in bad. At a time when they are earning record high farm income, it makes little sense for them to be the main beneficiaries of national farm policy.

Government has directed schools to serve children healthier meals, and when possible to source more of the foods used in child nutrition programs from local and regional producers, mostly small to medium-size producers. This merits much stronger support from policymakers. Not only would it benefit children, including low-income children, but also a great many farmers and their communities, reviving a connection between agriculture and rural development that once was much stronger.

Included in the 2012 Hunger Report is a proposal to restructure the current farm safety net. Income-support programs should be replaced by a more efficient system of revenue insurance, and support should be available to all farmers and based on principles of fairness and shared responsibility.

1 in 7 PEOPLE in the world is chronically **HUNGRY.**

9 billion
Population estimates suggest that by 2050 the planet will be home to 9 billion persons, up from the current population of 7 billion. This represents a 30% increase in less than 40 years.

Chapter 2:
Fortifying the U.S. Nutrition Safety Net

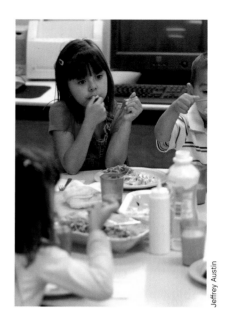

Preventing people in the United States from going hungry is the single most important objective of federal nutrition programs. In times of high unemployment and reduced incomes, government spending on nutrition programs increases to help people cope with these difficult economic conditions.

In the past three years, since the country plunged into a severe recession, participation in nutrition programs has skyrocketed. The economy continues to stumble. Millions of people can't find work or can't find sufficient work to support their families. The programs are doing precisely what they're designed to do: counteract the impact of the recession on families and help prevent the recession from getting worse. Once the economy begins growing again at a steady and sustainable rate, the number of people eligible for nutrition programs will be closer to what it usually is.

Federal nutrition programs go a long way towards reducing hunger, but they accomplish much less by way of ensuring a healthy, well-balanced diet. This is especially troubling since more than half of all participants in nutrition programs are children. Dietary habits form early in life and tend to last a lifetime. Rates of obesity and other diet-related health conditions are soaring, and the medical costs associated with obesity have risen to hundreds of billions of dollars a year. Thus, nutrition programs need to make greater efforts to enable low-income families to overcome barriers to purchasing healthy foods.

In the upcoming farm bill, policymakers have an opportunity to make the needed improvements to nutrition programs. The nation's largest nutrition program, the Supplemental Nutrition Assistance Program (SNAP), formerly the Food Stamp Program, is reauthorized in the farm bill. Most importantly, SNAP benefits must be maintained.

In addition, SNAP should continue to scale up incentives to use benefits to purchase healthy foods. The farm bill can also provide more healthy foods to schools and daycare centers. Allowing schools to purchase more locally or regionally sourced foods when possible would benefit struggling small farmers and rural communities.

About 1.4 million
The estimated total number of hired crop workers in the United States.

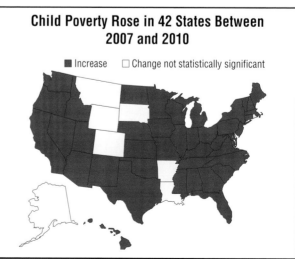

Child Poverty Rose in 42 States Between 2007 and 2010

■ Increase   □ Change not statistically significant

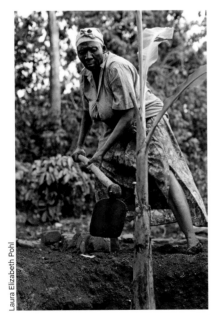

Chapter 3:
Farm Workers and Immigration Policy

For more than a century, agriculture has been an entry point into the labor market for immigrants in the United States. Presently, close to three-fourths of all U.S. hired farm workers are immigrants, most of them unauthorized. Their unauthorized legal status, low wages, and inconsistent and sometimes unpredictable work schedules contribute to a precarious economic state.

Immigrant farm workers fill low-wage jobs that citizens are reluctant to take. Attempts to recruit citizens for farm worker jobs traditionally held by immigrants have failed. In the absence of immigrant labor, farmers would be forced to shift to mechanized crops or stop producing altogether. Domestic production of fruits and vegetables—foods Americans should be consuming more of—could decrease significantly without immigrant farm workers.

In spite of the key role they play in U.S. agriculture, unauthorized immigrant farm workers labor under increasingly hostile conditions. The Agricultural Job Opportunity, Benefits and Security bill (AgJOBS) was developed cooperatively by farmers and farm worker advocates to address the status of farm workers. Public concern about unauthorized immigration by and large has held up prospects of enacting the bill into law.

The status quo is unacceptable. Farm workers should be able to work without fear of deportation, and farmers need a steady source of labor and assurances they will not lose access to workers they depend on. It is up to policymakers to help the public see the importance of immigrant farm workers to the U.S. agricultural system.

AgJOBS—or any agricultural guest worker program that recruits from Mexico or Central America—should include development assistance to reduce poverty in rural areas where these workers originate. Rural development can provide poor people with alternative sources of livelihood than migrating to the United States.

Chapter 4:
Rebalancing Globally

The United States responds directly to hunger and malnutrition in the developing world with food aid and agricultural development assistance.

U.S. food aid programs and agricultural development assistance are increasingly focused on pregnant and lactating women and children younger than 2. Even brief episodes of hunger among people in these vulnerable groups are cause for alarm. A third of all child deaths are attributable to malnutrition, while survivors face lifelong physical and/or cognitive disabilities.

The United States should strengthen its traditional role as the largest provider of food aid, while also moving quickly to improve its nutritional quality. New mothers, young children, and other vulnerable people, such as those living with HIV/AIDS, can benefit from highly nutritious forms of food aid now available. These cost more than the foods normally included in U.S. food aid, but it is possible to reduce costs by purchasing in or near the countries where they are needed and by phasing out the inefficient practice of monetizing food aid to conduct development projects.

The United States should strengthen its commitment to Feed the Future, the innovative U.S. Global Hunger and Food Security Initiative critical to long-term progress against hunger and malnutrition. Feed the Future represents the U.S. government's strongest support in decades for agricultural development in poor countries. The focus on agriculture is especially valuable because the vast majority of poor people in developing countries earn their living by farming, and the majority of these farmers are women.

The United States must make larger investments in agricultural research to help meet the global need to produce crops that can feed a growing population, respond to shifts in dietary patterns, and adapt to changes in climate. Current funding for both U.S. research institutions and the international network of agricultural research centers is hardly adequate to meet these challenges.

All poverty-focused development assistance is instrumental in helping poor countries achieve the Millennium Development Goals. Cuts to U.S. foreign assistance, including USAID's operating budget, would harm efforts to make foreign assistance more effective, efficient, and sustainable.

MAIN RECOMMENDATIONS IN THE 2012 HUNGER REPORT

- Farm policies should lean more towards the production of healthy foods.

- Farm policies should help to build markets for domestic farmers to provide nutrition programs with healthy foods.

- Farm policies should be linked to local and regional development of rural areas.

- SNAP, formerly food stamps, should at least be able to protect all family members from hunger for the duration of their monthly benefits.

- SNAP should include incentive programs that make it easier for recipients to afford healthy foods.

- Child nutrition programs should provide meals that meet established dietary guidelines.

- Unauthorized farm laborers should have a legal means of being in the United States.

- An agricultural guest worker program should include support for rural development in migrant-sending communities of Mexico and Central America.

- The United States should strengthen its traditional role as the largest provider of food aid, while also moving quickly to improve its nutritional quality.

- The United States should strengthen its commitment to Feed the Future, the innovative Global Hunger and Food Security Initiative that is critical to sustainable progress against hunger and malnutrition.

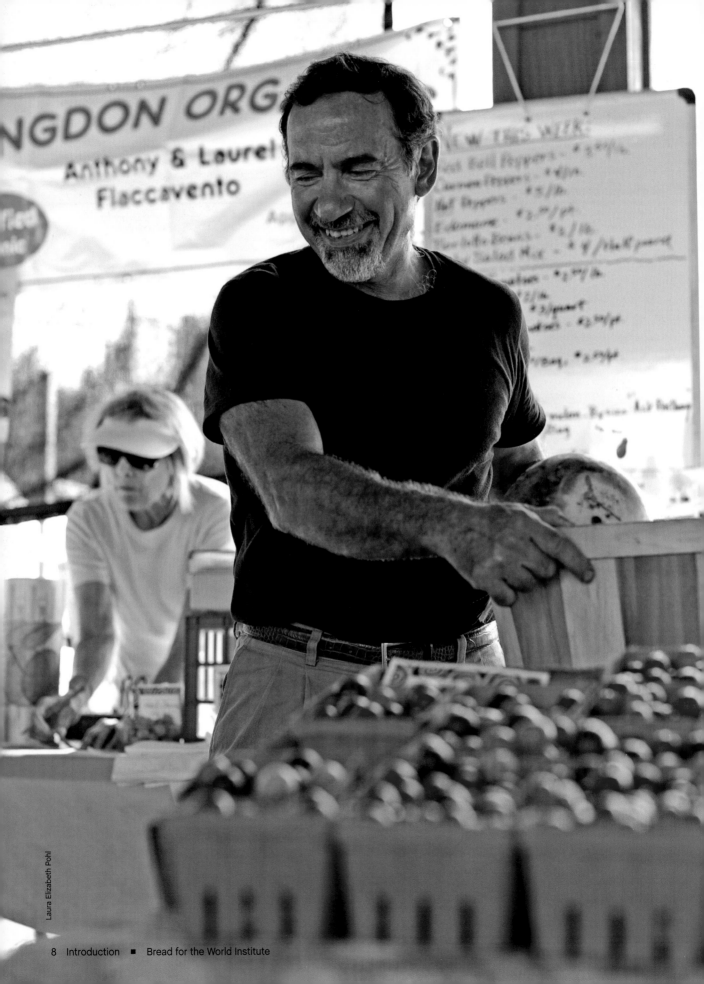

A Question of Balance

CHAPTER SUMMARY

The 2012 Hunger Report recommends ways for the federal government to better respond to the agriculture and nutrition challenges of today and tomorrow.

With one in four Americans participating in a federal nutrition program, the nation's nutrition and farm policies absolutely need to be aligned. Farm policy should significantly increase production of healthy foods. But farm policies alone can't automatically improve nutrition among low-income families. Nutrition programs need to do more than provide food for hungry people; they must ensure that healthy food is available to all.

The 2012 Hunger Report recommends ways for U.S. development assistance and food aid programs to work together more efficiently. Food aid programs should follow the lead of Feed the Future—the new U.S. Global Hunger and Food Security Initiative—by focusing more deliberately on improving nutrition outcomes for the most vulnerable people, especially pregnant and lactating women and children under the age of 2. This will help achieve the strongest possible nutrition outcomes with the limited resources available.

On the eve of 2012, Congress is negotiating dramatic cuts in the federal budget. Cuts to programs designed to overcome the effects of poverty are in neither the short- nor the long-term interests of the nation. The recommendations in the 2012 Hunger Report are all the more relevant because the budget decisions are so urgent.

People may disagree about what items in the federal budget are necessary for the public good, but we take for granted that it's in everyone's interest for the government to fight hunger. In fact, there should be zero tolerance for hunger— no matter what the size, ideology, or other responsibilities of the government may be, it must do what is necessary to keep people from going hungry.

Global hunger and U.S. hunger rarely converge as closely as they do in the farm bill. Normally, change in food and farm policy occurs incrementally. The 2012 Hunger Report calls for bolder, more determined thinking about how U.S. food and farm policies can meet the global and domestic challenges of the 21st century.

Introduction

Recommendations

- Domestic nutrition programs serve in both the country's short- and long-term interest by protecting people against hunger and by reducing the cost of treating diet-related health conditions.

- U.S. food aid and development assistance that helps poor countries to reduce poverty and hunger also can benefit domestic farmers by cultivating new trading partners for higher value U.S. agricultural products.

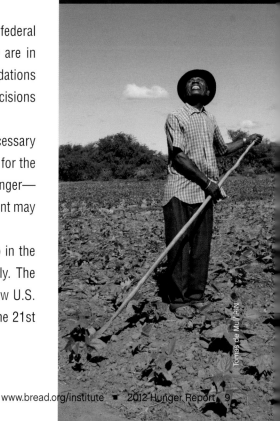

Tomás de Mul/IRIN

Policymaking is always a question of balance: balancing interests near and far, in the present and future, in the world as it is and the world as it should be. Soon Congress will begin writing the next farm bill, which must rebalance U.S. food and farm policies in ways that link agriculture with nutrition and health and promote viable, sustainable livelihoods for farmers—both in the United States and in developing countries. The 2012 Hunger Report aims to show how U.S. food and farm policies can achieve these objectives.

2011 brought Americans little peace of mind about the nation's economy. On the eve of 2012, Congress is negotiating dramatic cuts in the federal budget. Bread for the World and other anti-hunger groups are working hard to fight cuts that would harm people living in poverty. This report lends support to that effort by explaining how food and farm policies are inseparable from the problems facing people in poverty.

The recommendations in the report are all the more relevant because the budget decisions are so urgent. Cuts to programs designed to overcome poverty are in neither the short- nor the long-term interests of the nation. The report makes clear the costs of jeopardizing long-term benefits to the nation to lower the current budget deficit: it would be a Pyrrhic victory. For a less costly and more sustainable way to reduce federal budget deficits, the government should follow policies that promote economic growth, such as those included throughout this report.

Drought in the Horn of Africa forces people to flee their homes in search of food. Famine conditions persist in areas of Somalia.

As surprising as it may sound in view of recent political rhetoric, the budget challenges today pale in comparison with far more serious long-term challenges. Around the world, land and water resources are becoming scarcer because of climate change and unsustainable farming practices. Agricultural productivity may not be able to keep up with global population growth, in part because agricultural research has been starved for public support. Shrinking food supplies, and the use of food crops to make biofuels, such as corn to make ethanol, are driving up the cost of food well beyond what people in poverty can afford, including people in some of the world's most volatile regions. The 2011 Horn of Africa famine is just one result.

The United States, too, uses unsustainable agriculture practices. In addition, the United

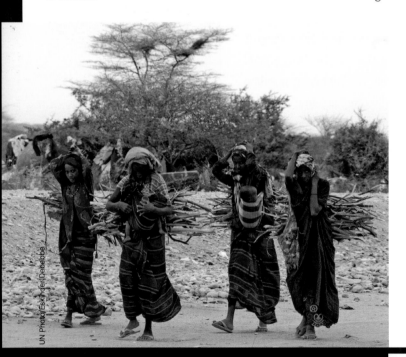

UN Photo/Eskinder Debebe

13 million

The number of people in the Horn of Africa affected by drought and/or conflict in Somalia.

Sub-Saharan Grain Yields are Lowest in the World

Tons per hectare

World

North Africa

Latin America & Caribbean

Asia

Sub-Saharan Africa

1990 92 94 96 98 2000 02 04 06 08

States faces an epidemic of obesity and the health problems associated with it. These are significant contributors to the spiraling healthcare costs that are the country's single biggest fiscal challenge. In fact, unless we get healthcare costs under better control—which will require lowering obesity rates—the U.S. government will have fewer and fewer resources available for other, non-healthcare-related needs.

The 2012 Hunger Report takes up these challenges and shows how to address them.

Public Goods Are Public Sector Priorities

As Congress and the White House debate over which programs to cut, we might take a moment to consider why it is necessary to use government resources to meet challenges like those just mentioned. Let's assume most of us agree that government resources should be used for public goods (things that are in the public interest), especially when the private sector has no inherent reason to provide these. Food security is a public good: people may disagree about what items in the federal budget are necessary for the public good, but we take for granted that it's in everyone's interest for the government to fight hunger. In fact, there should be zero tolerance for hunger—no matter what the size, ideology, or other responsibilities of the government may be, it must do what is necessary to keep people from going hungry.

The optimal solution to hunger is a good job that pays well enough for an individual or family to survive without help from public resources. But when the U.S. economy doesn't have enough such jobs—and is producing few jobs of any kind—the most direct way to prevent hunger is with federal nutrition programs. These include the Supplemental Nutrition Assistance Program (SNAP), formerly food stamps; the Special Supplemental Nutrition Program for Women, Infants and Children (WIC); and the school lunch and breakfast programs. Sometimes people find themselves in need of help from nutrition programs for longer than they ever expected, such as when long-term unemployment is at an historic high—meaning now. At such times, programs need

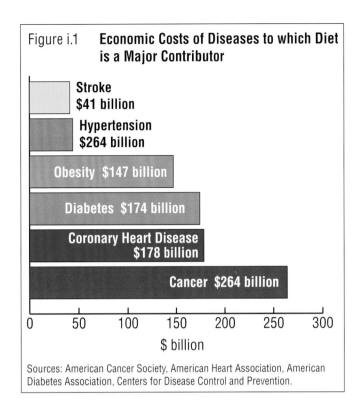

Figure i.1 **Economic Costs of Diseases to which Diet is a Major Contributor**

Stroke $41 billion
Hypertension $264 billion
Obesity $147 billion
Diabetes $174 billion
Coronary Heart Disease $178 billion
Cancer $264 billion

$ billion

Sources: American Cancer Society, American Heart Association, American Diabetes Association, Centers for Disease Control and Prevention.

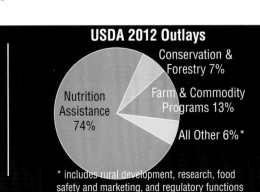

$98.5 billion of agricultural exports in 2009 produced a total domestic economic output of nearly **$227.6 billion** and **828,000 jobs.**

USDA 2012 Outlays

Conservation & Forestry 7%
Farm & Commodity Programs 13%
All Other 6%*
Nutrition Assistance 74%

* includes rural development, research, food safety and marketing, and regulatory functions

to do more than provide food for hungry people; they must ensure that the food is healthy.

Hunger is a direct threat to health. In fact, people who are hungry are by definition people in poor health. There is only a difference of degree: the severity depends on how long a person has been hungry. Even intermittent hunger can be harmful to human health.

In addition to fighting hunger, federal nutrition programs work against the related threat of obesity. The obesity epidemic in the United States is widespread, and its causes range beyond not being able to afford healthy foods. But this is a significant contributor to obesity; households that qualify for nutrition programs have higher obesity rates than middle- or upper-income households. It is also a cause that the United States should be able to eliminate through nutrition programs. In reality, however, sometimes the programs come up short.

The prevalence of obesity across income groups tells us something troubling about the U.S. food system writ large. Farm policies are implicated in this: they are designed to support a handful of commodities in producing an abundance of calories. Technology has enabled agribusinesses to process cheap commodities into more and more low-nutrient, calorie-dense food products; they can then sell them to consumers for lower prices. Mean-

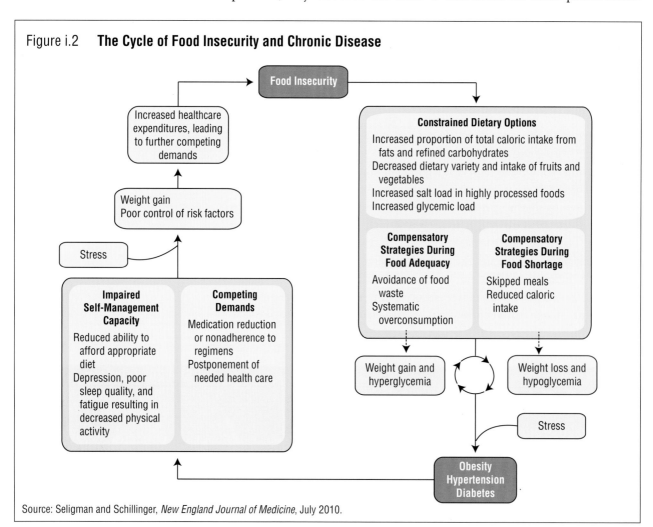

Figure i.2   **The Cycle of Food Insecurity and Chronic Disease**

Source: Seligman and Schillinger, *New England Journal of Medicine*, July 2010.

while, federal farm policies give virtually no support to crops with more diverse and healthy nutritional content. The policies have, in short, worked against a healthier diet for Americans nationwide.

In 2009, the Centers for Disease Control and Prevention estimated the medical costs of obesity at $147 billion per year.[1] A 2007 study sponsored by the Sodexho Foundation made a conservative estimate of the health-related expenses of hunger in the United States: $67 billion per year.[2] Undoubtedly, both figures have risen still higher since these studies came out. There is thus ample evidence that the cumulative costs of obesity and hunger are incredibly high. We can't afford them. This is why farm policies should focus on doing everything in the agriculture sector's power to contribute to better health outcomes—and therefore help reduce healthcare costs.

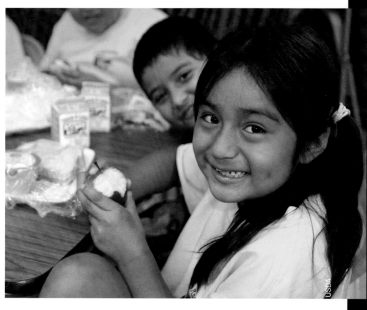

The National School Lunch Program serves 31 million children per day, two-thirds of whom qualify for free or reduced-price meals.

The 2012 Hunger Report is not recommending that farm policies directly subsidize production of healthy foods such as fruits and vegetables. Rather, policymakers should drop the current restrictions on farmers that discourage or prevent them from including these crops in their production plans. We recognize that production agriculture—the primary beneficiary of today's U.S. farm policies—has made significant contributions to reducing hunger by lowering the price of food. This report proposes reforms to federal farm policy that will help improve Americans' diets and equip the federal government to better respond to the agriculture and nutrition challenges of today and tomorrow.

Farm policy reform could significantly increase the nation's production of healthy foods. But farm policies alone can't automatically improve nutrition among low-income families. Two problems that fall within the purview of nutrition policy and programs must also be resolved: higher costs and less access. Healthy foods such as fresh produce still cost appreciably more than unhealthy foods such as fruit drinks and potato chips. It is also more difficult to find healthy foods in low-income neighborhoods than in wealthier communities, and these neighborhoods have a higher concentration of fast food outlets with cheap, unhealthy menu choices.[3]

Federal programs implemented through institutional structures such as schools can help solve these problems. The National School Lunch Program and the School Breakfast Program can provide children with healthy foods that otherwise might be inaccessible at home and in their communities. Late in 2010, passage of the Healthy, Hunger-Free Kids Act—the legislation that reauthorized federal child nutrition programs—signaled that lawmakers have this intention. Child nutrition reauthorization improved nutrition policies, but it would have a much stronger impact if the full weight of farm policy were also working toward the goal of better child nutrition. The 2012 Hunger Report shows how the two could work together to improve foods served in school-meal programs.

Focusing on school meals is particularly important. Far more frequently among children than among adults, obesity is correlated with one's family income. Also, research shows that dietary habits are formed early in life and are much harder to change when people get older.[4] But as we work to create incentives for healthier food choices among school-age children, we must also protect SNAP (the Supplemental Nutrition Assistance Program, formerly food stamps) and WIC (the Special Supplemental Nutrition Program for Women, Infants and Children). They must continue to work as intended, meaning that participation in the programs should rise in difficult economic times, when more people are in need.

Helping Ourselves by Helping Poor Countries

Some U.S. policymakers are convinced that rising federal deficits outweigh the value of U.S. investments in overseas development assistance. But evidence would suggest otherwise. In the long run, the U.S. economy benefits more by helping developing countries to reduce poverty, so that these countries become trading partners with us.

A few decades ago, the countries that are some of our strongest trading partners in Asia (South Korea, Taiwan, and Singapore, to name a few) had economies that were veritable basket cases—South Korea's economy was weaker than North Korea's at the time of partition[5]—yet these countries developed rapidly by historical standards, and their own efforts were facilitated by steadfast assistance from the United States.

At the time of this writing, the United States is on the verge of signing a free trade agreement with South Korea that is described by Democrats and Republicans alike as crucial to the growth of the U.S. economy. It's just one example of how consistent investments in overseas development pay off in the end, both for our partners and for us.

It's worth noting that U.S. development investments in these countries began in the agricultural sector.[6] The poorest countries are always agriculture-based economies, and the largest share of poor people earns a living in agriculture. When development occurs from the bottom up, the tide of progress carries poor people along with it. Growth spurs investments in education. Children can go to school rather than to the fields to support their family's subsistence-level earnings. Education makes it possible for countries to participate more fully in the global economy, investing in technology (much of it purchased from the United States) to expand their industrial capacity.

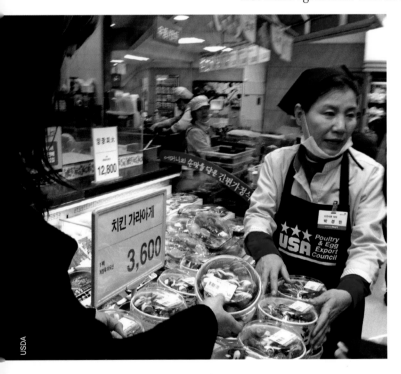

U.S. grain exports to South Korea began as food aid in the 1950s. The United States continued to provide food aid to South Korea through the early 1980s. Today, South Korea is a top commercial market for U.S. agricultural products.

U.S. investments in agricultural development through the Feed the Future initiative are helping partner countries that today resemble the South Korea of half a century ago. The initiative focuses most of its resources on Africa, targeting assistance to countries whose governments have a track record of matching donor assistance with investments of their own. Feed the Future builds on lessons learned in the Millennium Challenge Account and PEPFAR programs by providing incentives to national governments that work together with private sector and civil society groups to solve problems. The U.S. government works with its own domestic partner organizations in a similar way.

African governments recognize that agriculture is a sector that they themselves must invest in to catalyze economic growth. Before Feed the Future, many countries had already begun to do so, taking steps to realize the vast potential of their collective agricultural resources through greater regional integration of their economies.

Donors realized their neglect and began to catch up when a surge in food prices woke them up to the critical role of agriculture in development. In a matter of months, more than 100 million additional people fell into hunger because the prices of staple grains rose so dramatically. In 2009, in the aftermath of the worst hunger crisis in history not related to a famine, the U.S. government established Feed the Future. In 2011, volatile food prices again drew international attention to the plight of the world's billion chronically hungry people. Food-price volatility has become the new normal. (See Figure i.3.)

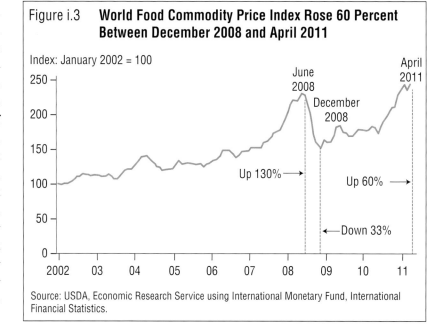

Figure i.3 World Food Commodity Price Index Rose 60 Percent Between December 2008 and April 2011

Index: January 2002 = 100

Source: USDA, Economic Research Service using International Monetary Fund, International Financial Statistics.

In our 2011 Hunger Report, we applauded the U.S. government for responding forthrightly to the hunger crisis. In the 2012 report, we emphasize how this is no time to pull back on the investments the U.S. government pledged in Feed the Future. It is also no time to pull back on food aid. Nothing the United States does for people in crisis situations around the world is more of a lifeline than food aid, a $2 billion annual investment that keeps nearly 50 million people each year from going hungry.[7] In the 2012 Hunger Report, we recommend ways for Feed the Future and U.S. food aid programs to work together more efficiently.

For example, we recommend that food aid programs follow the lead of Feed the Future by focusing more deliberately on improving nutrition outcomes for the most vulnerable people—who are pregnant and lactating women and children under the age of 2. In recent years, research has shown that nutrition interventions occurring at key times in people's lives—especially during the first 1,000 days from pregnancy to the second birthday—dramatically improve their developmental potential for their entire lifetimes.[8] All U.S. development programs should seize on these findings and incorporate them appropriately. In particular, the United States should coordinate the two areas most specifically focused on fighting hunger: the one-two punch of food and farm policies in the developing world. This will help achieve the

BOX i.1 STARVATION IN THE HORN OF AFRICA

by Faustine Wabwire
Bread for the World Institute

A catastrophe that was long forewarned is unfolding right before our eyes. The current drought in the Horn of Africa is the worst in 60 years, and the refugee situation is the world's worst humanitarian crisis. A combination of high food prices, failed rains, and continued conflict and displacement has put more than 12 million people on the brink of starvation.

By September 2011, the United Nations officially declared a state of famine in six areas of Somalia.[11] Among the worst-affected people are small farmers and agro-pastoralists who have no more stocks of cereals and cannot afford to purchase staple foods.

History teaches us that food shortages may be triggered by drought, but famine is not the inevitable result. For a famine to occur, it usually takes a combination of drought, extreme poverty, and, above all, political instability and weak governance.

Somalia has experienced several years of civil war and has been without a central government since 1991. In 2009, 3.2 million people were in need of food assistance as a result of internal displacement, conflict, and drought. The same combination of causes is responsible for the current tragedy, only this time it is much worse because food is so much more expensive.

In Somalia, prices of the two major commodities that are produced domestically, red sorghum and white maize, have increased by 30 to 240 percent and 50 to 154 percent in one year,[12] respectively, across the country. Prices of imported food commodities, such as rice, sugar, wheat flour, and vegetable oil, are also higher than a year ago.

Despite early warnings of looming food shortages as far back as August 2010, the World Food Program remained 60 percent underfunded by March 2011, and had to cut back its feeding programs in Somalia and Ethiopia. The value of early warning systems is rapidly eroded if not matched by a sufficient political commitment to early action.

The situation in the Horn of Africa underscores the importance of one of the recommendations in the 2012 Hunger Report—to take greater advantage of prepositioning food aid in areas where it is known it will be needed. It's better and cheaper to prevent calamities than to respond to hunger emergencies. Often, though, funds for preparedness and contingency planning are in short supply, while large amounts of money are spent on post-disaster responses.

In the Horn of Africa, long-term solutions are needed to mitigate the impact of future droughts due to the changing climate in the region. Focus on diversifying livelihoods and supporting indigenous crops will cushion vulnerable populations against climate shocks. Providing drought-tolerant seeds and livestock breeds that can withstand dry-land conditions can improve food security. Experience shows that long-term development requires sustained commitment from national governments and the international donor community.

The U.S. Global Hunger and Food Security Initiative, Feed the Future, is an important step forward in U.S. policy to support sustainable agricultural development in food insecure nations. But for programs like that to work in countries like Somalia, which are war-torn and without any government structures, it is vital to help restore stability. This will require stepped-up diplomatic efforts on the part of the international community, including the United States, combined with efforts to foster economic and social development.[13]

Faustine Wabwire is a policy analyst in Bread for the World Institute.

UN Photo/Stuart Price

strongest possible nutrition outcomes with the limited resources available, getting the biggest bang for the buck.

Over the next 50 years, Africa's population is expected to grow by more than that of any other continent. Quantifying the benefits of reduced global poverty for the United States is not easy. But, for example, 50 years ago China's per-capita income was roughly the same as the countries of sub-Saharan Africa.[9] Yet in the past 15 years, exports of U.S. soybeans to China have increased 26-fold.[10] As we help African countries participate more fully in the global economy, we help our own country by cultivating more significant trading partners.

Rebalancing and the Farm Bill

Global hunger and U.S. hunger rarely converge as closely as they do in the farm bill. As the 2012 farm bill reauthorization approaches, Congress confronts an environment dramatically different from the lead-up to the 2008 farm bill. The world has experienced many changes that bear directly on issues members of Congress will be deciding (see Box i.2).

The farm bill gives policymakers the opportunity to help solve both short- and long-term challenges to global and domestic food security. Provisions could include investing in agricultural research at U.S. land-grant colleges to develop ways to grow food in changing climate environments; helping farmers sell their products directly to consumers to earn higher incomes—including sales to millions of low-income consumers who now lack access to healthy, nutritious foods in their communities; rewarding farmers who put in place sustainable and responsible environmental practices; and, in international policy, allowing greater flexibility in food aid procurement and improving the nutritional quality of the foods the United States provides as humanitarian assistance.

Normally, change in food and farm policy occurs incrementally. Given all that has happened recently and all that continues to happen, however, we need bolder, more determined thinking about how U.S. food and farm policies can be reformed to better meet the global and domestic challenges of the 21st century.

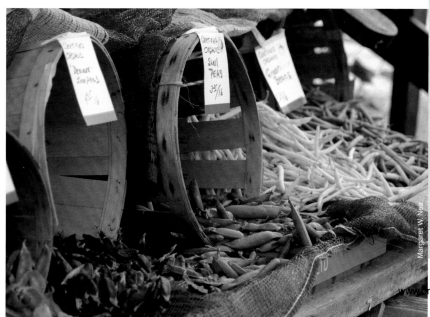
Margaret W. Nea

BOX i.2 A WORLD OF CHANGE SINCE THE LAST FARM BILL

- Volatile food prices and their disquieting effects on poor people and on geopolitical stability.

- Surges in food prices in 2007-2008, and again since 2010, which have exposed the deficiencies in the ability of the global trading system to deal with such shocks.

- Corn-based ethanol becoming a major contributor to food-price volatility.

- Growing concern about how the world will feed 9 billion people by 2050.

- Better understanding of the impact of climate change on agriculture and of how agriculture contributes to climate change and could potentially slow its impact.

- Better understanding of the importance of nutrition in human development in the 1,000 days between pregnancy and age 2, and the economic consequences of early malnutrition over a person's lifetime.

- Better understanding of the role of agriculture in promoting nutrition and health—and of the importance of linking these sectors through policies and programs.

- Rising public concern about hunger and obesity that is directing attention to policies that affect food production and consumption.

THE GOOD FOOD MOVEMENT

by Ken Cook
President, Environmental Working Group

"Food is *hot*."

I get that a lot these days.

Local food, organic food, slow food, whole food, real food, sustainable food; foodsheds, food deserts, regional food; food patriotism, food justice, food rules, fair food, peak food; industrial food, genetically modified food, superfood, food sovereignty, food celebrity, Food Network; Know your farmer, Know your food: it's all hot.

You don't have to be a foodie to know that even raw food is hot.

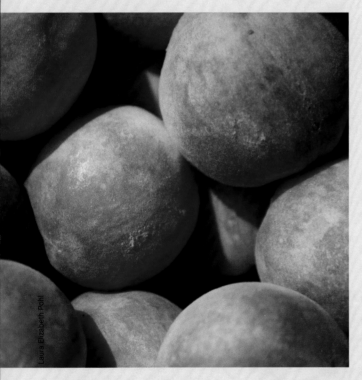

Laura Elizabeth Pohl

So what's not hot about food? The politics of it. The politics of food are barely warm.

Consider all the attention paid in recent years, from the White House to Wal-Mart, to the need to reduce the damage the American diet is doing to our spreading girth and diminishing health. Heart disease is on the rise, diabetes is epidemic. Most disturbing of all, America's kids are increasingly both overweight and malnourished.

Children in low-income households have a very good chance of being both hungry and obese.

This past year we had a remarkable opportunity to intervene as a society and get our kids hooked from the start on healthy food and healthy eating when the school lunch program was up for review in Congress. An intervention would have cost money—billions of dollars more per year than we're spending now, so that we could serve kids lunches with more fruits, vegetables and other healthy fare. But we would have saved many more billions than we invested, because healthy school lunches will reduce the lifetime medical costs of diet-related illness and boost the economic productivity that comes with a healthier workforce. En route to those long-term gains, we'd have kids who are happier and perform better in school—especially poor kids, for whom school lunch is often the only reliable daily meal.

So what happened? Congress did pass a new school lunch law, and that law did make some laudable improvements. But funding for the legislation was woefully short of what was needed to fix school lunch.

And how did Congress come up with the modest amount of money that it did add to the school lunch program budget?

By cutting the budget of the Food Stamp Program—known now as SNAP (Supplemental Nutrition Assistance Program). While benefits were largely preserved, the cuts still weakened a program that now serves a record 45 million Americans, almost half of whom are children—the very same children the school lunch program is intended to help.

Where was the food movement when this momentous policy opportunity slipped through our fingers faster than a canapé of sautéed ginger prawn on an heirloom-potato latka with mango-avocado purée and just a hint of sea salt? Where were the legions of passionate locavores when local kids had a shot at

THE GOOD FOOD MOVEMENT

tasting local greens from a school salad bar, instead of a ladleful of over-salted slop from the lunchroom steam table? Where were the critics of industrial agriculture and factory farms when the freezer truck backed up to the grade school cafeteria loaded with chicken nuggets, mystery meat, surplus cheese, and chocolate milk?

Where were we? Why, we were right there in the fight—on the merits, in spirit, in our hearts, maybe even on our blogs. It's just that not nearly enough of us rang the phones, fired off emails or darkened the doorsteps of the politicians who ultimately decided that America couldn't afford to feed kids well at school—poor kids in particular—beyond a bit of money scraped together out of another program that feeds those same poor kids. Another thing those politicians thought they couldn't afford? Offending the vested interests that benefit from keeping the school lunch program as it is.

We face the same disconnect between the broadly shared values within the food movement and our ability to give political voice and power to those values in the looming federal budget fights. What is at risk? Federal nutrition assistance programs for low-income Americans, international food aid, food safety enforcement, an array of programs that support local food initiatives, conservation of land and water, the survival of small and medium-size family farms…just about any policy or program you could think of that is in support of the "good food movement" is on the chopping block.

If you were to interview any food shopper, whether strolling through a farmer's market or a supermarket, or if you surveyed the leaders of any of the hundreds of public interest organizations working to reform our food system, I'm betting they would agree with every one of the following values—and probably many more.

No child should go to bed hungry or poorly nourished, at home or around the world. We should be safe from foodborne illness, know where our food comes from, and we have a right to know what's in it. Our food and diets should be a source of health and well being, not ill health and disease. The food economy should be one of opportunity, and its workers should be fairly compensated. Farm animals should be treated humanely. Agriculture should regenerate and protect the environment, not degrade it. Fresh, local, affordable food should increasingly be a commonplace, not a novelty, in American agriculture.

In order for the food movement to find the political voice we still clearly lack, we have to find ways to work together on the many values that unite us. Public interest institutions in the food movement have a special obligation to make this effort. It isn't easy or without risk. We have to fight our way out of issue silos that separate us and institutional habits that frustrate collaboration.

To my mind, if any organization is going to provide the leadership we need to capture the energy and passion of this new food movement and its shared values, it's Bread for the World. Bread for the World? No, actually, it's not that artisanal bakery in Sausalito where everyone goes for the fabulous rustic country 27-grain, gluten-free boule on the way to Pilates.

Bread for the World is a place where your heart meets your mind, introduces it to your spine, causing you to get off your duff to think and do something about the food someone else does not have—at all. Someone you've never met. Someone who's hungry, and who quite probably is just a child.

And then, after perhaps some prayer and reflection, Bread for the World is a place that helps you do something about it with like-minded friends.

That's the food movement I wish to be part of.

Ken Cook is president and co-founder of the Environmental Working Group (EWG), a public interest research and advocacy organization focused on protecting human health and the environment.

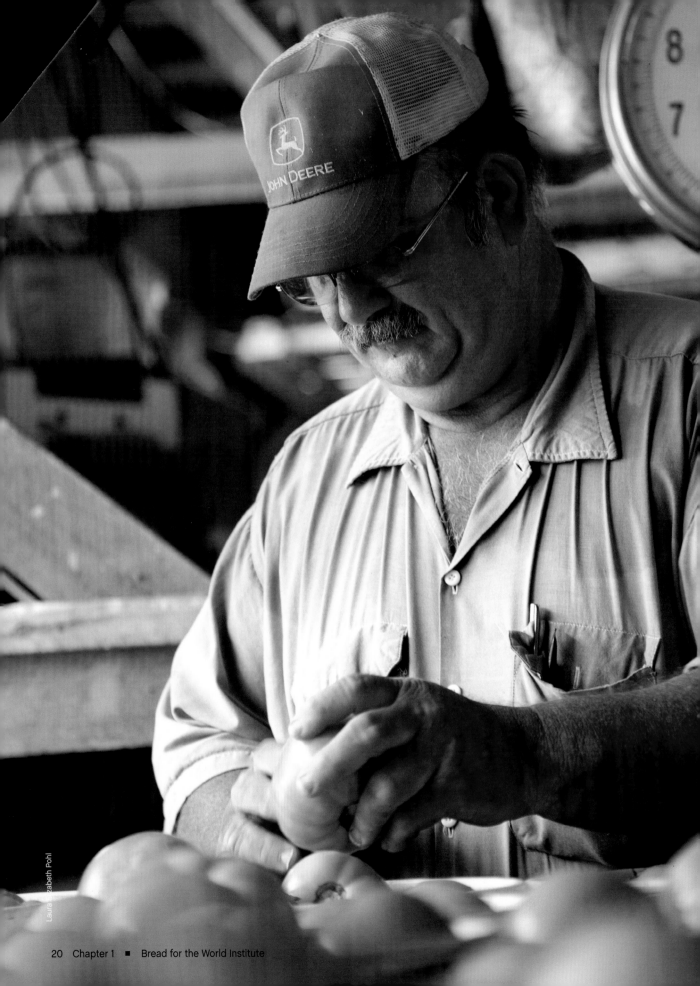

Farm Policies for Today and Tomorrow

CHAPTER SUMMARY

America's farmers and the federal government are natural allies in the fight against domestic hunger and malnutrition—and this alliance is enshrined in the nation's farm policies. The U.S. public needs farm policies to ensure a safe and affordable food supply, to protect the sustainability of vital natural resources that agricultural production depends on, and to produce well-balanced, nutritious foods.

A cursory look at the U.S. food system reveals the latter—producing well-balanced, nutritious foods—as badly in need of attention. Rising healthcare costs associated with chronic diet-related diseases should lead policymakers to reassess the balance of farm policies. Current policies favor production of calories, not nutrients. Today, the United States does not produce enough fruits and vegetables for Americans to meet the recommended daily allowances (RDAs) of vitamins and minerals. Thus, farm policies should lean more towards the production of healthy foods.

A rapidly growing segment of the U.S. population is demanding healthy, sustainably produced foods. Small and medium-size producers, the farmers best suited to meet this demand, receive virtually no support from U.S. farm policy. The largest, wealthiest producers of a limited number of crops are the biggest beneficiaries of government support. At a time when they are earning record high farm income, it makes little sense for them to be the main beneficiaries of national farm policy.

Government has directed schools to serve children healthier meals, and when possible to source more of the foods used in child nutrition programs from local and regional producers, mostly small to medium-size producers. This merits much stronger support from policymakers. Not only would it benefit children, including low-income children, but also a great many farmers and their communities, reviving a connection between agriculture and rural development that once was much stronger.

Included at the end of this chapter is a proposal to restructure the current farm safety net. Income-support programs should be replaced by a more efficient system of revenue insurance, and support should be available to all farmers and based on principles of fairness and shared responsibility.

Chapter 1

Recommendations

- Farm policies should lean more towards the production of healthy foods.
- Farm policies should be linked to local and regional development of rural areas.
- Shared responsibility, fairness, and efficiency should define how government partners with farmers on risk management.

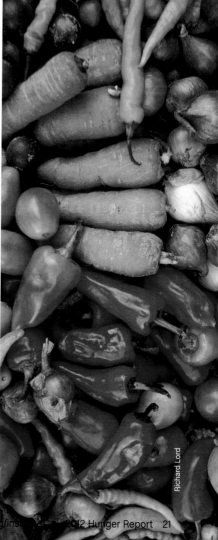

Richard Lord

Revisiting Rural Priorities

In recent years, the U.S. farm sector has recorded its highest growth rates since the 1970s.[1] At the time of this writing, 2011 looks set to be the most prosperous year of all.[2] The rise in global grain prices has been very good for the U.S. farm sector, and the U.S. Department of Agriculture (USDA) forecasts a rising demand for U.S. grain for years to come.[3]

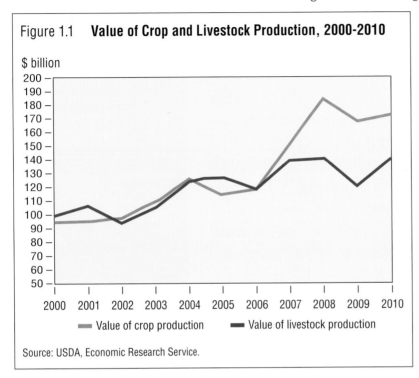

Figure 1.1   Value of Crop and Livestock Production, 2000-2010

$ billion

— Value of crop production   — Value of livestock production

Source: USDA, Economic Research Service.

It is no wonder the U.S. farm sector is prospering. The United States has been blessed with some of the most productive farmland in the world. U.S. agricultural producers are thriving as more people around the world escape poverty and seek to improve their diets, usually by adding animal products. By far the largest share of U.S. farm income comes from sales of feed grain and what are called "value-added products," meaning the cattle, hogs, poultry, and other livestock that consume the feed grain.

From 2007-2010, U.S. agricultural exports averaged more than $100 billion annually.[4] Trade with emerging markets has been fueling this higher level of exports—particularly trade with China, now the top export destination of U.S. agricultural products.[5]

While the U.S. economy as a whole has run trade deficits since the 1970s, the agricultural sector has bucked this trend by posting steady surpluses.[6] Between 1996 and 2011, soybean exports to China alone increased an astounding 26-fold.[7]

Outside the metropolitan centers where most of the U.S. population resides, hundreds of millions of acres of farmland stretch across the countryside. More than 40 percent of the U.S. landmass is farmland.[8] Yet most Americans live far from where the food they eat is produced and know little about the farm sector or the role of the government in supporting farmers.

Federal farm policy can be traced back to the Great Depression. The U.S. Agricultural Assistance Act of 1933 was in effect the first farm bill. Farm

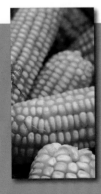

Between 2000 and 2009, corn used for ethanol increased by 3.7 billion bushels, while total corn production increased by 3.2 billion bushels. During this same period, U.S. ethanol production increased from 1.6 billion gallons to 10.8 billion gallons.

The farm share of every dollar spent on food is **15.8¢** and the marketing bill is **84.2¢**

policy during the Great Depression not only helped farmers keep producing the food needed to feed the country, but also kept rural America from sinking deeper into poverty. From 1929 to 1932, during the first years of the Great Depression, farm income plummeted by 52 percent,[9] so the 1933 act was much-needed. In the early years of farm policy, government support for farmers was the equivalent of rural development: the farm sector was indivisible from the rest of the rural economy.

Today, federal farm programs are still in place, but they no longer play much of a role in reducing rural poverty in the United States. This is because the face of rural poverty has changed since those early farm policies were established. Poor people in rural areas now work primarily in the service sector—much like poor people in metropolitan areas. Just 6.5 percent of the rural labor force works on a farm.[10] Farmers themselves are not often poor; the median income of farm households is higher than of U.S. households as a whole.[11] Some farming areas have high rates of poverty, particularly the Deep South and parts of the West, but it's unusual for people who earn a living farming to be in poverty. The major exception is immigrant farm workers, whose experiences of poverty in America are some of the harshest.

Farm policies that support the incomes of American farmers seem unnecessary at this point. And, in fact, most farmers don't receive any direct support from the U.S. government. Among those who do, there are gaping inequalities—the largest, wealthiest farms receive much more than everyone else. It is hard to make a case that this is fair under any circumstances, but particularly at a time when elected officials are scouring the budget to eliminate wasteful spending. This is an optimal time to rethink U.S. farm policy.

Reforming farm policy does not mean eliminating support. Farming is a risky undertaking, and all farmers need a guarantee of government protection in the event of a catastrophic loss in revenue. Tornadoes, droughts, floods, heat waves, frost, erratic markets, tit-for-tat trade policies: these are only some

People who earn their living as farmers have a unique role in society as stewards of an essential public good—an agriculture system that feeds and nourishes everyone.

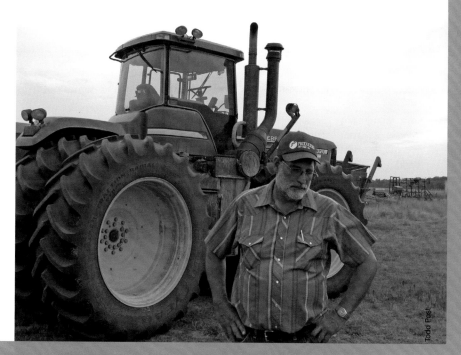

Todd East

Nearly half of the nation's 2,050 nonmetropolitan counties lost population between 1988 and 2008; for more than 700 counties, this loss exceeded 10 percent.

$167.3 billion

Commodity subsidies in the United States totaled $167.3 billion from 1995-2010. The top 10 percent of recipients were paid 76 percent of commodity payments.

of the systemic risks that are beyond the control of individual farmers and justify a government safety net. But what kind of safety net, who is included, and how and when to use it, are the questions that make all the difference.

At the end of this chapter, Bread for the World Institute proposes revamping the farm safety net to make it a better deal for the vast majority of U.S. farmers and a better deal for taxpayers.

People who earn their living as farmers have a unique role in society as stewards of an essential public good—an agriculture system that affects the health and well-being of everyone. Like anyone else, farmers need to be able to provide for their families and support their communities; it is important that farming allows them to earn a decent living. The thrust of this chapter is to improve farm policies, not to jettison policies that work well to serve the public good.

Production Agriculture—Taking the Farm to Scale

Few images are more iconic of U.S. agriculture in the 20th century than a farmer seated on a tractor. But how much do we know about agriculture today? The latest tractors come equipped with global positioning systems (GPS) so sophisticated that they can tell farmers where to plant seeds within a fraction of an inch to maximize yield.[12]

Consider the following ad for a new line of tractors in development. "The day may not be far off when a farmer does his spring planting, not from the driver's seat of a tractor, but from his office desk. And instead of driving a single tractor, he will be able to monitor several automated units at once, as they till fields, plant seeds, dispense fertilizer, and harvest crops." This ad for Robotic Tractors comes not from John Deere or another farm equipment manufacturer, but from the website of Intel, the chipmaker.[13]

On a shelf alongside the kitchen table in his home, Arlyn Schipper has a collection of miniature scale models of all the farm tractors he's owned since he started farming almost four decades ago. Schipper farms 6,000 acres of corn and soybeans in central Iowa. With so many acres, he is considered a large operator even by Iowa's farm-size standards. The model tractors illustrate how technology has transformed the U.S. agricultural sector over the last half-century—and they also explain why Schipper has built a farm operation of 6,000 acres. When modern tractors allow him to plow 6,000 acres as easily as 600, and a single tractor puts him hundreds of thousands of dollars in debt, it makes sense to try to use the investment to its full potential.

As a board member of Foods Resource Bank, a U.S. based anti-

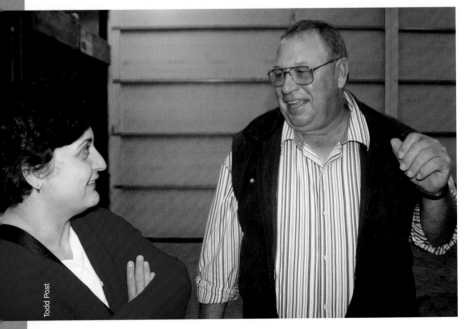

Iowa farmer Arlyn Schipper talks with Mannik Sakayan, deputy director of government relations at Bread for the World.

Todd Post

hunger organization (and a sponsor of this report), Schipper volunteers with other U.S. farmers from the Midwest to share some of what they've learned about farming with smallholders in the developing world. On a trip to Zambia in the winter of 2011, he couldn't resist the urge to strap himself to a mule and plow a row of corn as farmers do in the village he was visiting. One row was enough for him.

Since the beginning of the 20th century, breakthroughs in agricultural technology have transformed farming in the United States, making possible astonishing increases in productivity and efficiency. Productivity gains in agriculture have coincided with farms getting bigger.[14] The data show that each U.S. farmer is now producing enough to feed 155 people—compared to 19 people in 1940.[15] Arlyn Schipper has never tried to calculate how many people his farm feeds, but he takes immense pride in the fact that the food he produces prevents people in the United States and around the world from going hungry.

Consumers in the United States spend a lesser share of their incomes on food than

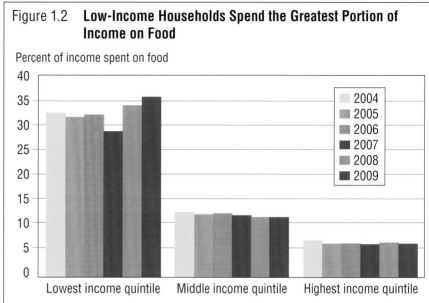

Figure 1.2 **Low-Income Households Spend the Greatest Portion of Income on Food**

Percent of income spent on food

Note: Average annual incomes for the quintiles in 2009 were $9,846 for the lowest, $46,012 for the middle, and $157,631 for the highest.

Source: U.S. Bureau of Labor Statistics.

people in any other nation. Leaving aside issues of quality for the moment, everyone in the country benefits from low food prices. Low-income households, with the least to spend on food, perhaps benefit the most. (See Figure 1.2.) Production agriculture—the kind done by Schipper and other large-scale operators—is crucial to maintaining U.S. food security and preventing hunger. This does not mean hunger has been eradicated in the United States—not as long as its underlying causes, primarily poverty, persist—but hunger rates would surely be higher if not for the relatively low cost of food.

Schipper hopes to see the family business he has built over decades carried on by his son, Brent, who is now farming alongside his father. At this stage of Brent's career, it is impossible to overstate the benefits of having a parent as successful as Arlyn. His father's mentoring alone is priceless. A more tangible benefit is the physical assets, such as tractors and land, Brent stands to inherit. In Iowa, the cost of raising a conventional crop of corn or soybeans ranges from $600-$800 per acre.[16] This does not include the cost of the land itself—and in 2011, the price of an acre of Iowa farmland passed the $10,000 mark.[17] In 1982, 12 percent of Iowa's farmland was owned by someone age 75 or older. By 2007, that figure was 28 percent.[18]

When grain prices are high, as they've been for most of the past decade, farmland prices soar; this makes it much harder for beginning farmers to gain a toehold in the land market. Banks are less inclined to offer credit to

BOX 1.1   U.S. AGRICULTURE HAS TO BECOME MORE PRODUCTIVE AND SUSTAINABLE

By 2100, the global population is expected to peak at 10.1 billion.[23] According to the United Nations Food and Agriculture Organization (FAO), agricultural productivity will need to increase by 70 percent to keep up with the growing population.[24]

Malthusian predictions that population will outstrip food production have been proven wrong ever since Malthus himself made this argument in the 19th century. But climate change could make for a different outcome in the 21st century. The U.S. Global Change Research Program, a consortium of 13 government departments and agencies, reports that climate-change impacts can already be observed in major crop-producing areas of the United States. Over the past 30 years, the Midwest and northern Great Plains have experienced increases in average winter temperatures of more than 7 degrees Fahrenheit.[25]

Responding to climate change alone would be a significant challenge, but there are additional reasons to be concerned about whether the production agriculture system that provides us with plentiful, affordable food is sustainable.

Agricultural production depends heavily on fossil fuels—non-renewable resources. David Pimentel of Cornell University estimates that the U.S. food system consumes 19 percent of the fossil fuels used in the United States. When forestry is added, the figure rises to 24 percent—the same as U.S. automobiles use.[26] It would be hard to imagine a future in which automobile manufacturers will not need to become more energy efficient—and agricultural producers are no different.

Other stark challenges include:

- **Erosion.** The United States is losing soil 10 times faster than it can be replenished naturally.[27] In 2007, topsoil was eroding at a rate of 200,000 tons an hour.[28]

- **Water pollution.** Agriculture is the leading source of pollution in the nation's rivers and lakes and a major source of pollution in estuaries. This pollution comes mostly from fertilizer application and from animal waste produced in feedlots.[29]

- **Greenhouse gases.** Agriculture is the largest emitter of nitrous oxide, one of the most potent greenhouse gases contributing to climate change. Again, this comes mainly from fertilizer application.[30] On a per-molecule

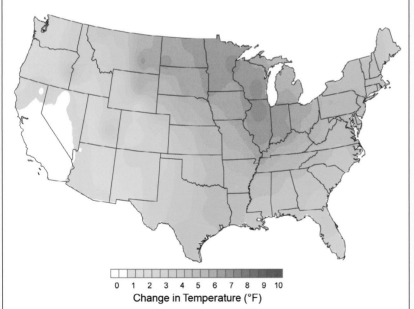

Figure 1.3   **Winter Temperature Trends, 1975 to 2007**

0 1 2 3 4 5 6 7 8 9 10
Change in Temperature (°F)

Temperatures are rising faster in winter than in any other season, especially in many key agricultural regions. This allows many insect pests and crop diseases to expand and thrive, creating increasing challenges for agriculture. As indicated by the map, the Midwest and northern Great Plains have experienced increases of more than 7°F in average winter temperatures over the past 30 years.

Source: National Oceanic and Atmospheric Administration, National Climate Data Center.

basis, nitrous oxide is 300 times more potent than carbon dioxide.[31]

- **Pesticide exposure.** U.S. agricultural producers use more than 500 million pounds of pesticides each year.[32] Pesticide exposure is harmful to humans, animals, and the environment.[33]
- **Resistance to antibiotics.** Recent studies indicate that 80 percent of all antibiotics in the United States are given to farm animals, mostly to prevent disease outbreaks in feedlots. Overuse of antibiotics in farm animals is contributing to increasing resistance to antibiotics among disease-causing pathogens.[34] These are antibiotics also used to treat humans.

There are farm policies in place to reduce pollution and promote the conservation of natural resources. In recent farm bills, funding for conservation has increased faster than for other farm programs,[35] and more farmers are able to participate in conservation programs than ever before. That's good, but a serious shortcoming is the lack of monitoring and evaluation in conservation programs. The public should know what it is getting for tax dollars spent on these programs, but currently, farmers are under no obligation to disclose which anti-pollution practices they are implementing or whether these are benefiting the environment.[36] In general, U.S. farm policy relies on voluntary approaches to solving environmental problems. At a minimum, farm runoff should be regulated under the Clean Water Act, and feedlots—the largest source of toxic ammonia emissions—should be regulated under the Clean Air Act.

The daunting challenges of rising population and climate change mean that every farmer who receives government support should be required to operate more sustainably. Farmers surely understand that it's in their own best interest to be good stewards of the natural resources they depend on for their livelihood.

a farmer without sufficient capital to back up a loan. Policymakers need to be concerned about rising land prices and other capital costs facing farmers who are just starting out. According to government figures, U.S. farmland values roughly doubled in nominal terms between 2000 and 2010; they rose by 58 percent in real terms (after accounting for inflation).[19] USDA's Farm Service Agency (FSA) has traditionally been the lender of last resort.[20] The 2008 farm bill affirmed the role of FSA in supporting beginning farmers and enhanced other supports for them, but it's not clear that these provisions are enough to stay ahead of the cost curve.[21]

New farmers are needed to help feed growing U.S. and global populations. By 2050, the U.S. population is expected to increase by nearly a third. Meanwhile, the average age of American farmers continues to climb—currently it is 57,[22] the same age as Arlyn Schipper. The issues associated with production agriculture, particularly the difficulties facing beginning farmers, must remain a priority of policymakers for some time to come.

Against the Grain—The Value-Added of Small and Medium-Size Farmers

Rising commodity prices do not translate into higher profits for all U.S. farmers. As commodity prices rise, so do the costs of fuel, fertilizer, seed, and other inputs. Scaling up the size of a farm operation mitigates the effects of rising input costs, but not all farmers are in a position to increase the size of their operation.

Farmers with hundreds rather than thousands of acres are considered medium-sized producers.[37] For these farmers, and for small-scale producers who farm less than 100 acres, the challenge is to figure out how to succeed in a system geared to larger producers.

Tim Nissen is considered a medium-sized producer. A decade ago, he was farming 700 acres of conventional corn and soybeans in eastern Nebraska. In Bread for the World Institute's 2007 report, *Healthy Food, Farms and Families*, Nissen explained why he got out of farming these crops. Without government support, he was barely able to survive. Nissen wanted to be more entrepreneurial, and he found farming conventional corn and soybeans too constraining. Once he was no longer forced to follow the rules required for recipients of government payments, he diversified his farm operation by adding fruits and vegetables, including grapes to establish a winery. At the time we met, the winery was about a year away from beginning production.

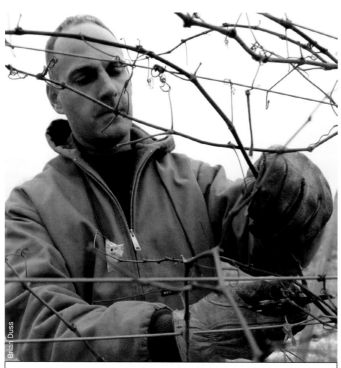

Nebraska farmer Tim Nissen used to raise conventional corn and soybeans, but now he is farming organically.

The winery is now producing. Through the Nebraska Department of Tourism, Nissen has arranged for the wines to be publicized along the 231-mile Outlaw Trail, a scenic byway that promotes the state's natural resources, history, and culture. He sells to wholesalers, liquor stores, and restaurants across Nebraska. But his most financially successful venture so far comes not from buyers of his wine, but from people willing to pay him for bottling wine. Many people produce wine as a hobby but would rather let someone else do the bottling. Once Nissen learned the necessary skills, he began operating a mobile bottling facility. For several weeks of the year, he travels across much of the Midwest. In one four-state region, Nissen offers the only such mobile service, so he has this niche market all to himself.

By diversifying his operation, Nissen is managing risk the way farmers used to, before farm policy turned risk management upside down and made it reasonable for farmers to grow just two crops. In addition to fruits and vegetables, he raises organic feed grains for niche livestock markets.

Nissen is regarded as an oddity by his neighbors. When we last spoke with him in 2011, the price of corn had climbed to the highest level in decades. Many of his neighbors have cashed in on the ethanol boom ever since the mid-2000s, when Congress mandated dramatic increases in biofuel production. Would he have stuck with growing conventional corn if he'd known the ethanol boom was coming? He says definitely not. "Corn is going to be replaced by other feedstocks," he says, "and when that happens, the boom will turn to bust." He thinks the future is much brighter for organic producers. In the last decade, sales of organically produced foods grew by double digits every year, and there's little sign that this trend is waning.[38] (See Figure 1.4.)

Nissen isn't opposed to using government support as a matter of principle; he receives support from U.S. conservation programs to improve his stewardship of water and soil quality. He also got a "value-added producer" grant to assist his transition to organic production. Establishing the winery is an example of adding value to the production of grapes. The grant program gives priority to small and medium-sized producers as well as to beginning and/or disadvantaged farmers and ranchers,[39] and is designed to help them succeed in niche markets. For

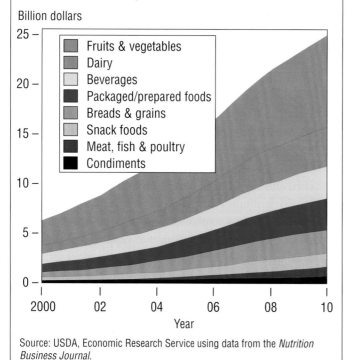

Figure 1.4 **U.S. Organic Food Sales Estimated at Nearly $25 Billion in 2010**

Billion dollars

Legend:
- Fruits & vegetables
- Dairy
- Beverages
- Packaged/prepared foods
- Breads & grains
- Snack foods
- Meat, fish & poultry
- Condiments

Year: 2000, 02, 04, 06, 08, 10

Source: USDA, Economic Research Service using data from the *Nutrition Business Journal.*

small and medium-sized producers, the truth may be that adding value is their best chance to survive in a system that favors large producers.

Profitability doesn't always require that farmers own lots of acres. Alex and Betsy Hitt, owners of Peregrine Farm, earn $27,000-$28,000 an acre on the five acres they farm outside Chapel Hill, North Carolina.[40] They've grown many different crops, depending on the season, the profitability of the crops, their personal preferences, and the markets available to them. Like Nissen, diversification is a fundamental part of the Hitts' business strategy, as is direct sales to consumers.

USDA reports that for every dollar spent on food, the farm's share averages 15.8 cents; the rest goes to marketing.[41] When farmers take on more of the marketing and selling of their products, they earn a larger share of these dollars. But most don't market or sell their products. Farmers generally prefer to do what they know how to do best: farm.

Program Crops versus Rural America

"The future of U.S. farm policy must grapple with two fundamental questions," says economist Robert L. Thompson, co-chair of the Agricultural Task Force for The Chicago Council on Global Affairs and a professor of agricultural economics at the Johns Hopkins School of Advanced International Studies. "Of the federal dollars allocated to agriculture and rural America, how much should go to farmers as individuals and how much should be invested for the greater good of agriculture and rural America?" asks Thompson. "Of the fraction that goes to farmers as individuals, how much should be linked to the production of specific commodities and how much should be decoupled from what the farmer produces?"

In the early years of farm policy, there was scarcely any room for doubt about the relationship between farm policy and the greater good of agriculture and rural America. When the Agricultural Assistance Act of 1933 was written, farmers made up half the rural population. Today, farm policy exists primarily to enhance the incomes of individual farmers, and any ripple effects for the rest of the residents of rural communities are less than apparent.

In the years since Arlyn Schipper and his wife started their family, they've seen the population of their county—one of the most productive farm counties in Iowa—shrink by what they estimate is two-thirds. Population loss is inevitable in farm communities when farms get bigger by buying smaller farms. Communities can withstand a certain amount of population loss, but when schools

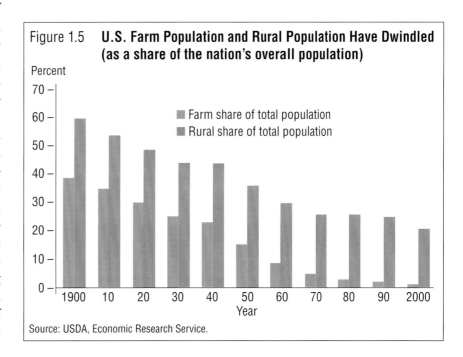

Figure 1.5 **U.S. Farm Population and Rural Population Have Dwindled (as a share of the nation's overall population)**

Percent

Farm share of total population
Rural share of total population

Year

Source: USDA, Economic Research Service.

BOX 1.2   RETHINKING U.S. BIOFUEL POLICY

Some policymakers praise biofuels as a way to reduce dependence on foreign oil and cut the greenhouse gases (GHGs) responsible for climate change. However, not all biofuels are able to accomplish these things: success ultimately depends on the choice of feedstocks to produce the biofuel.

In the United States, the dominant biofuel is ethanol made from corn. So far, corn-based ethanol has not moved the United States closer to using less foreign oil or reducing greenhouse gases[42]—even though about half of the corn grown in the United States is now used to produce ethanol.[43]

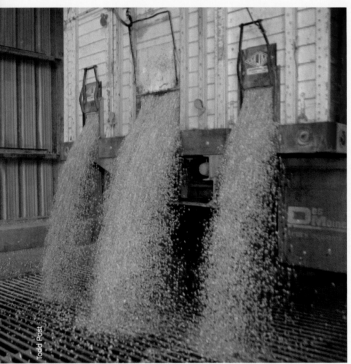

Corn unloaded from truck to begin the process of converting into ethanol at the Lincoln Energy Plant in Iowa.

A 2011 report by the International Energy Agency argues that by 2050, more than a quarter of the world's transportation fuel could be biofuels.[44] But realizing this potential will require much greater support for "advanced biofuels"—something altogether different than from the corn-based ethanol produced in the United States.

Advanced biofuels can be made from many types of materials, such as wood chips, grasses, waste, and even algae. The United States has the potential to produce abundant quantities of advanced biofuels,[45] but this potential won't be realized as long as corn dominates the biofuel sector.

The greatest deterrent to the development of advanced biofuels in the United States is current biofuel policies, which are tilted so heavily toward ethanol that they discourage research and development of advanced biofuel options. From 2005-2011, taxpayers paid for more than $30 billion in subsidies for corn-based ethanol. Most of this came in the form of tax credits to the oil industry to blend ethanol with gasoline—a nearly incomprehensible use of public resources since blenders did not need an incentive to use ethanol. Ethanol was already in use as an additive to gasoline—and, in fact, the only possible alternative additive had been phased out by 2006.[46]

In addition, Congress set renewable fuel standards in 2005 and 2007 mandating aggressive increases in biofuel consumption. Because most biofuels produced in the United States are corn-based ethanol, the standards only reinforced ethanol's domination of the renewable fuels market.

Finally, an import tariff on ethanol protects U.S. producers from foreign competitors—most notably Brazil, the other major ethanol producer. In Brazil, ethanol is produced with sugarcane.[47] "The presence of the tariff," writes Christopher Knittel of the Massachusetts Institute of Technology, "strongly suggest[s] that the main motivation behind ethanol-related policies is likely to protect farmer profits, rather than reduce GHGs or our dependence on foreign oil."[48] Thanks to the triple incentive of subsidies, a production mandate, and a protective tariff, the corn-based ethanol industry has grown so much that the United States is now a net exporter of ethanol.

How does ethanol affect hungry people? Corn-based ethanol is one factor in the sharp rise in global grain prices that plunged more than 100 million additional people into

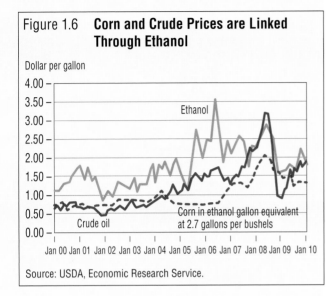

Figure 1.6 Corn and Crude Prices are Linked Through Ethanol

Dollar per gallon

Ethanol

Crude oil

Corn in ethanol gallon equivalent at 2.7 gallons per bushels

Jan 00 Jan 01 Jan 02 Jan 03 Jan 04 Jan 05 Jan 06 Jan 07 Jan 08 Jan 09 Jan 10

Source: USDA, Economic Research Service.

hunger in 2008 and tens of millions more in 2011. In an effort to rebut the argument that ethanol displaces corn that could be used for food,[49] the ethanol industry frequently points out that it can produce ethanol and feed grain together in the same manufacturing process. This technology does exist, but ethanol is not off the hook as a contributor to global hunger. Since 2005, when the biofuel policies discussed above were adopted, the price of corn has been hitched to the price of crude oil. As crude prices rise, so does demand for ethanol. In other words, as world oil prices rise, so do corn prices. Figure 1.6 illustrates this relationship. Historically, oil has been a much more volatile commodity than grain.[50] Not any longer, it appears.

One of the U.S. motivations for expanding corn-based ethanol was the hope that it would lead to energy independence and increase national security. But in light of ethanol's contribution to food-price volatility, and to the political and economic instability that accompany it, efforts to replace oil with corn through biofuel policies threaten to replace one national security threat with another.

close because there aren't enough kids to teach and businesses move out because there aren't enough customers, it's difficult to argue that farm policies that encourage consolidation are supporting rural development or the health of communities.

The main reason for farm consolidation is the improvements in agricultural technology that enable large farms to realize significant economies of scale. But technology isn't developed in a vacuum. When Earl Butz, Secretary of Agriculture during the Nixon administration, exhorted America's farmers to "get big or get out," he wasn't merely voicing an opinion. Information available in recent years leaves little room for doubt that Butz was directly telegraphing the future of farm policy. From 1995-2010, the largest 10 percent of farms got 76 percent of the $262 billion the federal government spent on farm support. Their average annual payment was $30,751—while the bottom 80 percent of farms that received support got an average of $587.[51]

Five crops—corn, soybeans, wheat, cotton, and rice—get the largest share of government support.[52] In farm policy jargon, these are referred to as program crops. They are also sometimes called commodity crops or row crops—picture row upon row of a single crop, stretching out toward the horizon. Corn, soybeans, and wheat get the most government support in absolute dollars, while rice and cotton receive more dollars per acre. Does the U.S. government support for program crops help spur broader rural development? One way to answer this question is to look at regions of the country where farmers get payments to grow rice and cotton. Arkansas leads the nation in rice production, Texas in cotton. Many of the counties in Arkansas and Texas that receive significant farm support have the dubious distinction of being "persistent poverty" counties—meaning that they have had high poverty rates for decades.

In Woodruff County, Arkansas (population just over 7,000), rice producers received $191 million in farm program support between 1995 and 2009. During that same period, the county's poverty rate averaged 26.5 percent and unemployment averaged 8.6 percent.[53] Food prices are low in Woodruff County, as they are in general for Americans. Low food prices may help the county's poor people get by, but the best anti-hunger program is a well-paying job. By that measure, farm support policies have failed to deliver. The investment of billions of dollars a year has generated little economic development in places where it is needed most.

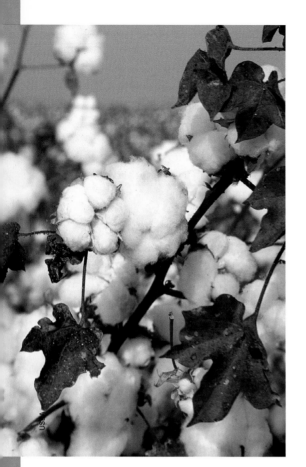

Cotton is one of the most heavily subsidized crops in the United States. From 1995-2010, U.S. cotton farmers received $31 billion in government subsidies.

Farm Policies and Poverty

Thompson's second fundamental question about farm policy asks whether it should be based on production and decoupled from which crops farmers produce. Basing farm support payments on production is problematic for several reasons. When commodity prices are high, farmers still get government support to produce crops, even though the market is providing plenty of encouragement. When commodity prices are low, farmers get government support to produce—and overproduce—when there is no market signal to do so. These subsidies distort trade.

In fact, production subsidies violate World Trade Organization (WTO) rules that the United States agreed to follow. If the government fails to change these trade-distorting policies, U.S. exports—agricultural *and* non-agricultural—could face stiff penalties in international markets.[54] Production subsidies also benefit the largest farms disproportionately because of these farms' tremendous economies of scale. Farm policies based on production should be eliminated. Conservation subsidies do not distort trade and could be distributed more equitably among farms of all sizes. Box 1.1 explains why farm policy should treat conservation as a top priority.

As the Doha Round, the current round of WTO negotiations, stumbles along with little progress in sight, it is important to remember what it was intended to achieve. When the round opened in 2001, in the wake of the 9/11 terrorist strikes in the United States, it was billed as a "development round." In the world's least developed countries, agriculture is how the vast majority of the population earns a living, and agricultural development is the most accessible path to wide-scale poverty reduction. Since the start of the round, we have witnessed the effects of highly volatile markets for agricultural commodities: they drive up hunger rates in poor countries around the world. A successful conclusion to the Doha Round has the potential to create a more stable environment and smooth out a portion of this volatility.[55]

Past rounds of multilateral trade negotiations have helped developing countries get access to manufacturing and service markets that were once closed to them. But agricultural trade remains a sticking point. Developing countries will only see progress as a result of the Doha Round if developed countries commit to liberalizing markets for the products that are the developing countries' comparative advantage: raw commodities. The round is likely to remain stalled as long as U.S. agricultural policies are in violation of WTO rules.

Turning to the United States, it's clear that farm policies also affect Americans living in poverty. As health problems related to diet become more and more common, farm policies have come under much greater scrutiny.[56] Two-thirds of Americans are overweight or obese, and this condition is linked directly to dietary choices.[57] If current trends continue, obesity and overweight will account for one-fifth of all healthcare expenses by 2020.[58]

Poor diets increase the risk of cardiovascular disease, cancer, diabetes, and hypertension. People living in poverty suffer disproportionately from all of these diet-related health conditions. While food prices in this country were falling throughout the 20th century, the prices of fruits and vegetables did not fall nearly as quickly as the prices of subsidized program crops. Hence, relative food prices have moved directly against a healthier diet, and consumption patterns clearly reflect this trend.[59] (See Figure 1.8, next page.)

In 2011, USDA issued new guidelines on the recommended daily allowances (RDAs) of vitamins and minerals in diets. People cannot meet most of the new RDAs without consuming more fruits and vegetables, yet the United States *does not even produce enough fruits and vegetables to meet the RDAs*.[60] The number of acres devoted to production of fruits and vegetables is roughly 2.5 percent of the total U.S. cropland under production.[61]

Farmers' choice of crops to grow is driven by what U.S. farm policies favor. Consider the Direct Payments program, a lump sum payment provided to owners of farmland with a history of raising program crops. Seventy percent (220 million acres) of all harvested cropland is eligible for the program.[62] Farmers who receive direct payments are under no obligation to plant anything on this land. But if they do raise a crop, it must be a program crop. If they attempt to divert even a single acre to grow fruits and vegetables, they risk losing government support for all the acres they qualify for.

One way to increase production of healthy foods—and make them more affordable to low-income households—would be to allow farmers to diversify their farm operations. Diverting just 1 percent of program crop acres to grow fruits and vegetables would increase U.S. fruit and vegetable production by a third.[63] A large farmer like Arlyn Schipper may not be interested in diversifying, but medium-sized farmers struggling to survive and dependent on government subsidies may well find this a compelling option.

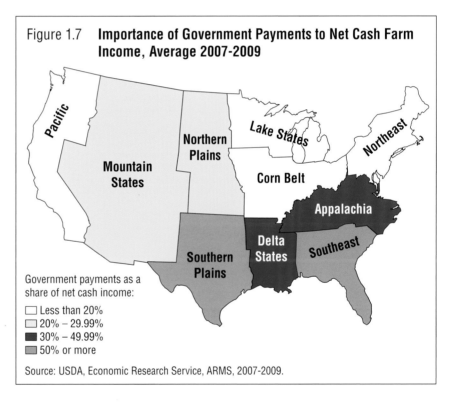

Figure 1.7 **Importance of Government Payments to Net Cash Farm Income, Average 2007-2009**

Government payments as a share of net cash income:
- ☐ Less than 20%
- ☐ 20% – 29.99%
- ■ 30% – 49.99%
- ▨ 50% or more

Source: USDA, Economic Research Service, ARMS, 2007-2009.

The Direct Payments program has been costing taxpayers $5 billion every year—a figure that has made the program emblematic of government waste. At a time of record farm profits, it is difficult to understand why taxpayers should provide farmers with billions of dollars that come with no strings attached except a requirement not to grow fruits and vegetables (the healthy foods that USDA says Americans need to eat more of). The program became still more notorious once information became publically available showing that half of the payments go to landowners who are not farmers. Many are speculators who've never set foot on the farmland—thousands of residents of New York, Boston, Chicago, Miami, Los Angeles,

Seattle, and other metropolitan areas. Together, they own a significant share of U.S. farmland.[64]

Past farm bills have considered changes to the restrictions in the Direct Payments program on planting other crops. The 2008 farm bill included a pilot program to incorporate "flex acres," allowing farmers in six states to divert 75,000 acres from program crop production to raise vegetables for processing. A 2011 evaluation showed that only 13.6 percent of the flex acres were used to grow alternative crops.[65] A few factors that likely contributed to this low figure: one, unlike markets for fresh vegetables, the markets for processed vegetables have been stagnant for years; two, participating farmers found the rules of the program cumbersome; and, three, with record high grain prices, farmers have had less incentive to switch to other crops.

Fruit and vegetable growers have traditionally opposed easing the planting restrictions on program crops because it would create more competitors for them. They have argued that program crops already command a greater share of government support than fruits and vegetables, so it would be unfair to lift the planting restrictions.[66] They are certainly correct that program crops get a greater share of government support, but this is no reason to keep renewing a bad policy. Fruit and vegetable growers' concerns can be addressed in other ways. For example, policymakers could expand the purchase of fruits and vegetables in federal nutrition programs to help offset a loss of market share. For more on this and other options, see Chapter 2.

An Appetite for Sustainably Produced Foods Creates New Opportunities for Farmers

The percentage of Americans who smoke has been dropping for decades as a result of greater public awareness about the health risks of tobacco use.[67] Until recently, however, U.S. farm policies included support for tobacco farmers. In the 1990s, government support began to wane as the tobacco industry came under attack for marketing its products to children. Children were, in fact, the only subgroup of the U.S. population whose tobacco use had not decreased. In 2004, the government decided to get out of the business of supporting tobacco farming altogether.

Today, a growing share of the public opposition to farm subsidies stems from concerns about diet-related health conditions, including childhood obesity. As in the case of tobacco, aggressive marketing of junk foods to children has outraged parents and some policymakers. In the lead-up to the 2008 farm bill, the American Medical Association weighed in by calling for efforts "to ensure that federal subsidies encourage the consumption of products low in fat and cholesterol."[68] Congress did not heed the doctors' advice.

Figure 1.8 **Per Capita Annual Availability of Fruit and Vegetables Has Been Declining**

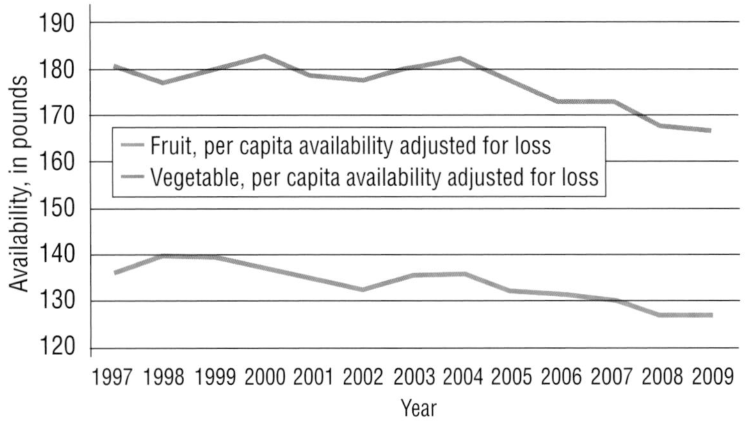

Availability, in pounds

— Fruit, per capita availability adjusted for loss
— Vegetable, per capita availability adjusted for loss

Year

Source: USDA, Economic Research Service.

It is premature to project the fate of federal support for tobacco onto corn—the crop most associated with junk foods because of high fructose corn syrup—but concerns about increasing childhood obesity and healthcare costs are not going away. If farm subsidies—for corn or any other crop—were to be eliminated, farmers who had been dependent on them might learn something about how to adapt from a group of ex-tobacco farmers in southern Virginia and eastern Tennessee.

When Robin Robbins was a little girl, she used to help her grandfather farm tobacco in southwest Virginia and thought she wanted to be a farmer some day, too. Today, she farms a portion of her grandfather's land with her husband and daughters, but instead of tobacco, they raise fruits, vegetables, and horticultural products. Robbins also has a full-time job as the marketing and sales manager for Appalachian Sustainable Development (ASD), a nonprofit organization formed in 1995 for the express purpose of helping former tobacco farmers to diversify their crops.

This area of central Appalachia was once home to thousands of tobacco farmers, many of whom were living in poverty or near-poverty. The tobacco program was a quota and price support system. Government told farmers how much to grow, and the farmers knew exactly how much they would be paid each year.

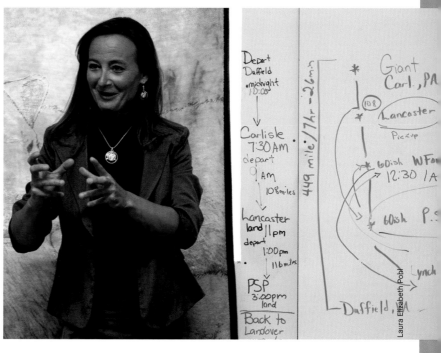

Robin Robbins is the marketing and sales manager for Appalachian Sustainable Development (ASD) in southwest Virginia. ASD has helped farmers who used to grow tobacco switch to sustainably produced fruits and vegetables.

ASD partners with 50 ex-tobacco farmers to supply local and regional markets with sustainably grown fruits and vegetables. Anthony Flaccavento, the founder of ASD and a farmer himself, trained his fellow farmers in how to produce these crops so that they meet food safety regulations. "With tobacco there was a tried and true recipe," says Flaccavento, "one that was supported by USDA extension. But when the farmers began to switch to fruits and vegetables, the extension agents around here had no experience with these crops." That has changed, according to Flaccavento, who credits the USDA extension offices with getting themselves up to speed quickly.

Robbins describes ASD's role as an aggregator. "It doesn't make sense for one farmer to try to sell five boxes of peppers to a grocery store a hundred miles away. But I combine that farmer's five boxes with another farmer's 10 boxes and another farmer's 20 and another's 20, and with that kind of volume we can reach markets they'd never be able to get to on their own."

ASD has an infrastructure to fulfill its orders that is matched by few of the other U.S. regions with burgeoning markets for local and regional foods. ASD has built a $750,000 processing facility where produce is washed, graded, and packed for distribution. Produce leaves the processing facility in one of ASD's two trucks. On a white board in her office at the processing center, Robbins has drawn flow charts of the routes the trucks take to reach customers. She knows exactly how long it takes for them to reach their destinations in every one of the markets they serve. ASD and its farmers supply major grocery chains like Whole Foods, Kroger's, and Food City.

The market for local and regional foods is small but growing rapidly.[69] One reflection of that growth is that Wal-Mart, the largest food retailer in the world, announced in 2010 that it plans to double its purchases of sustainable, locally grown produce in the United States by 2015.[70] Wal-Mart and other food retailers are responding to consumer demand for what marketers are calling "sustainability brand" products[71]—a demand that stems from a backlash against mainstream agribusiness and what is seen as the relentless production of highly processed, unhealthy foods.

Many in the local and regional food movement—a "movement" is a fair characterization at this point[72]—are seeking a more direct link to the farmers who produce the food they eat. Not only Wal-Mart but USDA has picked up on this desire. In 2009, Secretary of Agriculture Tom Vilsack launched the 'Know Your Farmer, Know Your Food' initiative, which could be the agency's most deliberate effort in decades to reestablish a linkage between agriculture and rural development. "Reconnecting consumers and institutions with local producers will stimulate economies in rural communities," said Vilsack. "American people [who] are more engaged with their food supply will create new income opportunities for American agriculture."[73]

Reconnecting Farm Policy with Nutrition

So far there is little evidence to suggest that low-income households are a significant part of the consumer demand for local and regional foods. Farmer's market purchases, for example, account for less than 1 percent of all SNAP redemptions.[74] Wal-Mart has been criticized as doing a disservice to farmers by lowering the prices of locally sourced foods,[75] but critics may not realize that people using SNAP benefits tend to shop at food outlets where they can find the lowest prices.[76]

The interests of low-income households would seem to be at odds with those of farmers, whose objective is to get the best prices for their products. There are hopeful signs that USDA is trying to work through these differences. We'll examine one of these efforts here. Farm-to-school programs are a way to ensure

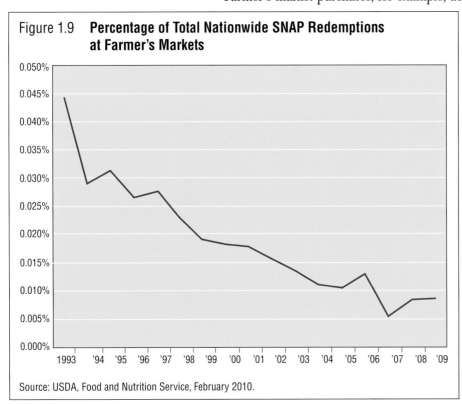

Figure 1.9 **Percentage of Total Nationwide SNAP Redemptions at Farmer's Markets**

Source: USDA, Food and Nutrition Service, February 2010.

that low-income households are not excluded from the goal of improving the country's food choices. Each day, more than 30 million students participate in the National School Lunch Program (NSLP); two-thirds of them receive free or reduced-price meals.[77] The NSLP is an ideal market for farmers' "seconds"—products that are of sound nutritional quality but unacceptable for sale in retail markets because of blemishes. Farmers are willing to sell these at a lower price because they would probably otherwise end up in the compost pile.

The NSLP was established in 1946 with the express purpose of improving national nutrition standards while increasing demand for domestic agricultural products.[78] In 1946, Americans' hunger problem was typically undernutrition, a result of chronic hunger.

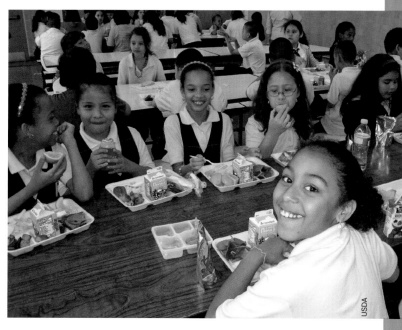

Schoolchildren at Bruce-Monroe Elementary School in Washington, DC, celebrate lunch after receiving a Gold Award of Distinction honor through USDA's HealthierUS School Challenge.

Farm policies encouraged production of fats and sugars because the understanding then was that in order to grow, hungry children needed foods high in fats and sugars.[79] America's farmers responded—and they continue to respond. Since 1970, the consumption of corn sweetener calories has increased by 359 percent. Fat calories, primarily from corn and soy, rose by 69 percent.[80] In contrast, per capita consumption of fruits and vegetables, after rising steadily from 1970-2000, has declined over the last decade.[81]

It is important not to lose sight of the historical relationship between nutrition programs and farm policy. We do not need farm policies that encourage farmers to produce more fats and sweeteners to feed hungry children. Rather, the childhood obesity epidemic has focused attention on improving the nutritional value of school meals. There is overwhelming support among healthcare professionals, including the Institute of Medicine's Committee on Nutrition Standards for National School Lunch and Breakfast programs,[82] for increasing the amount and variety of fruits and vegetables served in school meals.

In April 2011, Secretary Vilsack announced plans to begin sourcing more foods locally as part of a joint effort to improve the quality of school-meal programs and support economic development in rural communities.[83] Vilsack's focus on improving the quality of school meals advances the agenda laid out in the 2010 reauthorization of child nutrition programs, the Healthy, Hunger-Free Kids Act. This legislation governs the National School Lunch and Breakfast programs and several other programs that benefit school-age and preschool children. Passage of the Healthy, Hunger-Free Kids Act was one of the few examples of bipartisanship in the last Congress. A significant share of the credit for this achievement is due to the tireless efforts of anti-hunger and pro-nutrition groups, including Bread for the World, who worked patiently to bridge partisan differences.

The childhood obesity epidemic has focused public attention on improving the quality of foods served in school-meals programs. Farm-to-school programming is not the cure-all the nation has been looking for. It is one tool—and at present, one small tool. For farm-to-school initiatives to become more than a small improvement in child nutrition programs, the U.S. government will need to resolve the problems that now pose major barriers to local producers' participation. The government reimburses schools for the foods they purchase, but the reimbursement rates are so low that in most cases, schools must choose providers based on cost rather than quality. This puts local producers, whose value-added is the higher quality of their produce, at a disadvantage compared to large-scale food service operations with their economies of scale.

Another challenge is infrastructure. Working with fresh foods in school cafeterias requires cooking skills. But the longstanding trend in school-meal programs has been to reduce the amount of scratch cooking. Fresh ingredients have been replaced by heat-and-eat meals that are designed to save money by requiring fewer staff. Seasonality poses yet another challenge. Millions of school meals are served each day, *every* day of the school year.

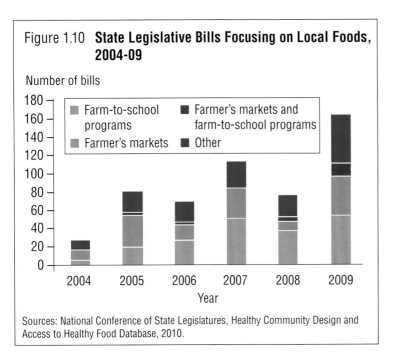

Figure 1.10 **State Legislative Bills Focusing on Local Foods, 2004-09**

Number of bills

Legend:
- Farm-to-school programs
- Farmer's markets
- Farmer's markets and farm-to-school programs
- Other

Sources: National Conference of State Legislatures, Healthy Community Design and Access to Healthy Food Database, 2010.

Greenhouses can extend growing seasons, but this doesn't change the fact that months go by when the fields are not producing but children are eating lunch at school. Seasonal constraints can be partly overcome using light processing. But, like the rest of the agricultural sector, food processing has become more concentrated, leaving whole areas of the country without local processing facilities.[84]

None of these challenges are insurmountable, but they require action. Under the 'Know Your Farmer, Know Your Food' Initiative, USDA's Rural Development Agency has dedicated funds to the processing, distribution, aggregation, and marketing of locally or regionally produced food products—another positive sign that USDA is thinking broadly about lowering the barriers between food producers and low-income consumers.

The United States is not the first country to see farm-to-school programs as a way to link rural development with improvements in child nutrition—many other nations, both rich and poor, have had the same idea. The Ghanaian government, for example, uses local farmers as much as possible to supply food to its national school feeding program. Infrastructure is a weak link in Ghana as in the United States, but the farm-to-school program has prodded the government to strengthen the supply chains needed for the program to succeed. The benefits to the farmers and their communities multiply as roads are built and as less food is wasted because adequate storage systems have been put in place. Perhaps most importantly, the infrastructure improvements spur job creation and more income in rural areas. The United States could realize similar benefits.

A Farm Policy that Creates Jobs and Helps Rebuild Struggling Economies

Michigan's economy had plunged into a deep recession well before the rest of the United States followed in 2008. From 2000-2009, Michigan led the nation in job losses: nearly one of every four jobs lost was in Michigan.[85] The manufacturing sector has been the mainstay of Michigan's economy ever since Henry Ford and the rise of the U.S. auto industry. Despite the recent hard times, manufacturing is still a significant sector. As in much of the rest of the Rust Belt, many manufacturers in Michigan have scaled back production, moved overseas, or simply gone out of business.

Few sectors of Michigan's economy have shown more potential to get people back to work than agriculture. Agriculture is now the second most-productive sector of the Michigan economy, behind what remains of the once-dominant manufacturing sector. Sen. Debbie Stabenow (D-MI), chair of the Senate Committee on Agriculture, Nutrition and Forestry, is keen to point out that agriculture in Michigan is a $71 billion industry and provides one of every four jobs in the state.[86] This is especially noteworthy because Michigan agriculture receives much less federal support than states dominated by program crops. Over the last 30 years, as most Midwestern states were losing rural population, Michigan led the region in rural population gains.[87]

Michigan's agricultural sector is defined by its diversity. The state is second only to California in the number of crops it produces. In the southern part of the state, corn and soybeans are plentiful, and Michigan also has a thriving dairy sector. But what the state is mainly known for is the wide variety of fruits, vegetables, and horticultural products grown there. USDA refers to these as specialty crops (as opposed to program crops). The federal government supports specialty crops mainly through conservation programs and investments in agricultural research and extension. With these crops, technology plays a less important role in determining the sector's production capacity. Rather, specialty crop production is labor intensive—and therefore creates many more jobs than program crops.

Mark Coe is one of the many Michigan residents who have found a niche in agriculture after major upheaval in their previous industries. Coe owned a photography development business in Mount Pleasant, MI, a bustling city compared to his hometown, Kaleva, a small town where he grew up surrounded by farms. The digital revolution in photography swept in so fast that it put Coe and most of his competitors out of business. In his early 40s, he moved back to Kaleva to care for his aging mother and mull over how to put his career back on track. Calvin Lutz, a childhood friend and the owner of Lutz Farm, asked him if he would be interested in helping out part-time with managing the farm. Lutz, a third-generation farmer, raises an assortment of fruits, vegetables, and Christmas trees on 1,800 acres.

Coe had been around farming all his childhood, but he didn't know the business from the inside. Yet he needed work and told his friend he'd try. Seven years later, he's still managing Lutz Farm, now full-time. Since Coe started working for Lutz, the farm has prospered and he has helped it expand into new markets. One of the markets Coe is most excited about is farm-to-school.

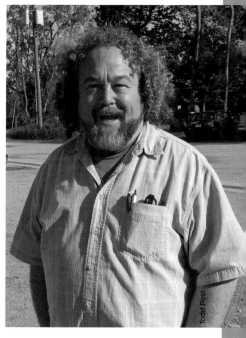

Michigan farmer Mark Coe is an enthusiastic supporter of farm-to-school programs in his state.

BOX 1.3   EAT WELL & CREATE JOBS

A study by Michigan State University found that if Michigan residents ate just 20 percent more fruits and vegetables produced in-state, it would create $200 million in farmer income and almost 2,000 additional off-farm jobs. "It is clear that relatively small changes in individual eating habits across a state's population can have significant direct and indirect impacts on employment and income," said Michael Hamm, one of the authors of the study. "In a sense, the figures we came up with are conservative in that they don't account for the economic benefit resulting from improved nutrition and health."[91]

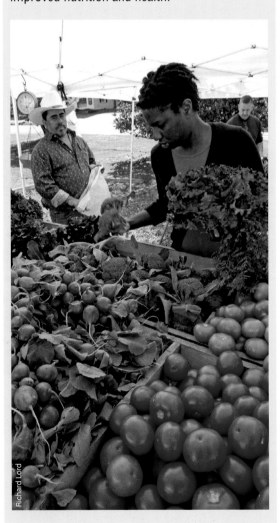

Richard Lord

"I was invited to a meeting about farm-to-school programs and thought this sounds interesting," he explained. "After all, my job is trying to figure out new markets—but there were the infrastructure hurdles to overcome. About a year later, I had a distributor come to me and say, 'We have a deal with Chicago Public Schools and they need peaches, can you fill an order?' I loaded up a truck with peaches and sent it off to Chicago. A couple of days later, I started getting phone calls from school administrators in Chicago telling me how much the kids loved the fresh peaches. They'd never had a fresh peach before. I thought this is cool—and could be something big."

Coe is now helping to develop farm-to-school programs in northwest Michigan and looking for investors to build a processing center on Lutz Farm so that he and other farmers in the region can supply their crops to schools throughout the year. He says that not all the infrastructure challenges have been solved yet, but he's impressed that Michigan is emerging as a national leader in farm-to-school programs and feels confident that public officials are going to help resolve the challenges.

"There are obstacles everywhere you look in farming, and farmers figure out how to overcome them every day," he says. One of the biggest obstacles he sees is getting local farmers to work together. "Farmers don't usually like to share information about who they're selling to," he explains. In this case, though, their mutual interests in helping kids eat better and supporting local and regional economic development has united them. Coe believes that identifying these shared goals will have ripple effects in local communities, sustaining partnerships that are dedicated to a common vision of community development. His can-do attitude reflects, above all, his faith in his community.

Farm policy and rural development have been on divergent paths for decades, but Michigan may be showing the whole nation how to bring them closer together again. The policy environment is crucial: do farmers believe that government is a partner, or just another obstacle for them to overcome? In Michigan, Governor Rick Snyder has said he wants to build up industries that are already strong.[88] In agriculture, this means building new markets for farmers.

Farmers need partners at both the state and federal levels. Sen. Stabenow has said, "I'm focused on continuing to support the great men and women of our state who work so hard, day in and day out, to produce a safe and abundant food and fiber supply that powers our nation's economy."[89] The Michigan senator is talking about her own state, but others stand to benefit if she is correct in her assessment; federal legislation is not written for the benefit of a single state. "When we talk about the farm bill," she has said, "we are really talking about a jobs bill."[90]

Bread for the World Institute

Congress is scheduled to rewrite the farm bill in 2012 in the midst of a bipartisan push to reduce the federal deficit. Above all, the emphasis will be on eliminating unnecessary programs.

The U.S. Department of Agriculture website lists 11 major risk management programs,[92] including crop insurance, which includes multiple products of its own.

The current patchwork of programs could be replaced with a comprehensive system of revenue insurance. It could cover all crops and all farmers (eliminating the current bias against fruits and vegetables), provide more help to the farmers who most need help (instead of sending the biggest checks to the most affluent landowners), and do more to encourage environmental protection.

One well-designed program to help farmers manage risk would provide them with all the support they need from government. It could also save taxpayers billions of dollars.

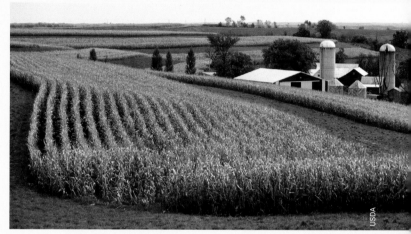

Risk management is a core competency of any farmer.

Revenue Insurance for the Whole Farm

A farmer's revenue is determined by what he earns from all his farm activities. Every farmer has a break-even point, and everyone's is different.

A farmer mainly needs government assistance to protect against severe losses in revenue. An unexpected price shock or weather event can be devastating. Farming is a capital-intensive enterprise. Equipment requires large capital investments to purchase and maintain. Inputs like seeds and fertilizer, and fuel to run equipment, are other production costs incurred annually. Land prices must also be accounted for.

What farmers do not need is income support. This is a crucial point because most farm policies are designed to help farmers manage risk by subsidizing income—for example, the Direct Payments program. Farmers are under no obligation to produce a crop to receive this support, which comes to nearly $5 billion per year for all program participants.

With farm household income consistently exceeding average household income over the last several decades, there is no justification for income support. Decades ago, when farm household income was much lower than average household income, subsidizing farmer incomes made more sense. Agriculture was once the main driver of rural economies, but that is not the case any longer in many parts of the country.

Revenue-based protection is not a new concept. More than half of all government crop insurance programs are considered revenue-based (as opposed to yield-based). Several revenue-based proposals have been put forward during previous farm bill reauthorizations. Revenue-based support has won more attention than ever in 2011 because a substantial restructuring of farm policies appears inevitable as the 2012 farm bill draws near. In 2011, some of the largest commodity groups, such as the

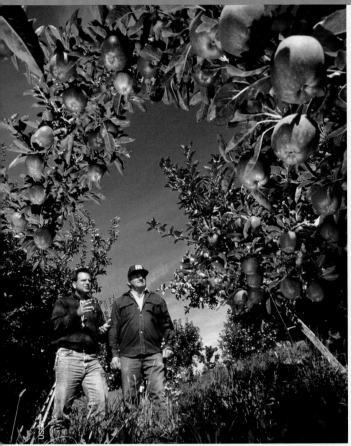

From 1995-2010, U.S. apple producers received $262 million in government support. Compare this to what corn producers received. See photo caption on page 43.

corn, soybean and cotton growers, have put forward their own versions of a revenue insurance package.

In September 2011, a revenue support plan was proposed by Senators Brown (D-OH), Thune (R-SD), Durbin (D-IL), and Lugar (R-IN). The Aggregate Risk and Revenue Management Act of 2011 (ARRM) aims to replace several of the current risk management programs. The Congressional Budget Office scored ARRM as costing $28.5 billion over 10 years, a savings of $19.8 billion compared to preserving the status quo.[93] While ARRM is a laudable effort to consolidate existing programs into a more efficient risk management system, it could go further in key respects—as could the other revenue-based systems mentioned above. The fact that ARRM saves $19.8 billion underscores how much could be saved by restructuring the existing risk management system. It is possible to achieve even greater efficiency and still provide farmers with adequate protection.

Revenue insurance should cover the whole farm enterprise. A whole-farm approach covers all activities from which farmers generate revenue. Most government crop insurance programs that are revenue-based apply to single crops rather than the whole farm. Whole-farm insurance is currently available under the federal crop insurance program, but it has been only lightly used.

Not only are farmers able to insure crops separately, they can also insure all the different fields they farm separately. Farmers with lots of land tend to farm multiple fields. Fields may be located miles apart, sometimes counties apart. As their enterprises grew in size, they may have had little choice but to farm this way. Land becomes available where it is, not always where the farmer wants it to be. If farmers weren't forced to expand this way, most would likely choose such an approach anyway as part of a risk management strategy. Diversification is an axiom of risk management, but since most large farm operations are not diverse in terms of the variety of crops they produce, they diversify by managing noncontiguous fields. It makes sense when you consider that a hailstorm could wipe out a farmer's crop on one field and not touch another less than a mile away.

While it may make sense to farm this way, it makes very little sense to insure parts of the enterprise when a farmer's revenue (and his financial well-being) is ultimately determined by the sum of his activities. A whole-farm approach to revenue insurance is critical to achieve a higher level of efficiency.

Government Support that is Trade Compliant

World trade has been moving inexorably toward more openness, and U.S. agriculture has benefited greatly and stands to benefit still more if the trend continues. Open markets benefit consumers, too. In a period when agricultural markets have become more volatile, trade liberalization can help to smooth out some of the volatility. That's especially important in poor countries, where large portions of the population spend most of their income on food.

Decoupled support is favored by economists because it is the least trade-distorting. Decoupling means support is not linked to production of particular commodities.[94] Programs that are coupled with production provide farmers incentives to produce when prices are low. This production then drives prices still lower and thus distorts the market. U.S. farmers have every reason to embrace the principle of decoupled support. U.S. policymakers should too, because the opening of markets in other countries depends to some extent on the willingness of the United States to lead by example.

Trade compliance is an issue for all farm programs. The United States is a member of the World Trade Organization (WTO) and like all members must comply with WTO rules. In 2003, Brazil brought a case against U.S. cotton subsidies, arguing U.S. programs coupled with production were distorting trade and harming Brazilian cotton producers. Through every step of the process, the WTO ruled in favor of Brazil. With the appeal process exhausted in 2009, the United States was faced with a choice of either reforming the cotton program or accepting WTO's ruling, permitting Brazil to raise tariffs on a range of U.S. exports. Rather than reforming the cotton program, the U.S. government negotiated a settlement with Brazil that costs U.S. taxpayers $147 million a year. The U.S. government is calling this a temporary fix until the next farm bill, but for the past two years the United States has been subsidizing the Brazilian cotton industry so that the Brazilian government will allow the U.S. government to continue subsidizing its own cotton producers.

Those familiar with current farm programs are likely aware that the Direct Payments program is considered decoupled support. The Direct Payments program provides a lump sum to owners of farmland with a history of raising certain crops. The program was established 15 years ago with the publically stated intention of helping to wean farmers off government subsidies, but it has morphed into something altogether different. Much of the money is transferred to investors rather than farmers, largely through an increase in the value of the farmland they own. The program rewards landowners, not the farmers who work the land. In some cases these may be the same people, but every year billions of dollars are transferred to landowners who are not farmers. While it may help some farmers to manage risk by smoothing cash flow, it is a terribly inefficient way to do so, giving much of the program's resources to people with no direct involvement in agriculture.

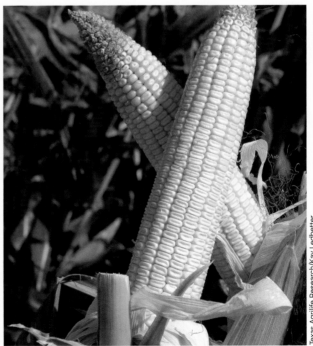

Corn subsidies, through a combination of income-support programs, totaled $77.1 billion from 1995-2010.

Texas Agrilife Research/Kay Ledbetter

A COMPREHENSIVE RISK MANAGEMENT SYSTEM

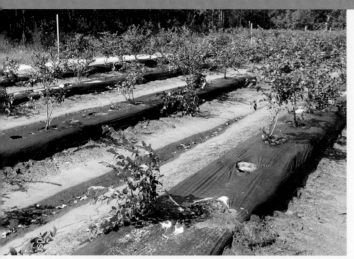

Blueberry crop damage in North Carolina from Hurricane Irene in August 2011.

The Direct Payments program should be eliminated. The fact that the Direct Payments program is decoupled from production—and therefore trade compliant—doesn't compensate for its other flaws. It doesn't provide benefits to all farmers, so it is essentially unfair. Whole-farm revenue insurance should be able to preserve the decoupling concept.

Shared Responsibility and Fairness

The principle of shared responsibility is paramount to how government and farmers work together to manage risk. For farmers, managing risk is about assuring their livelihoods. 2011 was a banner year for the U.S. farm sector, bringing some of the highest crop prices in a generation. In Kansas, Oklahoma, and Texas, however, 2011 also brought some of the worst drought conditions to that region since the Dust Bowl in the 1930s. Hurricane Irene pulverized farms up and down the East Coast, wiping out tens of thousands of acres of crops in late August. Every year, somewhere across the United States, farmers suffer losses because of adverse weather conditions they cannot avert.

Natural disasters such as droughts, hurricanes, floods, and tornadoes are referred to as systemic risks because they typically affect large geographic regions. For national

governments, it would be politically infeasible not to provide support. Disaster assistance has hardly ever faced widespread public opposition. The public understands that the food that ends up on its tables originated in some farmer's field. When government comes to the aid of ruined farmers, it is in a sense providing assurance to the public that its food security will not be undermined.

The government's responsibility is to provide support to farmers as protection in the event of a loss. Losses vary in nature. In the event of large losses due to systemic risks, such as natural disasters, the public should pay the greater share. (See the box below for more clarity about systemic risks). To cover more isolated risks, farmers ought to pay a commensurate share of the cost in insuring themselves. The federal government should define a level of coverage that it would pay for entirely, and then if the farmer wanted a higher level of coverage, she could pay for that additional increment of coverage unsubsidized. For a whole-farm revenue insurance program to qualify as nontrade distorting under WTO rules, the share of revenue insured by the government cannot exceed 70 percent.

The farmer would be able to supplement government support by purchasing a suitable complementary insurance product according to his own tolerance for risk

Systemic risks aren't solely weather-related. Crop prices may soar this year, but they could plummet in another year due to an economic recession or devaluation of currency in a key foreign market. No matter how well farmers manage their operation, they do not have influence over the rise and fall of crop prices in global markets. Variable input costs are another risk. Every farmer's revenue is affected by input costs, especially fuel costs. Crude oil prices could rise or fall suddenly depending on events in another part of the world that have nothing to do with how a farmer runs his or her business.

exposure. This is consistent with the principle of shared responsibility and leaves individual farmers with plenty of flexibility. ARRM contains a similar provision: "While this new program would provide critical revenue protection when needed, participants would rely on current private revenue insurance to manage greater losses that occur on their individual farms."[95] However, it should be noted that ARRM is not a whole-farm revenue program; it covers crop revenue on a crop-by-crop basis.

In exchange for public support, it is reasonable that farmers should comply with good environmental stewardship practices. No doubt most farmers are already good stewards of the environment. It is in their own best interest to be. Compliance should require little more, if anything, than what they are already doing of their own volition. The Direct Payments program (and nearly every other farm support and farm loan program) requires farmers to prevent soil from eroding from their land. This feature of the program should be preserved. There are currently no such requirements for crop insurance.

In addition, farmers must be able to demonstrate they are operating a viable enterprise. Viability can be measured in terms of average revenue over the course of a span of years. Naturally we realize that ups and downs occur in all industries. Indeed ebbs and flows in economic activity are the very definition of a business cycle. But if a farm is suffering revenue losses year after year, this does raise the question of whether it is a viable enterprise. It also raises legitimate questions as to whether the land being farmed should be used for agricultural production.

All farm enterprises should be eligible for public support—this ensures that one fundamental standard of fairness is met—but fairness is also a function of targeting and how people who need help the most are treated. Public support based on revenue treats low-income farmers (especially those for whom farm revenue makes up a significant share of household income) much fairer than income-support programs.

Conclusion

Policymakers have created an assortment of programs over many farm bill reauthorizations to help farmers. But it is not easy to tell why so many programs are needed. Invariably systems like this are inefficient, and the current risk management system lives up to that expectation.

Farming is a risky enterprise. Some kind of risk management system is necessary. The system outlined above would be more efficient than what exists now. Overall government spending on farm programs should fall by consolidating all existing risk management programs into a single revenue insurance program. Efficiency is a virtue under any circumstance. Given the pressures policymakers are under to reduce government spending, it cannot be overstated how much efficiency should be prized.

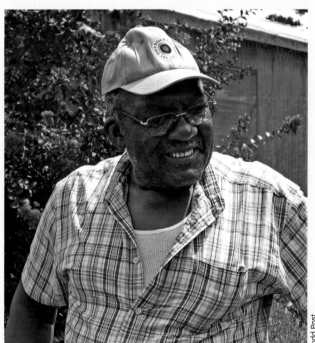

Todd Post

Under the risk management system proposed here, all farmers, regardless of income, would be eligible for support.

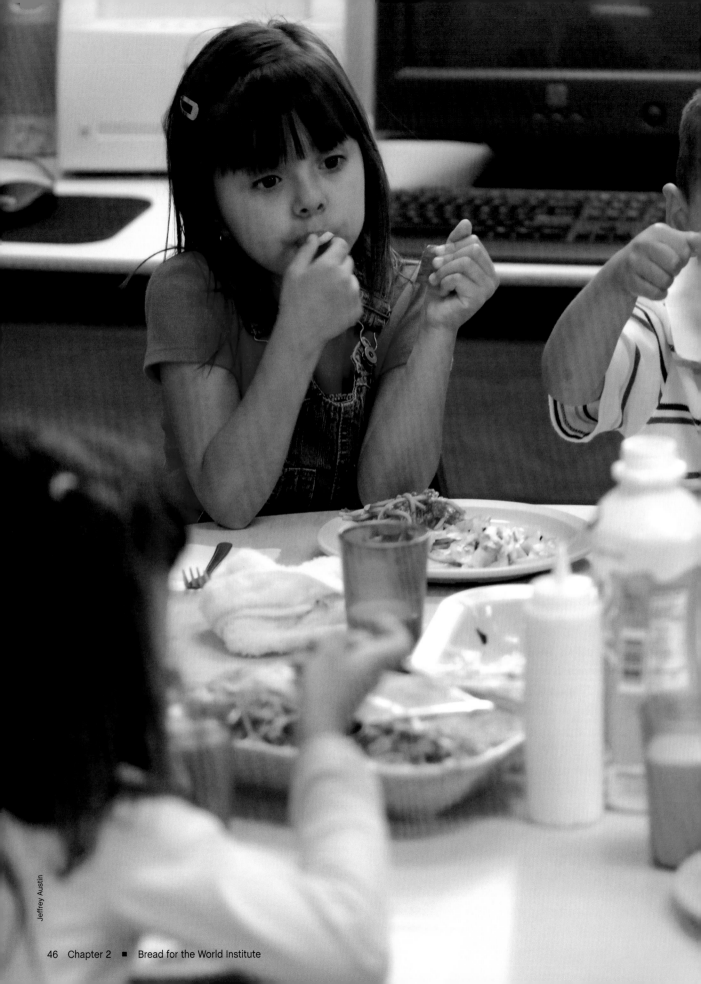

Fortifying the U.S. Nutrition Safety Net

Chapter 2

Recommendations

- SNAP, formerly food stamps, should be able to protect all family members from hunger for the duration of their monthly benefits. SNAP should also include incentive programs that make it easier for recipients to afford healthy foods.

- Child nutrition programs should provide meals that meet established dietary guidelines.

- Farm policies should help to build markets for domestic farmers to provide nutrition programs with healthy foods.

CHAPTER SUMMARY

Preventing people in the United States from going hungry is the single most important objective of federal nutrition programs. In times of high unemployment and reduced incomes, government spending on nutrition programs increases to help people cope with these difficult economic conditions.

In the past three years, since the country plunged into a severe recession, participation in nutrition programs has skyrocketed. The economy continues to stumble. Millions of people can't find work or can't find sufficient work to support their families. The programs are doing precisely what they're designed to do: counteract the impact of the recession on families and help prevent the recession from getting worse. Once the economy begins growing again at a steady and sustainable rate, the number of people eligible for nutrition programs will be closer to what it usually is.

Federal nutrition programs go a long way towards reducing hunger, but they accomplish much less by way of ensuring a healthy, well-balanced diet. This is especially troubling since more than half of all participants in nutrition programs are children. Dietary habits form early in life and tend to last a lifetime. Rates of obesity and other diet-related health conditions are soaring, and the medical costs associated with obesity have risen to hundreds of billions of dollars a year. Thus, nutrition programs need to make greater efforts to enable low-income families to overcome barriers to purchasing healthy foods.

In the upcoming farm bill, policymakers have an opportunity to make the needed improvements to nutrition programs. The nation's largest nutrition program, the Supplemental Nutrition Assistance Program (SNAP), formerly the Food Stamp Program, is reauthorized in the farm bill. Most importantly, SNAP benefits must be maintained.

In addition, SNAP should continue to scale up incentives to use benefits to purchase healthy foods. The farm bill can also provide more healthy foods to schools and day care centers. Allowing schools to purchase more locally or regionally sourced foods when possible would benefit struggling small farmers and rural communities.

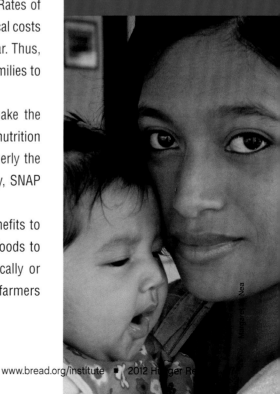

One in Four

At this point, it is hard to imagine the United States without a federal nutrition safety net. Still reeling from the worst economic crisis since the Great Depression, the country has millions of people who are out of work or working for far less money than before. Families have lost homes, depleted savings, or put dreams like purchasing a home or enrolling in college on hold. Hunger lurks in our nation's distressed communities. Nutrition programs like SNAP, National School Lunch and Breakfast programs, and WIC (for pregnant women, babies, and young children) help keep hunger at bay.

In May 2011, the number of people receiving SNAP benefits, already at an all-time high of more than 44 million, climbed by another million. It was the largest single-month increase since September 2008, when the Wall Street firm Lehman Brothers collapsed and the country spiraled into financial crisis.

In April, tornados pulverized sections of the country, destroying homes and property in areas that were already struggling. SNAP participation in Alabama increased by 102 percent, mostly because of a powerful tornado that touched down in Birmingham, the largest city in the state, destroying homes and businesses.[1] Just one month after the increase in participation, the number of SNAP participants in Alabama fell by 37.5 percent, as people affected by the storm started to recover and no longer needed assistance.[2]

When drought or floods destroy crops, Americans expect the federal government to be there to help farmers recover, and the government comes through. When natural disaster wipes out communities, Americans also count on government to be there to help families and businesses recover. The nutrition programs are one of the fastest, most effective lines of disaster response.

Few people realize that *one in four Americans* participated in a federal nutrition program in 2011.[3] Nutrition programs pay for food purchased in grocery stores and at farmer's markets; served in schools, day care, and senior centers; provided at food banks, food pantries, and soup kitchens; prescribed to women by their doctors for pre- and postnatal care.

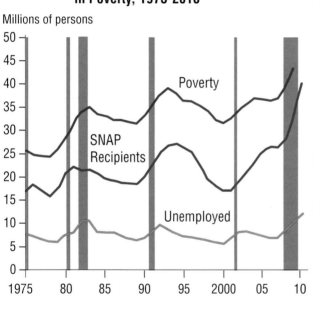

Figure 2.1 Number of SNAP Recipients, Unemployed People, and People in Poverty, 1975-2010

Millions of persons

Note: Vertical bars indicate recessions.

Source: USDA, Economic Research Service.

$731
The average monthly gross income for all SNAP households in 2010.

In 2010 the majority of SNAP participants were children or elderly. Nearly half (47 percent) of SNAP participants were under age 18 and another 8 percent were age 60 or older.

In 2010 the official U.S. poverty rate was 15.1%

Nutrition programs fortify America's families, students, and workforce. They keep families together, children learning, and the economy going. Without them, millions more households would be struggling to put food on the table.

There are undoubtedly holes in the safety net. Not everyone who needs help is eligible to participate in the programs. Some families aren't prepared to spend all their savings to meet the low asset limits that program participants are allowed. As noted earlier, federal nutrition programs could do more to help people eat healthy foods as well.

However, improvements in child nutrition programs as part of the Healthy, Hunger-Free Kids Act of 2010 are making it possible to reach more low-income children and to raise the nutritional quality of the food served. Bread for the World members and many partner groups pushed for these and other improvements—the most significant in 16 years. In spite of this success, much more progress is possible and needed, particularly at a time when more children than ever before depend on these programs as their primary source of a healthy diet.

In recent years, health professionals in the developing world have concluded that nothing is more important to human and social development than good nutrition at critical stages of a person's life, especially in childhood. Countries that have expanded nutrition programs, such as Bangladesh, Brazil, and Ghana, have made extraordinary progress in areas ranging from children's health and school performance to national economic growth and political stability. The United States, too, has used national nutrition programs to fight malnutrition. The first major U.S. nutrition program, the National School Lunch Program, was authorized in 1946, following World War II, when officials realized how many would-be soldiers had been rejected for military service because of malnutrition.[4]

Clearly, conditions in the United States today are much different than in developing countries. But the United States, like other countries, must sustain the progress it has made and adapt to changing circumstances. "Obesity is now the leading medical reason why young Americans today are unable to qualify for the armed forces," reads a statement signed by dozens of retired generals and other senior Armed Forces officials and sent to leaders of Congress in 2010, on the eve of the most recent child nutrition reauthorization.[5] The statement urged policymakers to support robust improvements in child nutrition programs. "At least 9 million young adults, or 27 percent of all young Americans ages 17 to 24, are too overweight to enlist," they noted.[6]

Childhood obesity and hunger both demand our attention since they carry serious consequences for individuals and for the country as a whole. The two

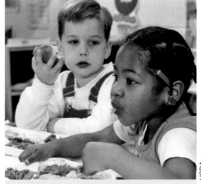

USDA

Highlights of Healthy, Hunger-Free Kids Act of 2010

- Makes significant nutrition improvements in school meals.

- Prevents junk foods from being sold in vending machines on school grounds.

- Reduces red tape so schools can serve more free and reduced-price meals to low-income children.

- Makes it easier for nonprofits to serve more children in Summer Food programs.

- Makes it easier for parents and childcare providers to obtain nutrition education resources.

- Allows state agencies to serve children in WIC for a full year, rather than six months.

- Expands the Afterschool Meal Program to 50 states, up from just 13 states.

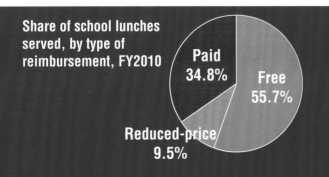

Share of school lunches served, by type of reimbursement, FY2010

Paid 34.8%

Free 55.7%

Reduced-price 9.5%

14.5% or 17.2 million households were at risk of hunger in 2010.

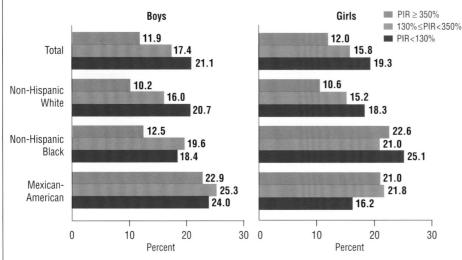

Figure 2.2 **Prevalence of Obesity Among Children and Adolescents Aged 2-19 Years, by Poverty Income Ratio(PIR), Sex and Race and Ethnicity, U.S. 2005-2008**

Legend:
- PIR ≥ 350%
- 130% ≤ PIR < 350%
- PIR < 130%

Boys

	PIR ≥ 350%	130% ≤ PIR < 350%	PIR < 130%
Total	11.9	17.4	21.1
Non-Hispanic White	10.2	16.0	20.7
Non-Hispanic Black	12.5	19.6	18.4
Mexican-American	22.9	25.3	24.0

Girls

	PIR ≥ 350%	130% ≤ PIR < 350%	PIR < 130%
Total	12.0	15.8	19.3
Non-Hispanic White	10.6	15.2	18.3
Non-Hispanic Black	22.6	21.0	25.1
Mexican-American	21.0	21.8	16.2

Poverty income ratio: The ratio of a family's income to the poverty threshold defined by the U.S. Census Bureau that applies to the family's composition.

Source: CDC/NCHS, National Health and Nutrition Examination Survey, 2005-2008.

problems are frequently interconnected. Philadelphia, for example, is one of the poorest cities in the United States, which makes it one of the hungriest as well. The obesity rate of Philadelphia's poor children is higher than that of children who are not poor.[7] In this, Philadelphia is not atypical but representative. According to a national survey of children's health, "The odds of a child's being obese or overweight were 20–60 percent higher among children in neighborhoods with the most unfavorable social conditions." *Unfavorable* social conditions, in plainer language, are the many problems that add up to what it means to live in a poor neighborhood. These include high levels of food insecurity, intermittent hunger, and limited access to supermarkets or to easy transportation to higher-income neighborhoods where healthy foods are readily accessible.[8]

Shopping for Healthy Foods—Access Barriers in Low-Income Neighborhoods

It's clear that the kind of food people eat, as well as whether they have enough, makes a big difference to their health. U.S. households purchase most of the food they consume in grocery stores, supermarkets, or superstores (e.g., Wal-Mart). This is particularly true of the 18.6 million low-income households participating in SNAP;[9] 90 percent of SNAP benefits are redeemed in grocery stores, supermarkets, or superstores.[10] Program rules prohibit redeeming SNAP benefits in restaurants and fast food establishments.[11]

Good access to supermarkets is associated with a healthier diet and reduced risk of obesity.[12] But in low-income communities, supermarkets and superstores are scarce. Other food outlets, such as small groceries or corner stores, carry a limited selection of healthy foods, especially fresh fruits and vegetables. In the 1990s, the term "food desert" was coined to describe such communities. Food deserts are found in both urban and rural contexts.[13] The most obvious and dramatic cases are in remote rural areas–places such as Indian reservations where some homes are more than 100 miles from the nearest supermarket. In an urban food desert, the distances may be much shorter, but lack of transportation still poses a barrier to shopping for healthy foods.

In New Haven, CT, the West River and Dwight neighborhoods have gone from being a food oasis to a food desert and back again. These neighborhoods have a high concentration of low-income residents. When Shaw's Supermarket opened in 1998, it was the first full-service store seen in West River or Dwight in almost 20 years.[14] Shaw's closed in March 2010 as part of a decision by corporate headquarters to cut back the number of stores. Once again, it became difficult for thousands of low-income residents to gain access to a diverse selection of healthy foods. What occurred in the West River and Dwight neighborhoods is noteworthy because it illustrates so clearly the challenges low-income neighborhoods face in gaining access to a source of healthy foods and holding onto it once they have it.

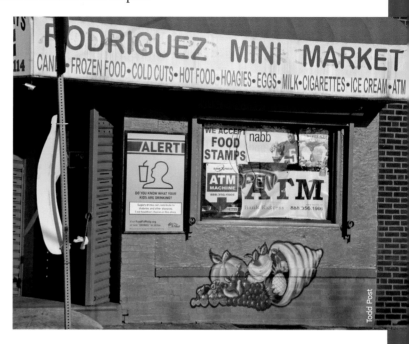

"Given that these neighborhoods aren't much more than a stone's throw from one of the world's wealthiest educational and medical complexes, Yale University, it was ironic that people in this low-income area had to endure such hardship to secure their daily sustenance," wrote Mark Winne, author of *Closing the Food Gap: Resetting the Table in the Land of Plenty* and cofounder of the Connecticut Food Policy Council. In the 1990s, Winne and the Food Policy Council supported the Greater Dwight Development Corporation (GWDC), a neighborhood nonprofit that led the effort to attract Shaw's to the neighborhood. GWDC also received support from Yale.

In a 2010 study on health conditions across the entire city of New Haven, the Yale School of Medicine found that residents of the West River/Dwight neighborhoods consumed more fruits and vegetables than people in other city neighborhoods. The study concluded, "This suggests that residents have benefitted from Shaw's and its closing will make it harder to find fresh produce in these neighborhoods."[15]

"It went beyond being a place to buy food," said Linda Thompson-Maier, a member of the GWDC when Shaw's opened and now the organization's president. "The supermarket provided a space in the community to see neighbors and socialize. There were few places elsewhere to do this. You could meet someone at the bakery counter or in the aisles and start a conversation that continued in the parking lot. Seniors came there during the day to use it as a gathering place."[16]

The store also brought the community together around food issues, Thompson-Maier told Bread for the World Institute. At the beginning of the month when SNAP/food stamp benefits were issued, store managers took advantage of this infusion of money into the neighborhood to promote certain foods, mainly junk foods. Customers found this practice distasteful and organized a petition to get the management to end such campaigns.[17]

GWDC persuaded the store's management to provide a share of store jobs to people from the community. The loss of the store was an economic blow to everyone, not just the employees who lost jobs. "Before the Shaw's

Nationally, low-income zip codes have 25 percent fewer chain supermarkets and 30 percent more convenience stores than middle-income zip codes. Convenience stores stock fewer healthy foods than supermarkets.

BOX 2.1 OBESITY AND THE FOOD ENVIRONMENT

Some communities have particularly high, concentrated obesity levels—nutrition experts call these obesogenic environments. Such environments are not confined to low-income areas, but they are more common there. Where there's a scarcity of full-service food outlets such as supermarkets, there are also fewer healthy food choices. A lack of places to shop is combined with a large number of fast food outlets—also common in low-income communities.

Fresh fruits and vegetables and other healthy foods tend to be more expensive than low-nutrient, calorie-dense processed foods. Low-income households are by definition those with fewer resources to spend on food, so healthy food choices are often simply out of reach. Buying less healthy food is dictated by economic conditions in the community. Food retailers in low-income communities understand this dynamic and select the products they will carry accordingly.

Nutrition programs help to bridge access gaps; for example, SNAP boosts the purchasing power of eligible households. But participants who live in low-income communities still face the problem of finding places to shop that carry a broad selection of healthy foods.

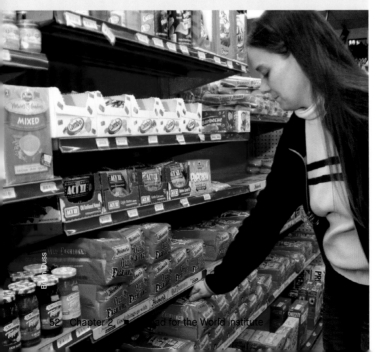

opened its doors, it was estimated that almost all of New Haven's $115 million in annual residential food expenditures were leaving the city for the suburbs," explained Winne. "By keeping a much greater portion of that wealth in neighborhoods that are starved for economic activity, the supermarket not only provided people with access to quality food at affordable prices but was also a good-size economic engine."[18]

Fortunately, this story ends on a positive note. In February 2011, the community succeeded in attracting another supermarket chain, Stop and Shop, to occupy the vacant space left by Shaw's.[19] Once again, GWDC provided the leadership and Yale offered support. It's important to note, though, that most low-income communities do not have such well-organized or powerful friends.

Philadelphia's Witnesses: Listen to the Voice of Hunger!

Funding for nutrition programs comprises 74 percent of the U.S. Department of Agriculture's (USDA) budget. These programs serve mainly families living in poverty or near the poverty line, helping them get the food they need to stave off hunger. Income determines eligibility. But it's more than lack of purchasing power that puts families at risk of hunger. The environments in which low-income families are forced to live pose additional risks.

In some neighborhoods of Philadelphia, as many as half of all residents live below the poverty line. Tianna Gaines-Turner and her family live in one of the most distressed neighborhoods in the city, the Frankford neighborhood in northeast Philadelphia. She and her husband are raising six young children, and the family is dogged by hunger most of the time.

The family moved here two years ago when they were offered subsidized housing after spending 10 years on a waiting list. On their first day in the new home, Gaines-Turner was sitting on the stoop with her children when a man approached from the sidewalk and told her to take the children and go inside. She understood what this meant and complied at once. Minutes later, the street exploded in gunfire.

The Gaines-Turner family has benefited from federal nutrition programs. Gaines-Turner has participated in WIC, her eldest child receives subsidized meals at school, and the whole family has participated in SNAP from time to time as their income fluctuates.

Currently, Tianna is the sole breadwinner in the family, working a combination of three jobs. Her husband, Marcus, was laid off during the recession and has not been able to find work.

Tianna Gaines-Turner was featured in a series of articles in the *Philadelphia Inquirer* about hunger in the city. She is part of *Witnesses to Hunger*, a research project developed by Children's HealthWatch and led by Dr. Mariana Chilton of the Center for Hunger-Free Communities at Drexell University's School of Public Health. *Witnesses* launched in 2008 with photographs taken and stories told by Philadelphia women living in poverty.

"Speak. Teach." read the invitation to participate in the project. "We want to learn from you." The women who participate in *Witnesses* know what it means to be hungry and are better teachers than anyone. As a Witness, Gaines-Turner has spoken a number of times to various groups of people who want to understand hunger in the United States.

The images that convey hunger to those who know it most intimately are often not the images that other people might associate with hunger. Hunger through a Witness' eyes may be a blood-soaked sidewalk, reflecting the dangers of walking from home to the grocery store. Hunger could be a triptych of bus stops, because that's what it takes to get to a store with healthy food choices.

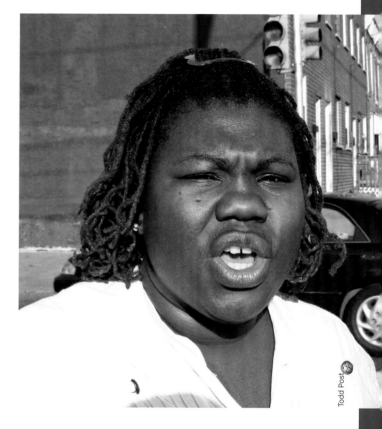

Philadelphia resident Tianna Gaines-Turner of *Witnesses to Hunger* has appeared on national television and in other major media to discuss her experience of being hungry.

Many of the *Witnesses* volunteers were born into poor families where hunger was a constant presence. In many ways, hunger stole their childhoods from them, and now as adults, they are raising families that continue to battle hunger. "They are the ones who actually have the answers," said Chilton. "Families are not just passive recipients of aid and advice. They are purposeful agents [who] want to break the cycle of poverty and despair, and they have a variety of needs."

Witnesses was born out of Children's HealthWatch, a multi-city research project that is studying the effects of hunger on the health and well-being of young children.[20] Chilton serves as the principal investigator of its Philadelphia site. The project screens children in emergency rooms and ambulatory care clinics at five medical centers around the country—good places to initiate contact with the children and their parents since undernourished children have higher rates of hospitalization. At each Children's HealthWatch site is a GROW Clinic, which treats children with "failure to thrive," the clinical term for a child who is severely underweight for her age.[21] If failure to thrive goes untreated, the consequences are lifelong, because so much of brain development occurs in the first years of life.

"In the GROW Clinic," says Chilton, "there is a pediatrician, nutritionist, psychologist, and social worker on staff, and the social worker and psychologist are the most important members of the team."[22] She cites a Children's HealthWatch finding that children in families on a waiting list for a housing subsidy were 52 percent more likely to be underweight than those whose families had the subsidy.[23] "Hunger is about so much more than food," she says. And it is more than physical anguish; it punishes its victims mentally, emotionally, and spiritually. "It's horrible when you see your kids not eating," says Tianna Gaines-Turner, "and you say to them why aren't you eating and they say because we want to make sure you can eat, Mommy."

"The idea that children are somehow protected from food insecurity by parents is a myth," says Ed Frongillo, professor of public health at the University of South Carolina. "Children are aware of the inadequate quantity or quality of food, the struggles that adults are going through to meet food needs, and the limitations of resources for meeting those needs."[24]

The effects of multiple hardships on children have been well documented by Frongillo, Chilton and her colleagues at Children's HealthWatch,[25] and researchers elsewhere—and portrayed more bluntly in the images and words of *Witnesses to Hunger*. Violence, evictions, parental anxiety rising to crescendo as the month comes to an end and the refrigerator empties—the list goes on.

There is only so much any one program can do to soften the effects of these problems on children. But an analysis by the Center on Budget and Policy Priorities shows that SNAP lifts more families with children out of poverty than any other assistance program except the Earned Income Tax Credit (EITC).[26] (See Figure 2.3.) About half of all Americans will receive SNAP benefits at some point before age 20. Among African-Americans, the figure is 90 percent.[27]

The EITC offers a tax refund, a lump sum payment that comes once a year and is ideal for paying down debt, fixing a busted car, dealing with a lingering medical problem, or other such expenses. Low-income working families find it difficult or impossible to budget for these items, because all their resources are simply consumed by day-to-day needs. SNAP and other nutrition programs, on the other hand, come through for low-income families all year long. They also help the many people who have short-lived scrapes with hunger without experiencing the other hardships of poverty. This is why programs such as SNAP are so vital to meeting the needs of all families, regardless of the harshness of their environment.

Nutrition Programs Struggle to Stave Off Cuts—Despite Success and Public Support

Each year, USDA updates the official data on hunger in the United States in a report, *Household Food Security in the United States*. It's based on the results of a survey conducted at the end of the previous year. The survey asks heads of household if during the past 12 months, due to economic hardship, they or any of their family members were forced to go without eating for any length of time or to reduce their food consumption to unacceptable levels. Those who respond affirmatively are considered "food insecure."

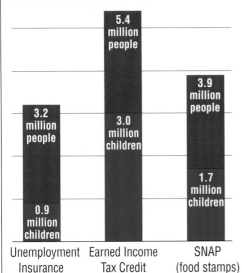

Figure 2.3 **Government Programs Kept Millions Out of Poverty in 2010**

People kept above the poverty line in 2010 when selected benefits are counted as income

Unemployment Insurance: 3.2 million people, 0.9 million children
Earned Income Tax Credit: 5.4 million people, 3.0 million children
SNAP (food stamps): 3.9 million people, 1.7 million children

Source: U.S. Census Bureau.

In 2008, 14.6 percent of all U.S. households were food insecure[28]—the highest rate since USDA began reporting food security data in the mid-1990s. One might have expected to see the percentage of food insecure households rise significantly in 2009 and 2010. But, in fact, there was no significant change—which seemed unlikely given the continued rise in unemployment.

Food insecurity did not rise dramatically *mainly because enrollment in SNAP increased*–by 25 percent in 2009. The average monthly participation in the program grew to more than 33 million people in 2009.[29] In 2010, enrollment climbed above 40 million people per month, and in 2011, it topped 45 million—about one in seven Americans.

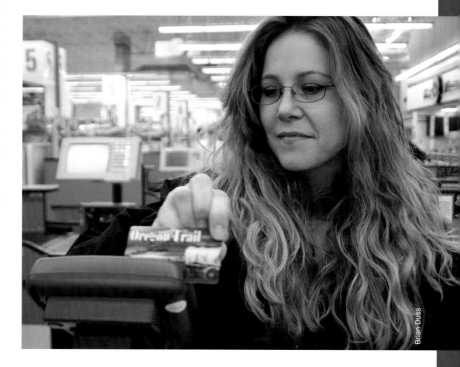

The American Recovery and Reinvestment Act (ARRA), enacted in February 2009, boosted monthly SNAP benefits by 13.6 percent. This meant that starting in April 2009, a family of four received an increase of approximately $80 per month.[30] The increase in benefits led to a 2.2 percent drop in food insecurity among low-income households that qualified for SNAP. But food insecurity did not decrease at all in low-income households just above the SNAP threshold,[31] which is 130 percent of the poverty level.

The Great Recession was the impetus for the increase in benefits, but it was long overdue in any case. Years before, USDA research on SNAP usage was already indicating that more than 90 percent of participating households run out of benefits well before the end of the month.[32] In households with children, it is common for parents to forgo food themselves so that children do not have to miss meals. Research points to this as a factor in why obesity occurs at higher rates among female heads of poor households. Periods of food scarcity lead to overconsumption once food becomes available again. This condition, known in clinical terms as "post-starvation hyperphagia," wreaks havoc on people's metabolism and makes them susceptible to weight gain.[33]

In 2010, as the news emerged that the boost in SNAP participation and benefits had done so much to hold the line against hunger in 2009, Congress was already in the midst of debating whether to cut the benefits back again. When Congress initially boosted monthly benefits, legislators decided to let inflation erode the value of the increase over time. First came an $11.9 billion cut in SNAP benefits to help pay for a $26 billion state aid package.[34] This decision made little sense for two reasons. The SNAP increase was, of course, intended to fill in the food gaps for households that come up short at the end of the month.[35] Unemployment was still hovering near 10 percent and was expected to remain high for some time. The additional resources meant that fewer parents had to make the choice to go without food to pro-

SNAP (or food stamps) participation has increased in part because of improvements in how the program is administered; for example, by providing benefits electronically through a debit card, as shown here, reducing stigma and lowering the cost of administering the program.

Matt Newell-Ching
Bread for the World

In Grant County, Oregon, it's expensive to be poor.

The average cost of a meal in the county is $2.83, which is 23 cents higher than the state average in Oregon, according to a 2011 study by Feeding America. For a family of four, this comes to an additional $82 per month.

Combine the high cost of food with unemployment averaging more than 13 percent in 2011, and it's easy to see why many of the 7,400 residents of this rural county tucked away in the mountains of eastern Oregon struggle against hunger. The food insecurity rate in the county is nearly 20 percent.

"There are a lot of isolated communities in Grant County that don't have access to affordable, nutritious food," said

Sharon Thornberry, community resource developer for the Oregon Food Bank. Residents in the most isolated parts of the county face the choice of paying higher prices for food that is closer or driving the longer distance and paying more for gas. "There's a Thriftway in John Day [the Grant County seat], but it's 70 miles south, or they can go 100 miles north to the next closest grocery stores," said Thornberry.

Through her work with the Oregon Food Bank, Thornberry is helping communities and towns across Oregon organize to increase their access to healthy, affordable food. This comes at a time when many groups around the country are reassessing their local

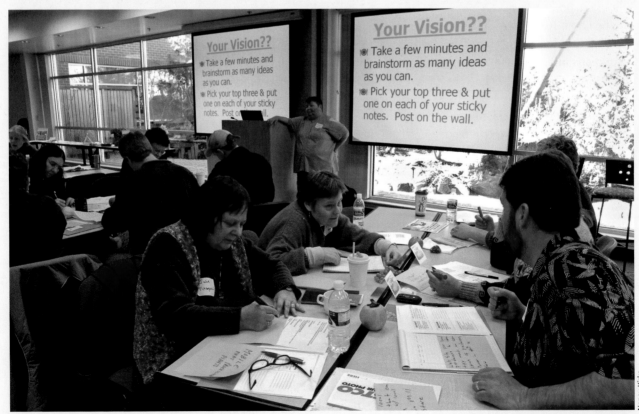

Nancy Kirks

food systems through a tool—the Community Food Security Assessment—offered on the website of the U.S. Department of Agriculture (USDA). Advocates can use the tool to analyze their community's food-related resources—from grocery stores to farms, soup kitchens, food pantries, and more—and evaluate residents' access to affordable, nutritious food. The only problem, according to Thornberry, is that many of these assessments have been completed but are now sitting on the shelf. The challenge is moving from assessing the needs to organizing for action.

Thornberry developed an organizing process for Oregon's communities called a Community FEAST (Food, Education, Agriculture Solutions Together). The idea is simple: bring together farmers, grocery store owners, emergency food providers, nutritionists, educators, community leaders, elected officials—as many stakeholders as possible—for a conversation about improving the local food system. At the end of the six-hour FEAST workshop, the seeds of a strategic organizing plan emerge.

One of the essential elements of the program is that it is led by a steering committee comprised of local stakeholders. "We [at the Oregon Food Bank] give advice," said Thornberry, "but it's the steering committee that continues the work long after the FEAST is done."

The efforts pay off. For example, before Grant County's FEAST in 2010, there was one emergency food pantry in the entire county and it was open only one day a month. Today, not only are there four food pantries, but a summer meals site, a community garden, and a farmer's market have recently been added.

Across the state, the idea is gaining traction. So far, 18 communities in Oregon and towns along state borders have held FEASTS, and 18 more have been planned for 2011 and 2012.

The first FEAST was held in 2009 in Clatsop County in the northwestern part of the state. Afterward, advocates formed a nonprofit called the North Coast Food Web with the goal of sustaining the work of the convening group. A newly formed farmer's market in the town of Astoria accepts SNAP benefits and has cooking demonstrations onsite. Workshops on seafood canning are also underway.

Elected officials are getting involved too. A city council member in the town of Klamath Falls came to the local FEAST and is now seeking grant funding to establish a downtown city food center. The entire city council of Forest Grove showed up for the community FEAST.

In 2009, Thornberry was honored as a Public Health Genius, an award given by the Oregon Community Health Partnership. She has her own personal experience of being hungry. In the late 1970s, she found herself homeless with two small children. "As a mother, there's no worse feeling than not knowing what to feed your kids. My motivation for this work is that no one should have to be in that situation," she said.

Matt Newell-Ching is an organizer in Bread for the World's western regional office.

Pictured on opposite page: Sharon Thornberry, community resource developer for the Oregon Food Bank, leads a FEAST in Lebanon, Oregon, in 2010.

tect their children from hunger. Second, the raise was intended to help state and local economies recover from the recession: every dollar spent on SNAP generates an additional $1.74 of economic activity.[36] The SNAP benefits moving through communities save jobs, making it possible for state and local governments to avoid layoffs of teachers, police officers, and other public employees, and preventing layoffs in the private sector as well.

A separate $2.2 billion in cuts to SNAP was the price of getting Congress to agree to the improvements in the Healthy, Hunger-Free Kids Act of 2010. Many viewed it as a quid pro quo, since the child nutrition programs benefit many of the same households that participate in SNAP. But according to Jim Weill, president of the Food Research and Action Coalition, this is not entirely true, because the money taken from SNAP had been benefiting whole families and would now be going primarily to school-aged children. Little was done to cushion the financial blow for infants, toddlers, and preschoolers,[37] for example—even though the most important developmental stage in life is early childhood.[38]

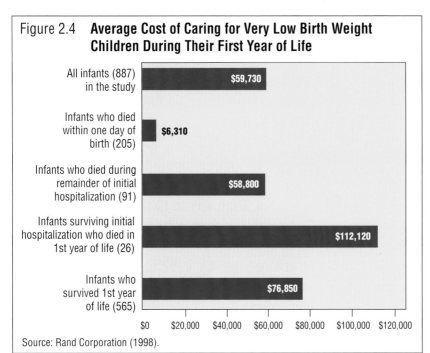

Figure 2.4 **Average Cost of Caring for Very Low Birth Weight Children During Their First Year of Life**

Source: Rand Corporation (1998).

Currently, all of the nutrition programs are at risk of additional cuts as Congress prepares to slash federal spending under the terms of an agreement forged with the White House in August 2011 to raise the government's debt ceiling. At the time of this writing, we do not yet know the breadth and depth of cuts or proposed cuts to nutrition programs. Many other programs that help low-income families, such as the EITC and other work supports, could also face cuts.

Thus far, SNAP as an entitlement program has managed to escape further cuts. WIC and other programs for low-income people have not been as lucky. In April 2011, $504 million was cut from WIC as part of a deficit reduction deal between the White House and Congress to avoid a government shutdown. Cuts to WIC are appalling considering all that is now known about the critical window of human development during the first 1,000 days of life. The nutritional status of the mother and child at this time makes all the difference for the rest of the child's life—from school achievements to work productivity.

Cutting WIC also makes little sense economically. In addition to providing foods needed for a healthy pregnancy and early childhood, WIC includes nutrition education and access to health care. The program has been proven to reduce rates of fetal mortality and low birth weight and to enhance the nutritional quality of a baby's diet.[39] A landmark study in 1991 showed that every dollar spent on WIC saves the government between $1.77 and $3.13 in Medicaid costs for newborns and their mothers. The findings in the study and the strong support for the program from doctors and other medical professionals[40] contributed to bipartisan support for steady increases in WIC funding to ensure that no family would be denied participation. But 20 years later—in spite of volumes of additional research that confirms the value of WIC[41]—it seems that ideological differences among elected officials threaten funding for a cost-effective program with broad public support (94 percent in a 2010 study).[42]

Cutting WIC, SNAP, and other nutrition programs goes against everything we know about the value of preventive care in saving on long-term healthcare costs. (See Figure 2.4.) Nutrition programs are one of the most cost-effective ways to control rising healthcare costs, which in the long run are a much greater threat to the nation's economy than the cost of nutrition programs. Hunger makes people more vulnerable to chronic health problems. Intermittent hunger also contributes to binge eating and overeating to cope with stress and depression. Hunger in babies wreaks havoc on their metabolism and makes them susceptible to obesity later in life. And hunger among children affects cognitive development and leads to lower academic achievement.[43]

Getting Serious About Obesity

SNAP is authorized through the farm bill, usually every five years. This is the most likely time for any significant changes to be made to the program. While deliberating the 2008 farm bill, members of Congress considered a proposal to ban the purchase of soda and other soft drinks with SNAP benefits. The proposal was ultimately rejected, but those who supported a ban pledged to try again during the next reauthorization.[44] Such restrictions are only one battle that defenders of SNAP will have to fight. There will also be fierce political pressure to reduce benefit levels in order to protect funding for farm programs.

SNAP doesn't have restrictions on food purchases, with the exception of prepared foods. Also banned are alcohol and cigarettes. What has led some legislators to consider soft drinks on a par with alcohol and cigarettes is an obesity epidemic that now claims more than a third of U.S. adults and 17 percent of children.[45] U.S. healthcare costs related to obesity are estimated to be $147 billion per year,[46] and there is no disagreement among public health specialists that overconsumption of soft drinks is a factor in soaring obesity rates.[47]

The farm bill is not the only time the subject of banning the purchase of soft drinks has arisen. States and municipalities that administer SNAP can seek a waiver from USDA to operate outside federally mandated rules. In 2010, New York City asked USDA for a waiver to ban purchases of soft drinks with SNAP benefits for two years in order to study the effects. As early as 2004, Minnesota sought a similar waiver to restrict purchase of soft drinks and other junk foods with food stamp benefits.[48] In both cases, USDA rejected the waiver request.

District of Columbia WIC Director Gloria Clark shown with DC's new mobile WIC clinic, which will travel to underserved parts of the city to provide needed services.

The New York and Minnesota decisions were the right ones. When the farm bill is reauthorized, Congress should resist public pressure to limit choices in SNAP. SNAP participants are an easy group to single out, because government benefits help them buy food, but changing SNAP rules is an ill-targeted way to try to reduce obesity. The obesity epidemic affects all income groups. In the last 20 years, obesity rates have risen among all demographic groups—*except* SNAP/food stamp recipients.[49]

Singling out SNAP participants for restrictions on purchases implies that SNAP contributes to obesity, but there is no such causal relationship. It's a logical leap to assume that SNAP contributes to obesity simply because many low-income households participate—on the contrary, research suggests that female SNAP participants have lower obesity rates than women who are eligible for SNAP but do not participate.[50] SNAP may in fact help fight obesity in low-income households.

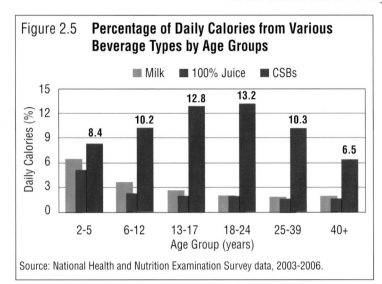

Figure 2.5 **Percentage of Daily Calories from Various Beverage Types by Age Groups**

Source: National Health and Nutrition Examination Survey data, 2003-2006.

We know that not all neighborhoods contain equally accessible amounts of healthy foods. We know that in low-income households, the quality of food too often must be sacrificed for quantity. Professor Christine Olson of Cornell University has spent much of her career studying food insecure families. She reports, "I can't tell you how many women say, 'I buy a 2-liter bottle of sugared soda for 99 cents, and that's what I consume for the day when things really get tight.'"[51] Angela Sutton, a volunteer for *Witnesses to Hunger*, puts her own situation in simple, stark terms: "I'm fat so I can make sure my kids have healthy foods."[52]

The nation is rightfully concerned about obesity, especially childhood obesity. Presently, children ages 2 to 5—from all income groups—get most of their beverage calories from calorically sweetened beverages (CSBs), as do all other age groups.[53] (See Figure 2.5.) Soda and other CSBs are the most popular beverages in all age groups, and Americans from all walks of life drink soda and other CSBs. They are considered normal beverage selections. Singling out SNAP participants as the only people soda is "bad" for would stigmatize them without confronting the nation's obesity epidemic. It could add to the number of eligible households who choose not to participate in SNAP—ironic since for years, USDA has worked to boost participation and reduce the stigma associated with food stamps/SNAP.

The soft drink industry spends more than a billion dollars a year marketing its products to Americans—with much of the advertising aimed at children.[54] The Federal Trade Commission said in a 2008 report to Congress that nearly two-thirds (63 percent) of the money spent marketing foods to children is used to sell soft drinks.[55] So far, Congress has allowed the soft drink industry to regulate itself. The industry has responded to public pressure by removing soda from vending machines in schools, but other CSBs, such as Gatorade and similar sports drinks, continue to be sold.

Researchers at Yale's Rudd Center on Food Policy and Obesity estimate that a one-cent-per-ounce tax on sugar-sweetened beverages would generate $79 billion in revenue between 2010 and 2015. It would also reduce soda consumption by about 24 percent and individuals' calorie consumption from sugar-sweetened beverages by an average of 150-200 calories per day.[56]

A tax on soft drink purchases would reflect the scope of the obesity epidemic—all who choose to consume soft drinks would help pay. Given the large amounts of soft drinks consumed in this country, the tax would also raise significant resources to aid in a national anti-obesity campaign.

Incentives to Help SNAP Households Purchase Healthy Foods

"Lower prices for some healthier foods, such as low-fat milk and dark green vegetables, are associated with decreases in children's Body Mass Index," concluded researchers at USDA in a 2011 report. "These results show that the effect of subsidizing healthy food may be just as large as raising prices of less healthy foods."[57]

Incentives make a lot more sense than restrictions if the goal is to encourage SNAP participants to choose healthy foods. As the research above suggests, for example, incentives could achieve the same goal intended by restricting soda purchases, but without stigmatizing families and making decisions on the details of daily life for working adults.

The 2008 farm bill authorized $20 million for a Healthy Incentives Pilot (HIP) to test whether SNAP households would take advantage of matching funds to purchase more fruits and vegetables.[58] State agencies from across the country were invited to compete to host the pilot. Hampden County, MA, was selected on the basis of a proposal submitted by the Massachusetts Department of Transitional Assistance.[59] Hampden County is home to two of the poorest cities in Massachusetts (Springfield and Holyoke) and has the second-highest obesity rate of the state's 14 counties.[60]

The pilot will begin in November 2011 and run for 15 months. For every dollar that SNAP households spend on fruits and vegetables, they will receive an additional 30 cents in benefits, up to a limit of $60 per month. "What this is doing is leveling the playing field for low-income folks, so that a healthier diet is within their reach," explains Julia Kehoe, state commissioner of the Department of Transitional Assistance.[61]

To stretch their food budgets, poor households have little choice but to sacrifice the quality of food. Healthy foods like fruits and vegetables are more expensive and less filling than calorie-dense, processed foods. The latter are simply better at keeping hunger pangs at bay. For example, a dollar's worth of potato chips buys five times as many calories as a dollar's worth of vegetables—and seven times as many as fresh fruit.[62]

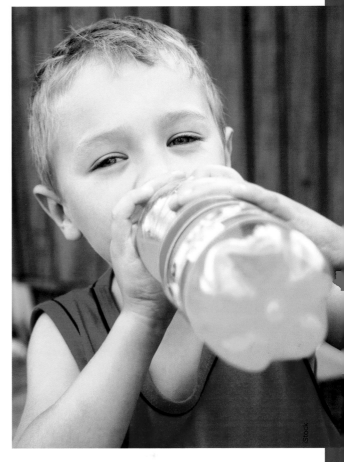

Nearly two-thirds of the money spent on marketing foods to children is for soft drinks.

In 2010, 43 percent of SNAP participants lived on incomes that were 50 percent or less of the poverty level[63]—the definition of "deep poverty" in the United States. For a family of four, 50 percent of the poverty line means $7.55 per person per day for all expenses: food, housing, transportation, utilities, healthcare, and everything else.[64]

Incentive programs within SNAP are not new. State and local governments partnering with private industry and nonprofits have tied "bonus bucks" to making purchases at farmer's markets. Wholesome Wave, a Connecticut-based nonprofit, sponsors an incentive program around the country to encourage SNAP recipients to shop at farmer's markets, including one in Abingdon, VA. "The incentives get people to the market," says Sara Cardinale, manager of the Abingdon Farmer's Market. "We know that people are coming back, so eating habits appear to be changing."[65]

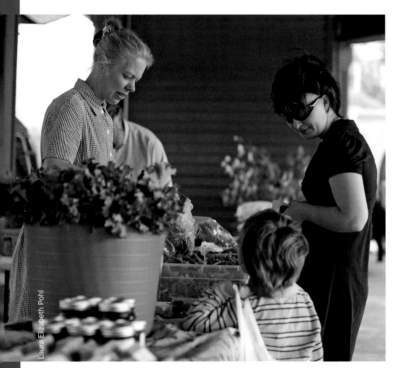

Marie Crise and her son Lee shop at the Abingdon Farmer's Market in Abingdon, VA, taking advantage of a "bonus bucks" program with their SNAP benefits to purchase healthy foods at a discount.

Marie Crise is one of those who uses her SNAP benefits at the Abingdon farmer's market. Crise's situation is all too common. She fled an abusive husband with her 4-year-old son Lee. Currently homeless, they are staying with a relative, using a "couch-surfing" approach until they can afford a room or apartment. Crise is a nursing student at the local community college and she understands how important good nutrition is for Lee at this stage of his life. The farmer's market is important to her because of the quality of the food. With the bonus bucks, she can feed her son well without having to sacrifice as much healthy food for herself.

After deciding how much she wants to spend from her SNAP benefits, Crise purchases tokens from the market's manager. For every $10 in SNAP benefits that she converts to tokens, she receives an additional $5 to spend at the market. The manager swipes the SNAP debit card through a wireless point-of-sales machine, the same one used to swipe customers' credit and bank debit cards.

Over the past decade, the Food Stamp Program/SNAP has made many changes to reduce the stigma once associated with the program. Perhaps the most significant has been the change from paper coupons to an electronic benefit transfer (EBT) card. At the grocery store, customers can access their SNAP benefits inconspicuously, as though they were using a bankcard. The EBT card has reduced the potential for fraud and the use of SNAP benefits for purposes other than food, but unfortunately the card has also made it harder for SNAP recipients to shop at farmer's markets. Purchases made with SNAP benefits at farmer's markets have plummeted since the introduction of EBT,[66] because most vendors at the markets still deal in cash only. The Abingdon Farmer's Market is among the small fraction able to handle electronic transactions.

Farmer's markets offer an ideal opportunity to strengthen the relationship between U.S. nutrition and farm policy. USDA offers help to farmer's markets that want to process SNAP benefits, but the technology to do so is expensive—the point-of-sales machine at the Abingdon Market cost $3,000—and the help USDA offers is mostly instructional, not financial. There are government programs that provide benefits for seniors and WIC families to shop at farmer's markets, but not yet a similar program for SNAP participants. The United States has more than 40 million people receiving SNAP benefits. If the program provided participants with greater incentives to shop at farmer's markets, markets across the country would have a powerful reason to invest in the necessary technology, while SNAP families would have more incentive to shop at farmer's markets.

Nutrition education is key to getting people to try new foods. Most people don't decide to improve their diets before they know what their options are. Farmer's markets are an optimal environment for nutrition education. In fact, most are already engaged in some form of it, such as offering samples and recipes—nutrition education by another name could be just plain direct marketing. For the best results, trained personnel should be leading outreach efforts. In 2010, USDA's Expanded Food and Nutrition Education Program (EFNEP) provided nutrition education to more than 600,000 adults and youths. The impressive results reported—at least 84 percent of adults and 57 percent of youth made improvements in diet, nutrition, and/or food savings—are typical for the program since its launch 40 years ago.[67]

Figure 2.6   2010 Impacts: USDA's Expanded Food and Nutrition Education Program (EFNEP)

Changing Adult Behavior

DIET QUALITY — 94% — Percentage of adults improving **diet**, including consuming an **extra cup of fruits and vegetables**

NUTRITION — 89% — Percentage of adults improving **nutrition** practices

FOOD SAVINGS — 84% — Percentage of adults bettering **food resource management** practices

Influencing Youth

DIET QUALITY — 61% — Percentage of 101,237 youth now eating a **variety of foods**

NUTRITION — 62% — Percentage of 132,250 youth increasing **essential human nutrition** knowledge

FOOD SAVINGS — 57% — Percentage of 103,943 youth increasing ability to select **low-cost, nutritious foods**

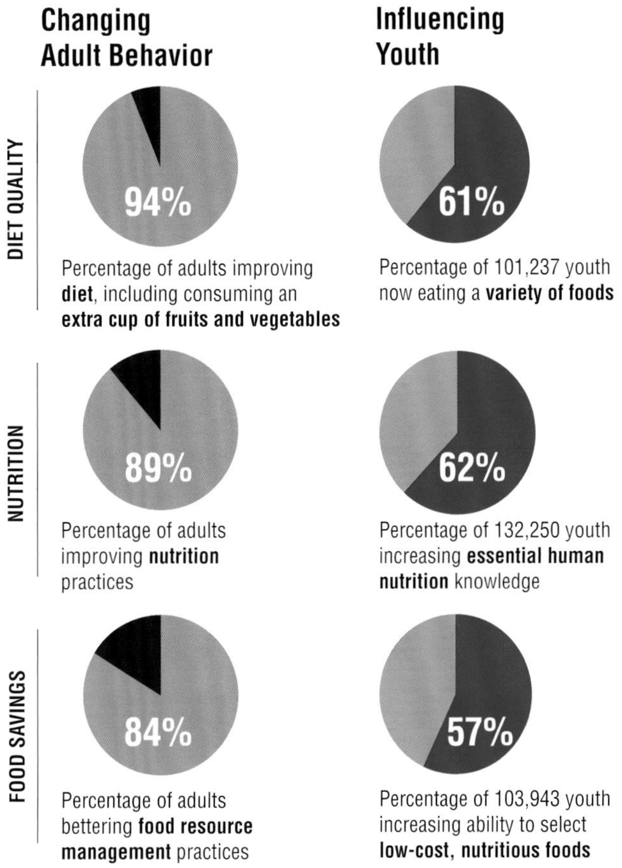

Source: USDA, National Institute of Food and Agriculture.

The School Cafeteria: Where the Healthy, Hunger-Free Kids Act and the Farm Bill Meet

Together with SNAP and WIC, the National School Lunch and Breakfast programs and the Child and Adult Care Feeding Program (CACFP) make up more than 90 percent of the federal funding for nutrition programs.[68] Schools and daycare centers play a central role in making sure healthy foods are available to low-income children. To do this, they depend on the foods provided through the National School Lunch and Breakfast programs and CACFP. The federal government became a much better partner with the passage of the Healthy, Hunger-Free Kids Act of 2010, which includes the first significant improvements to child nutrition standards in 16 years.

Improving the quality of meals served to U.S. children shouldn't end with the Healthy, Hunger-Free Kids Act, though. Additional improvements could be made through the farm bill. The Fresh Fruit and Vegetable Program, for example, is funded though the farm bill. It provides fresh produce to schools in neighborhoods where children might never have seen such foods before.

BOX 2.3   FARM-TO-SCHOOL PROGRAMS HELP KIDS EAT BETTER AND BENEFIT LOCAL FARMERS AND COMMUNITIES

At Platte River Elementary School in Benzie County, MI, 65 percent of the children qualify for free or reduced-price meals. And thanks to a farm-to-school program, children are also able to take fresh fruits and vegetables home with them.

The farm-to-school program also helps keep the school salad bars stocked. Twelve-year-old Alex Reed loves the salad bar at school. Fresh vegetables are rarely available at home for him and his five siblings because the family has trouble affording them. The family receives SNAP benefits to help pay for food. "A family of eight, you buy fresh fruits and vegetables and it is gone in a day and a half," says Alex's mother, Shannon Reed.[69]

Renee DeWindt (pictured below) came on board as food service director for Benzie County schools (and for two other districts in northwest Michigan) in 2005. Students at one of the middle schools had just gone on strike to protest the low quality of the meals served there.

On the day of the strike, not a single student went through the lunch line.

When the school superintendent hired DeWindt, he asked her to look into a new farm-to-school program. He'd learned about the fledgling effort from the Michigan Land Use Institute, which links local farms with cafeterias. There are two objectives: helping schoolchildren gain access to healthier food, and supporting local farmers and ranchers and their communities. Renee DeWindt was the right person for the assignment.

"The first thing people assume is [that] serving healthy, higher quality food costs more than schools can afford," she says. But it turned out to be the exact opposite. When she took over the management of the school food services budget in Benzie County, it was more than $100,000 in the red. DeWindt has turned it into a profit-generating enterprise—*and* the foods she serves are higher quality. Students and their parents are more satisfied, and the lunch lines aren't empty.

DeWindt's recipe for success comes down to cultivating strong partnerships with the children, their parents, and the local farmers she purchases food from. For example, a local dairy farmer had no market for some of his milk; he asked DeWindt if she could use it at a reduced cost since he would otherwise have to dump it. They worked out a deal: he provided her with a dispenser, and she now buys milk from him regularly. The milk is fresher than what she had been purchasing, and the children think it tastes better. In fact, the farmer told DeWindt that his customer base has grown because parents are buying it from him to give their kids at home.

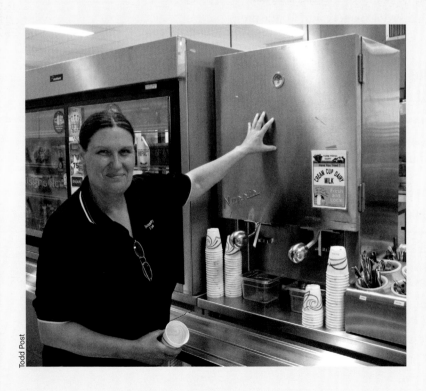

Todd Post

All schools are eligible to participate, but the program gives priority to those with the highest proportion of students eligible for free or reduced-price meals. The program was launched in the 2002 farm bill as a pilot in just four states. Because the pilot was a success and demand for the program began to come in from across the country, the 2008 farm bill made the Fresh Fruit and Vegetable Program permanent and available in all 50 states.[70]

Fresh fruit and vegetable consumption in schools has been on the rise for the past decade in Burlington, VT, where nearly half the children qualify for free or reduced-price meals. Burlington is one of 15 school districts in the nation to be named a USDA model farm-to-school program, an effort where local farms are tapped to provide a share of the foods served in schools.[71] Burlington's program has now grown beyond the cafeteria to bring healthy, fresh snacks into the classroom.

"If you put a bowl of grapes in a classroom, kids will eat them," says Doug Davis, food services director of Burlington Public Schools. "By the same token, if you put a bowl of chips there, they'd eat those too. But I'm not convinced that if you had a bowl of chips and a bowl of grapes, that they'd choose the chips instead of the grapes."[72]

Davis doesn't believe it's his job to stop kids from eating chips, or to get them to prefer grapes to chips. Instead, he wants to expose them to healthy foods they might not see at home. He sees that as his role as an educator. "In five or 10 years, these kids will be making their own food purchases. I hope when they go shopping for themselves or for their families, instead of two bags of chips they might decide to get a bag of grapes and a bag of chips. If we don't expose them to these foods early, we lose the opportunity to affect that decision."

Parents choose not to serve their kids certain foods for many reasons. For low-income parents, it may first be an economic decision: when food dollars are scarce, families simply can't afford to waste money on foods that kids might refuse to eat. Exposing children to healthy foods in the child nutrition programs reduces that risk somewhat. It can support parents who crave healthy foods but don't feel they can give themselves permission to buy them without knowing that their children will eat them—this lack of knowledge is part of what makes food choices tougher than they should be. Yet parental fruit and vegetable intake is one of the strongest predictors of fruit and vegetable consumption in young children.[73]

Fruits and vegetables are often spoken of in one breath as if they are one and the same, but research shows that children gravitate more naturally towards fruits than vegetables.[74] One way schools have gotten children to sample unfamiliar vegetables is by including them on salad bars. Schools that want a salad bar find they have a supporter in First Lady Michelle Obama, whose "Let's Move" campaign is championing public-

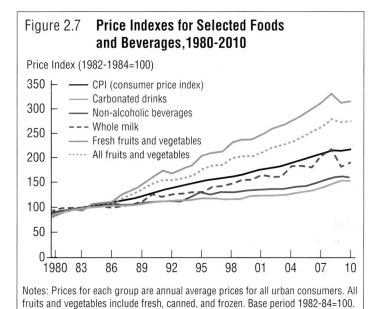

Figure 2.7 **Price Indexes for Selected Foods and Beverages, 1980-2010**

Price Index (1982-1984=100)

- —— CPI (consumer price index)
- —— Carbonated drinks
- —— Non-alcoholic beverages
- - - - Whole milk
- —— Fresh fruits and vegetables
- ······ All fruits and vegetables

Notes: Prices for each group are annual average prices for all urban consumers. All fruits and vegetables include fresh, canned, and frozen. Base period 1982-84=100. Source: National Health and Nutrition Examination Survey data, 2003-2006.

BOX 2.4

SMALL FARMERS CAN MAKE LOCAL FOOD SYSTEMS HEALTHIER

Joshua Cave of Cave Family Farm packs peppers at Pilot Mountain Pride Cooperative in Pilot Mountain, North Carolina. To provide an opportunity for predictable and sustainable income, Pilot Mountain Pride Cooperative, a local food movement group, provides a network of suppliers and end users. Hospitals, restaurants, and supermarkets in western North Carolina benefit from consistent delivery, better prices, certified safe handling, and a unified supply from a variety of local farmers. Pilot Mountain Pride was able to secure a Rural Business Enterprise Grant from USDA to purchase a refrigerated truck to distribute its produce. The grant program is an example of how USDA could scale up support for development of local food systems.

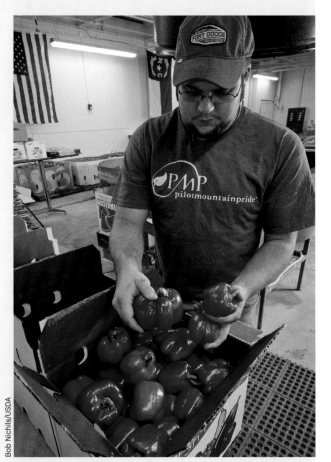

Bob Nichils/USDA

private partnerships to add thousands of new salad bars to school cafeterias.[75] A salad bar in every school may sound like a dream, but there are measures USDA can take to help make it a reality. The agency shouldn't relax its rules on food safety or ignore salad portion sizes, but it should work with food service directors to help them make rules and standards work "on the ground."

The Healthy, Hunger-Free Kids Act requires schools to add more fruits, vegetables, and whole grain products to their lunch and breakfast programs. The federal government has agreed to help by increasing reimbursements by 6 cents per meal. However, meeting the new nutrition guidelines carries an estimated cost of an extra 15 cents per lunch and 51 cents per breakfast.[76] The additional 6 cents provided by the government is helpful but leaves schools scrambling to come up with their share.

The farm bill includes some sources of additional funding that can be applied toward school meals. Section 32, a commodity distribution program, allows the Secretary of Agriculture to spend a little more than $1 billion on domestic nutrition programs,[77] including $400 million earmarked for fresh fruits, vegetables, and nuts.[78] Spending all the Section 32 funding on school meals wouldn't close the gap between what schools need to meet the new nutrition requirements and what the government has pledged to reimburse them, but it would help ease the burden. The problem with this idea, though, is that other institutions relying on the Section 32 program—such as food banks and daycare centers—would then be completely cut off from their funding.

Streamlining farm policies, as described in Chapter 1, would free up resources to improve school meal programs. The Environmental Working Group estimated that in 2009, California could have doubled the quantity of fruits and vegetables served in its schools for the equivalent of just 2 percent of the cotton subsidies received by farms in the state ($75 million).[79] Most of the cotton subsidies go to the largest and most profitable farms. With one in four Americans participating in a federal nutrition program, and farm income holding steady at the highest level in decades, it's harder than ever to argue that the most profitable farms are most in need of financial support. The poverty levels in our country today make it critical to align national farm and nutrition policies.

CHARITY CAN'T DO IT ALONE

Vicki Escarra
President and CEO, Feeding America

If you ask someone to imagine what hunger looks like, many people conjure up the images they have seen on TV—starving and malnourished children with distended bellies living in foreign lands. While hunger in the United States may not look the same as those images displayed on TV, hunger is an all too prevalent reality facing many of our neighbors right here at home. As Feeding America's recently published *Map the Meal Gap* study shows, hunger can be found in every county, congressional district, and state in the country.

According to the U.S. Department of Agriculture (USDA), the number of people at risk of hunger increased by nearly 12.6 million during the recent recession—from 36.2 million people in 2007 to 48.8 million people in 2010. This spike mirrored the dramatic rise in unemployment: the 111 percent increase in the number of unemployed people from November 2007 to November 2010 was mirrored by a 61 percent increase in participation in SNAP (formerly food stamps), the largest federal nutrition program, over that period. Likewise, food banks saw a 46 percent increase in clients seeking emergency food assistance between 2006 and 2010.

As a result of widespread unemployment, many people who previously considered themselves to be comfortably middle-class found themselves in need of assistance to provide enough food for their families. For many of those in need of food assistance, charity is often the first place they turn to for help. As the nation's leading domestic hunger-relief charity, Feeding America annually serves more than 37 million people through a national network of more than 200 food banks and the local agencies they support—more than 61,000 of them, including food pantries, soup kitchens, shelters, and others. Of these, 55 percent are faith-based. Together we now serve one in eight Americans.

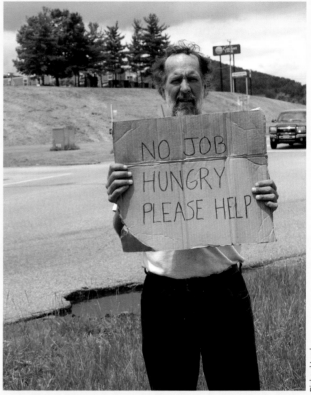

Richard Lord

Unfortunately, we are increasingly being called upon to provide more than short-term food assistance. Struggling families often turn to local charities as both the first line of assistance when they fall on hard times and the last line of defense when other supports are exhausted. As *Map the Meal Gap* shows, only about 55 percent of the food-insecure population have income levels eligible for SNAP. Newly unemployed people are often income eligible but exceed the limit on household assets to qualify for federal nutrition programs. Many working families have some employment, but lack the hours and wages necessary to be economically stable. These workers either do not qualify for federal nutrition programs, or do not qualify for enough assistance to fully meet their family's nutritional needs. In both cases, they have nowhere to turn but to the charitable food network to make sure their family has enough to eat.

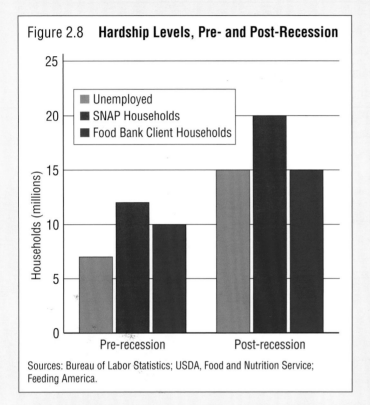

Figure 2.8 **Hardship Levels, Pre- and Post-Recession**

Legend:
- Unemployed
- SNAP Households
- Food Bank Client Households

Y-axis: Households (millions)
X-axis: Pre-recession, Post-recession

Sources: Bureau of Labor Statistics; USDA, Food and Nutrition Service; Feeding America.

While we rely heavily on generous charitable contributions, Feeding America would be unable to maintain its current levels of service without the support of federal nutrition assistance programs. The most critical program to food banks and the local agencies they support is **The Emergency Food Assistance Program (TEFAP).** TEFAP is a means-tested federal program that provides food commodities at no cost to low-income Americans in need of short-term hunger relief; it's distributed through organizations like food banks, pantries, kitchens, and shelters. Healthy and nutritious food commodities provided through TEFAP make up approximately 25 percent of the food distributed by Feeding America food banks; they are an essential resource for the emergency food system. Food banks combine TEFAP commodities with privately donated foods to maximize TEFAP benefits far beyond the budgeted amount for the program. In this way, food banks exemplify an optimum model of the public-private partnership.

Another critical federal nutrition program is the **Commodity Supplemental Food Program (CSFP)**, operated by more than one-third of all Feeding America food banks. CSFP provides nutritionally balanced food packages to approximately 604,000 low-income people each month, nearly 97 percent of whom are seniors with incomes of less than 130 percent of the poverty line (or approximately $14,000 for a senior living alone). CSFP provides important nourishment, helping to combat the poor health status commonly found among food-insecure seniors. CSFP leverages government buying power so that the $20 federal cost of each monthly food package provides a $50 retail value to participants. CSFP food packages are specifically designed to supplement nutrients typically lacking in participants' diets, such as protein, iron, and zinc; they play an important role in meeting the nutritional needs of low-income seniors.

An increasing number of Feeding America food banks are conducting outreach to inform clients of their potential eligibility for the **Supplemental Nutrition Assistance Program (SNAP)**. SNAP is the cornerstone of the U.S. nutrition safety net, ensuring families have adequate resources for groceries until their household economic conditions stabilize and improve. SNAP outreach connects clients who require more than short-term emergency food relief with the longer-term benefits they need. Were SNAP benefits not available, even greater numbers of people in this country would be at risk of hunger, and even greater numbers of people would be forced to rely solely on the charitable sector to meet their food assistance needs.

Feeding America food banks also operate an array

of programs aimed at the nearly one in four children at risk of hunger in this country, providing nourishment to children during out-of-school times when they might otherwise go without meals—after school, in the summer, on weekends, and during long school holidays. Many food banks receive federal funding for after-school and summer feeding programs. **The Child and Adult Care Food Program (CACFP)** and the **Summer Food Service Program (SFSP)** help defray the cost of providing meals and snacks, enabling food banks to leverage private resources to reach even more children and families in need of food assistance.

For the one in six Americans at risk of hunger, food banks and their local agency partners are truly the first line of defense, and many times the only resource standing between being able to put food on the family dinner table and going to bed with an empty stomach. However, the charitable food assistance network cannot meet the needs of these families alone. It is only through our public-private partnership with the federal government—through programs like TEFAP, CSFP, CACFP, and SFSP, and sustained support for SNAP and other programs in the nutrition safety net—that we are able to protect families from hunger.

Vicki Escarra is the president and CEO of Feeding America, the nation's leading domestic hunger-relief charity, serving 37 million people each year. The Map the Meal Gap *study can be found at www.feedingamerica.org/mapthegap.*

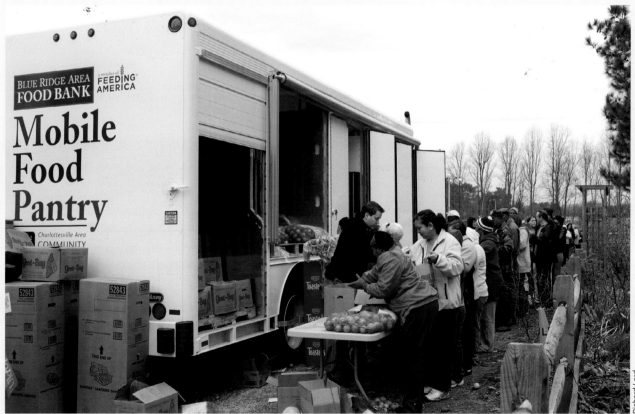

Richard Lord

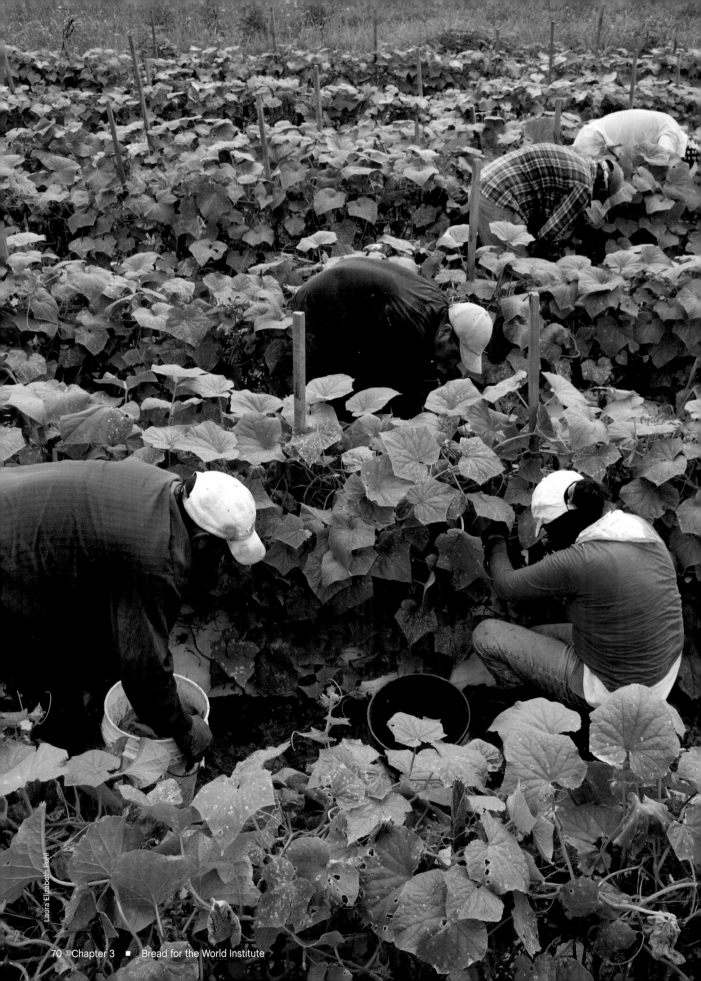

Farm Workers and Immigration Policy

CHAPTER SUMMARY

FOR MORE THAN A CENTURY, AGRICULTURE HAS BEEN AN ENTRY POINT INTO THE LABOR MARKET FOR IMMIGRANTS IN THE UNITED STATES. Presently, close to three-fourths of all U.S. hired farm workers are immigrants, most of them unauthorized. Their unauthorized legal status, low wages, and an inconsistent and sometimes unpredictable work schedule contribute to a precarious economic state.

Immigrant farm workers fill low-wage jobs that citizens are reluctant to take. Attempts to recruit citizens for farm worker jobs traditionally held by immigrants have failed. In the absence of immigrant labor, farmers would be forced to shift to mechanized crops or stop producing altogether. Domestic production of fruits and vegetables—foods Americans should be consuming more of—could decrease significantly without immigrant farm workers.

In spite of the key role they play in U.S. agriculture, unauthorized immigrant farm workers labor under increasingly hostile conditions. The Agricultural Job Opportunity, Benefits and Security bill (AgJOBS) was developed cooperatively by farmers and farm worker advocates to address the status of farm workers. Public concern about unauthorized immigration by and large has held up prospects of enacting the bill into law.

The status quo is unacceptable. Farm workers should be able to work without fear of deportation, and farmers need a steady source of labor and assurances they will not lose access to workers they depend on. It is up to policymakers to help the public see the importance of immigrant farm workers to the U.S. agricultural system.

AgJOBS—or any agricultural guest worker program that recruits from Mexico or Central America—should include development assistance to reduce poverty in rural areas where these workers originate. Rural development can provide poor people with alternative sources of livelihood than migrating to the United States.

Chapter 3

Recommendations

- Unauthorized farm laborers should have a legal means of being in the United States.

- An agricultural guest worker program should include support for rural development in migrant-sending communities of Mexico and Central America.

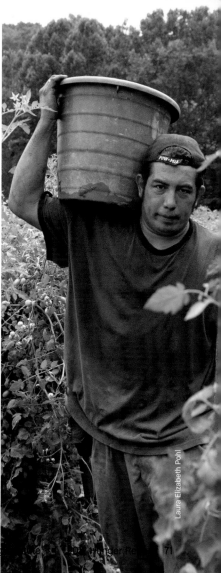

Laura Elizabeth Pohl

Maria's Story

Maria came to Florida *para salir adelante*—to get ahead. She arrived as a teenager in the mid-1990s, escaping a life of poverty on her family's Oaxacan corn patch.

Maria and her husband envisioned a future for their family that was out of reach in Oaxaca, one of the poorest states in Mexico. In south Florida, she worked seven days a week filling bins with squash, tomatoes, beans, and cucumbers. Neither of them enjoyed working in the Florida fields, but without papers it's all they could do. "That's why we came here—to work," said Maria, now 34 years old. "In the factories or restaurants they ask for papers, but in the fields no."

Although their lives were not easy, for years they felt they were moving ahead. But in 2008, the country plunged into a deep recession and agricultural work in Florida grew scarce. "For the past few years, we are working only to survive," Maria said. To supplement their income, the couple would travel north to plant tomatoes during the Florida off-season. In 2010, Maria couldn't go because she was pregnant, so her husband went to Ohio alone. The family has not been together since.

Traveling by bus on his way back to Florida, Maria's husband was stopped by immigration officials and deported to Mexico. "He wants to return, but it's very difficult," she said. "They charge $4,000 to $5,000 to cross the border. This is money I don't have."

Maria's husband is now in Mexico working to raise the money to return to the United States, but to earn what it costs is difficult for a laborer without a formal education or marketable skills.

Maria thought about going back to Mexico. For her U.S.-born children, Mexico is an unknown and unappealing destination; they're American in every sense of the word. Despite Maria's full-time job, the loss of her husband's income means that Maria's daughters, who are citizens, depend on federal nutrition programs to ensure they have enough to eat. Maria herself relies on support from civil society organizations like the Farm Worker Association of Florida. She continues to work in the bean fields. For the sake of her children, she's going to stay in the United States and hope for the best.

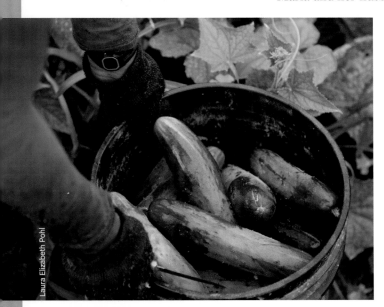

Laura Elizabeth Pohl

Labor-intensive agricultural commodities, primarily fruits, vegetables, and horticultural products, account for 35 percent of the value of all U.S. crops.

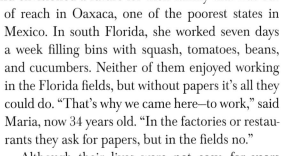

71%

The percentage of hired farm workers who are immigrants.

36 years
The average age of crop workers.

Number of unauthorized immigrants in the United States: **11.2 million**

The Agricultural Workforce

John Steinbeck's 1939 novel *The Grapes of Wrath* described the harsh working conditions of migrant farm workers from the Midwest. More than 70 years later, agricultural work in the United States is still often harsh and wages are low. But the composition of the farm labor force has changed. There are no more Okies. Instead, farm workers come from places like the Mexican states of Guanajuato and Michoacán. The majority of hired farm laborers in the United States are unauthorized immigrants (see Figure 3.1), and most unauthorized workers are from Latin America—particularly Mexico. Spanish is the lingua franca of farm labor; 71 percent of farm workers identify it as their primary language.[1]

U.S. agriculture has long been a point of entry into the labor market for immigrants, and the agriculture sector has been dependent on immigrant labor for more than a century. In the 1880s, 75 percent of seasonal farm workers in California were Chinese. In 1882, in response to pressure from working-class whites, Congress passed the first of a series of anti-Asian immigration laws that barred the entry of laborers from China. Field labor positions were subsequently filled by new waves of Asian immigrants: first Japanese and Filipinos, then laborers from British India. On the East Coast, French Canadians, Caribbean Islanders, and European immigrants, in addition to low-income native whites and African Americans, were part of the agricultural workforce.[2]

With the passage of legislation restricting immigration from Asia, farmers increasingly relied on a source of field labor that caused them much less grief. Mexico was a nearby source of workers, eager to escape poverty in their home country and often already familiar with farm work. The proximity of Mexico made it easier to expel these workers than Asians or Europeans.

During World War II, in response to reported labor shortages, the U.S. government made efforts to recruit Mexican farm workers. These efforts included a bilateral agricultural guest worker program which set the stage for the emigration of millions of Mexican agricultural workers (authorized and unauthorized) to the United States, both during and after the war.[3]

Figure 3.1 **Legal Status of Hired Crop Farm Workers, 1989-2006**

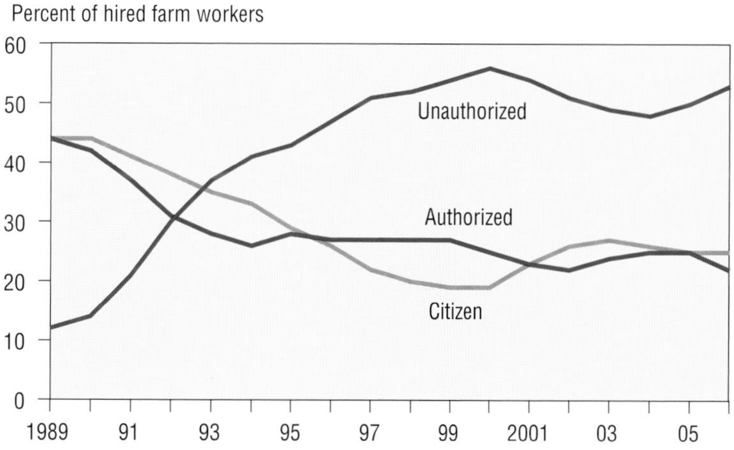

Percent of hired farm workers

Source: USDA analysis of National Agricultural Workers Survey data, 1989-2006.

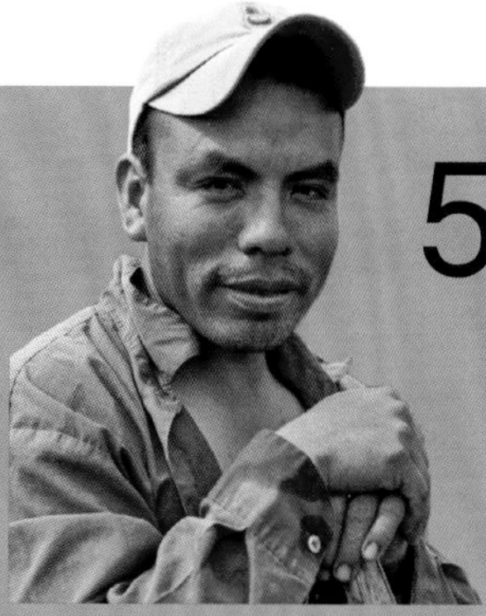

58% of all unauthorized immigrants to the United States are Mexican.

about ONE million Estimated number of crop and livestock workers who are unauthorized.

BOX 3.1 IMPORTING FARM WORKERS:
FROM BRACERO TO H-2A

As World War II intensified, the need to produce food for the troops helped overcome public opposition to Mexican agricultural guest workers. The Mexican government was also initially reluctant to allow its citizens to work in U.S. agriculture, but the Mexican Labor Program—commonly known as the "Bracero Program"—became the official Mexican contribution to the war effort.[4]

The Bracero Program operated from 1942 to 1964. Between 1 million and 2 million Mexican agricultural workers participated in the program, some going back and forth across the border several times for a total of 4.5 million admissions of workers to the United States. During the war years, the program required the U.S. Department of Agriculture to provide the Mexican workers with the same safety and health protections as U.S. agricultural workers. Employers had to pay migrant workers the prevailing wage so as not to undercut domestic farm worker wages. Other worker protections were also included. But the U.S. and Mexican governments failed to comply with key parts of the agreement—at the expense of Mexican workers.[5] During the 1950s, the effect of the Bracero Program was to suppress farm worker wages.

Although the program was initially slated to end after World War II, U.S. growers used their political clout to advocate for the program's continuation, claiming that eliminating it would cause labor shortages and end in disaster for U.S. agriculture.[6] The program eventually ended in 1964, after 22 years, in the midst of the Civil Rights Movement and under pressure from organized labor, the U.S. Catholic Church, and Mexican-American organizations that denounced exploitation and abuse within the program.[7]

Growers' predictions of catastrophe did not come to pass. The end of the Bracero Program brought changes that increased efficiency and improved working conditions. Agricultural economist Philip Martin explains that in lieu of cheap and abundant labor, growers began to use modern human resource methods to ensure that farm workers were deployed more efficiently. The most effective workers on each crop were identified and assigned to work in their areas of expertise, which led to more consistent production. Both workers and growers benefited financially from the increase in productivity.[8] Martin describes the post-Bracero era as the "golden age" for farm workers.

July 1942:
The United States and Mexico agree to the Mexican Labor Program (Bracero Program) to bring Mexican agricultural guest workers to the United States to fill seasonal farm worker jobs.

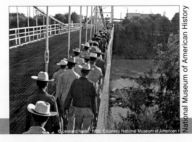

July 1942

September 1942:
First Bracero workers enter the United States in El Paso, TX, en route to Stockton, CA, sugar beet fields.

December 1952:
Immigration and Nationality Act creates the H-2 temporary worker program used mostly by East Coast growers (primarily hiring Caribbean temporary workers) while West Coast growers continue to rely on the Bracero Program.

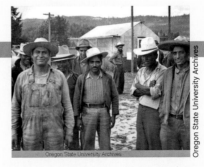

1956:
Annual Bracero admissions peak at 445,197.

BOX 3.1 IMPORTING FARM WORKERS:
FROM BRACERO TO H-2A

The end of the Bracero Program also meant increased mechanization. An industry that relied on immigrant labor had to adapt when the flow of legal immigrant workers stopped. Martin explains what happened using the example of tomatoes produced for sauces and other processed foods. These process-grade tomatoes were harvested by Bracero workers during the early 1960s. Within a few years of the program's end, harvesting was mechanized, the industry expanded, and tomato prices decreased.[9]

Farm workers became increasingly unionized in the late 1960s and the 1970s, since growers could no longer prevent labor strikes by threatening to replace striking workers with Mexican participants in the Bracero Program. From the end of the program in the mid-1960s through the 1970s, most farm workers were U.S. citizens. In 1965, farm labor leaders such as César Chávez organized boycotts of goods produced by growers that did not cooperate with farm worker organizations. Most growers were not directly affected by farm worker unions, but many raised their wage rates to discourage unionization; during the 1970s, farm worker pay was raised well above the federal minimum wage.[10]

But the golden age didn't last. Beginning in the early 1980s, economic crises in Mexico caused a surge in immigrant farm workers in the United States. The H-2A Temporary Agricultural Program was created in 1986, partly as a response to the increasing numbers of unauthorized farm workers. Today, H-2A remains the only legal means of employing foreign agricultural workers. But it is unpopular with both growers and farm worker advocates. Growers say it is too cumbersome to meet the needs of seasonal agriculture, while advocates say that its worker-protection provisions are not enforced effectively.

In theory, the H-2A program places no numerical limit on guest workers. In practice, about 100,000 long-season farm jobs—10 percent of all such jobs—are filled through the program.[11] H-2A has been growing in recent years; more growers are using this legal channel in response to the pressure created by more aggressive immigration enforcement.

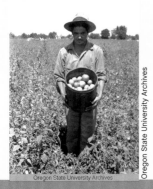

Oregon State University Archives

November 1986:
Immigration Reform and Control Act (IRCA) divides the H-2 program into the H-2A agricultural program and the H-2B non-agricultural program. The vast majority of H-2A workers are recruited from Mexico.

2011:
In response to immigration enforcement pressures, the H-2A program increases to about 100,000 workers annually, 10 percent of all long-season farm jobs.

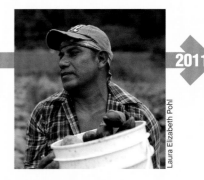

Laura Elizabeth Pohl

2011

December 31, 1964:
Bracero Program ends with a total of 4.5 million admissions since the program originated 22 years earlier. By the end, 2 million Mexicans have participated in the program (some for multiple years).

"The Most Economically Disadvantaged Working Group in the United States"[12]

Three-fourths of hired farm workers are immigrants, mostly from Mexico.[13] About half of all U.S. hired farm workers are unauthorized immigrants.[14] Although immigrant farm workers have higher incomes in the United States than at home, they don't always escape poverty as they had hoped.[15] Hired farm work is among the lowest-paid work in the country.[16] In 2006, the median earnings of these workers—$350 per week—were lower than those of security guards, janitors, maids, and construction workers. Only dishwashers were found to have a lower weekly median income.[17] (See Figure 3.2.)

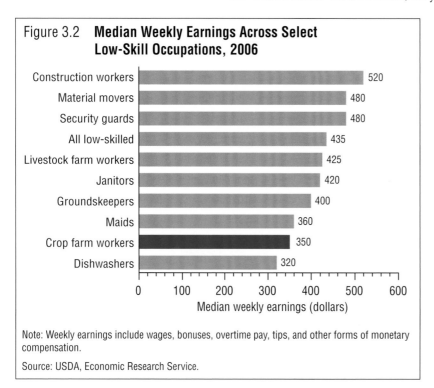

Figure 3.2   **Median Weekly Earnings Across Select Low-Skill Occupations, 2006**

Occupation	Median weekly earnings (dollars)
Construction workers	520
Material movers	480
Security guards	480
All low-skilled	435
Livestock farm workers	425
Janitors	420
Groundskeepers	400
Maids	360
Crop farm workers	350
Dishwashers	320

Note: Weekly earnings include wages, bonuses, overtime pay, tips, and other forms of monetary compensation.

Source: USDA, Economic Research Service.

Although the poverty rate of farm worker families has decreased over the past 15 years, it is still more than twice that of wage and salary employees as a group, and it's higher than that of any other general occupation.[18] A study commissioned by the Pennsylvania State Assembly found that 70 percent of the state's migrant farm workers live in poverty.[19] A 2008 survey in Washington state demonstrated the impact of poverty: 6 percent of farm workers reported being homeless—living in their cars or sheds.[20] In California, farm communities "have among the highest rates of poverty and unemployment in the state."[21] A study of Latino farm workers in North Carolina found that their level of food insecurity was four times higher than the general U.S. population. Nearly half—47 percent—of the Latino farm worker households in the study were food insecure; this proportion rose to 56 percent among households with children.[22] Another study found that 45 percent of all rural Latino families in Iowa were food insecure.[23]

A second cause of food insecurity—in addition to low wages—is the seasonal nature of some farm work. Families' average annual earnings decrease when laborers cannot find work throughout the year. In fact, farm workers' earnings average out to only about $11,000 a year.

Unauthorized legal status, low wages, and inconsistent, sometimes unpredictable work schedules add up to a precarious economic state.[24] In central Florida, where hurricanes and freezes can wipe out crops overnight, food insecurity is a perennial threat. In 2010, for example, a series of freezes destroyed the pepper, strawberry, and tomato crops that farm workers are needed for. "People are working a couple hours a day in some communities," said Bert Perry, a community organizer for the National Farm Worker Ministry in Florida.

Escalated immigration-law enforcement has injected fear into an already difficult economic situation. "There [in Mexico] we lived poor, but we lived peacefully," said a Mexican farm worker in Florida. "Here we live poor, but also in desperation." Fear sometimes deters farm workers from accessing nutrition and other federal programs they qualify for. In spite of their high poverty rates, 57 percent of all hired farm workers—a group that includes authorized as well as unauthorized workers—report receiving no public support.[25] Unauthorized farm workers, in particular, often rely on private organizations as their main source of support in emergencies.[26]

The Elusive Citizen Field Laborer

U.S.-born workers do not have much interest in farm labor, and it is not hard to understand why. Farm work is one of the most hazardous occupations in the United States.[27] Workers face exposure to pesticides and the risk of heat exhaustion, heat stroke, and/or repetitive stress injury. (See Box 3.2, next page.) Moreover, farm workers are not included in most minimum wage and hour guarantees. Most farm workers do not receive benefits, but some states with large numbers of farm workers, including California, Oregon, and Washington, provide wage and hour protections, as well as mandatory rest and meal periods over and above those mandated by federal law.[28]

Growers have a long history of successful advocacy for access to foreign agricultural labor. In the past, they have asserted—incorrectly—that without foreign workers U.S. agriculture would face disaster. But anti-immigration activists and some elected officials dispute the argument that U.S. citizens will not work as field laborers.

There is, in fact, ample evidence that U.S.-born citizens will not replace foreign-born farm laborers at any realistic wage. "There have been a number of efforts to recruit non-migrant workers ... and it has been very difficult to recruit and retain [them]," says Nancy Foster, president of the U.S. Apple Association. "Native workers do not show up for these jobs."[29]

In 2006, the Washington State apple industry launched a campaign to recruit U.S.-born field workers. State and county agencies set up advertising, recruitment, and training programs for 1,700 job vacancies. In the end, only 40 workers were placed.[30] Mike Gempler, executive director of the Washington Growers League, who helped run the recruitment program, said that the barriers to recruitment were simply part of the nature of farm work. "The domestic workforce ... found work that was inside, less physical, out of the sun. And [work] that wasn't seasonal so they didn't have to look for another job when the apples were off the tree ... [with] seasonal work you are always hustling to find the next job ... that's a stressor."

Following the 1996 Welfare Reform legislation, which required work as a condition of the new Temporary Assistance for Needy Families (TANF) pro-

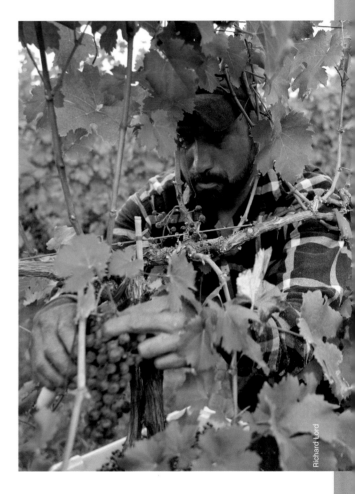

Richard Lord

Most wine grapes are harvested mechanically but some ultra-premium wines still employ farm workers for hand picking.

BOX 3.2   A CASE FOR ENVIRONMENTAL JUSTICE

by Jeannie Economos
Farm Worker Association of Florida

Do we really know the hidden cost of the food that we eat? Savoring strawberries or an orange, we generally think we are eating healthy fresh produce. Concepts such as Parkinson's syndrome, cancer, birth defects, autism, and Lupus are the farthest thing from our minds. Yet these are some of the realities that could be awaiting farm workers after a lifetime, or even after just a few seasons, of exposure to the toxic pesticides and fertilizers used today in U.S. fields and orchards.

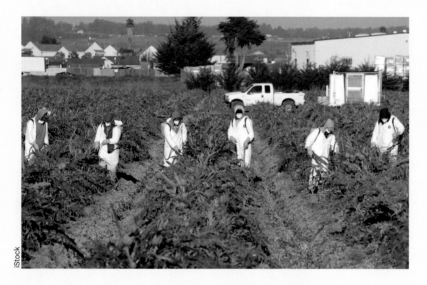

iStock

In addition to these long-term risks, the work that is vital to the production of our food also carries dispro-portionate risks of short-term health consequences. Hazardous and toxic pesticides can affect both workers and their families. Some of the immediate impacts of exposure to pesticides (within the first 12-24 hours) may include headaches, nausea, vomiting, dizziness, sweating, eye irritation, difficulty breathing, and skin rashes.

The Environmental Protection Agency (EPA) estab-lished the Worker Protection Standards to reduce the likelihood that farm workers would be directly or indirectly exposed to pesticides. But all too often, farm workers do not receive required training in pesticide health and safety protocols. The majority of farm workers today are immigrants who know little about their workplace rights and protections. Most speak limited English; this, coupled with fear of employer retaliation, may make them reluc-tant to discuss workplace dangers.

Organophosphates are chemicals commonly used in agriculture today, but they pose significant risks. One in particular, chlorpyrifos, has recently been linked to atten-tion-deficit hyperactivity disorder (ADHD) in children. While chlorpyrifos has been banned for residential use, it is still approved for use in agriculture, and farm workers' children often play or work in the fields alongside their parents.

As recently as 2007, the EPA approved the pesticide methyl iodide for use in agriculture, although it is a known carcinogen and groundwater contaminant. Safer and healthier alter-natives for pest control exist, but they have not been extensively studied or put into nationwide use. Until they are, farm workers will continue to be at serious risk from pesticide exposure.

Farm workers are often referred to as the "invisible ones." Though every one of us eats, few of us think about how and by whom our food was planted, tended, and harvested. And while there is information coming out regularly about the healthfulness of organic products, we hear virtually nothing about the health of families eking out a living in farm work while risking exposure to pesti-cides.

Jeannie Economos is the pesticide safety and environ-mental health project coordinator for the Farm Worker Association of Florida.

gram, Sen. Dianne Feinstein (D-CA) secured the passage of a program to place California's welfare recipients in farm jobs in the Central Valley. State and county workforce agencies and growers' associations collaborated to identify agricultural zones where welfare recipients could be channeled. But only a handful of potential participants were successfully recruited for farm labor.[31]

Manuel Cunha of the Nisei Growers League in California was involved in this recruitment drive. He explained, "There was a huge training program with the universities and the junior colleges to train these people [welfare recipients] in agriculture. Of 137,000 eligible workers, 503 applied and three actually went to work." Cunha echoed Gempler's comments on the barriers to recruiting citizens for farm work: "We are not going to train people in agriculture because it's seasonal and because it's too hard."

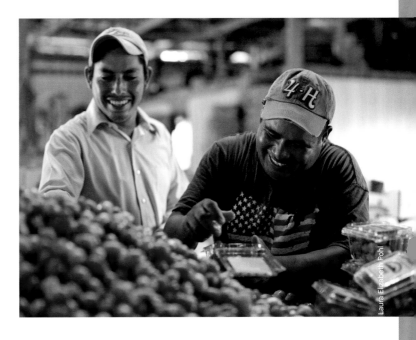

Miguel Baltazar Lorenzo (left) and Jesus Pulido Alejo sort and pack cherry tomatoes in Duffield, VA.

In short, there is no evidence that removing immigrants from farm labor would create job vacancies that unemployed citizens would fill. If immigrant farm workers were no longer available, growers would likely try to mechanize their crops or abandon labor-intensive agriculture, leaving the United States to fill the food gap with additional agricultural imports.

Farmers and Farm Workers

Even a cursory look at the intersection of the U.S. farm and immigration systems reveals a fundamental contradiction. While many farm operators depend on foreign labor, immigration law denies foreign workers legal status unless they arrive through the H-2A program. If a non-H-2A farm worker is in the wrong place at the wrong time, he or she can be expelled from the United States.

Growers have long urged authorities to look the other way as they employ a foreign-born, unauthorized workforce. But employers are now confronted with the possibility that using the E-Verify program for all new hires could become mandatory (see Box 3.3). With no viable alternative to immigrant labor, they are calling for reforms that would legalize their unauthorized workers.

The State Department has described poor working conditions on farms as "endemic," and the number of slavery cases involving farm workers demonstrates the extreme vulnerability of farm workers to the actions of those in positions of relative power.[32]

Florida has prosecuted several cases of abusive treatment of farm workers that met the legal definition of slavery. The Coalition of Immokalee Workers (CIW) played a key role in bringing these cases to light. Labor contractors, supervisors, and crew leaders are typically responsible for exploiting farm workers, although growers can use these intermediaries to try to shield themselves from charges of worker abuse by supervisors or of not intervening when abuse should have been suspected.

The most egregious abusers of immigrant farm laborers are sometimes unauthorized immigrants themselves. In one 2008 case, brothers Cesar and Giovanni Navarette and other members of their family—Mexican nationals— were found guilty of locking farm workers in trucks without running water or toilets, charging them $5 to wash using a garden hose, denying them pay, shackling them with chains, and slashing them with knives if they refused to work. Both Navarette brothers, as the leaders of this agricultural-worker slavery ring, pled guilty to charges of forced labor and other counts and received 12-year prison sentences.[33]

Not all relationships between farm workers and growers are adversarial. Many farm workers and growers have long-term relationships where both parties prosper. Today, farm worker advocates agree with growers on issues central to farm labor reform; both groups want a stable, legalized system of farm labor. Farmworker Justice, an advocacy organization based in Washington, DC, seeks to "empower seasonal farm workers" and finds itself working toward goals that growers also embrace. "[Growers] want access to their workforce without worrying about raids by Immigration, Customs and Enforcement (ICE)," says Farmworker Justice senior attorney Adrienne DerVartanian. California grower representative Manuel Cunha said that the increasing numbers of employment eligibility reviews conducted by ICE on farms have been "devastating to our industry."

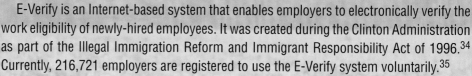

BOX 3.3   E-VERIFY

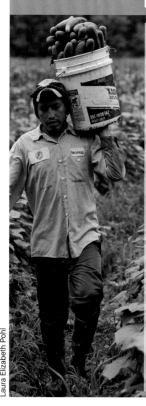

E-Verify is an Internet-based system that enables employers to electronically verify the work eligibility of newly-hired employees. It was created during the Clinton Administration as part of the Illegal Immigration Reform and Immigrant Responsibility Act of 1996.[34] Currently, 216,721 employers are registered to use the E-Verify system voluntarily.[35]

The "Legal Workforce Act," introduced in the U.S. House of Representatives on June 14, 2011, by Rep. Lamar Smith (R-TX), would mandate the use of E-Verify by every employer in the United States.[36] The act could directly impact the 1 million to 1.5 million unauthorized farm workers in the United States, their families, and their employers.

Smith and his supporters say that the program will clear unauthorized immigrants from jobs that should be filled by unemployed legal workers. "It addresses the jobs crisis and provides needed jobs for those who want them," Smith says.[37]

Growers say that mandatory E-Verify will deny them a labor force. "If it were implemented it would be … economically ruinous," says Washington Growers League President Mike Gempler.

The bill allows growers to count returning seasonal workers, those hired in previous seasons, as current employees who don't need to be verified.[38] Although this would provide some workers with a legal means of working, it provides little comfort to them outside of work, where they would still be considered illegal and, accordingly, subject to deportation.

A Specialty Crop Sector on Edge

Fruits, vegetables, and horticulture make up a class of agriculture known as specialty crops. More than 75 percent of all hired farm workers in the United States work on these labor-intensive crops.[39] The $51 billion specialty crop sector is increasingly a source of export revenue for the United States; between 1989 and 2009, exports of high-value agricultural products, including fruits and vegetables, more than tripled.[40] (See Figure 3.4, next page.)

While California and Florida remain the largest specialty crop producers, specialty crops are grown across the country, and many states depend on them to bolster their economies.[41] (See Figure 3.3. for states who use significant farm labor.) In the following sections, we consider how immigration issues are playing out in two of these states, Michigan and Georgia.

Michigan

Michigan is the second-most diverse agricultural state, after California, with commercial production of more than 200 commodities.[42] The resilience of its agricultural sector is particularly important for a state that has suffered long-term economic decline and job loss.

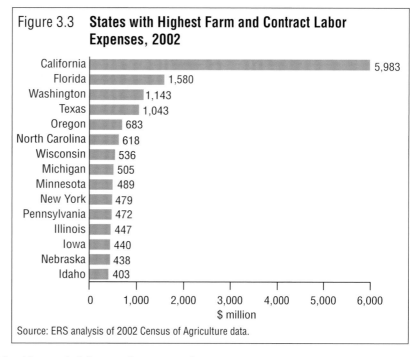

Figure 3.3 **States with Highest Farm and Contract Labor Expenses, 2002**

State	$ million
California	5,983
Florida	1,580
Washington	1,143
Texas	1,043
Oregon	683
North Carolina	618
Wisconsin	536
Michigan	505
Minnesota	489
New York	479
Pennsylvania	472
Illinois	447
Iowa	440
Nebraska	438
Idaho	403

Source: ERS analysis of 2002 Census of Agriculture data.

"Agriculture has been one of the real backbones [of the state's economy] as we've struggled with the manufacturing downturn," said Don Koivisto, director of Michigan's Department of Agriculture.[43] This is reflected in the state's population trends: while other Midwest states had shrinking rural populations, Michigan's rural population increased faster than its urban population during the three decades 1980-2010.[44]

Michigan's fruit and vegetable sector would be in peril without immigrant labor. According to a 2006 report from Michigan State University, crops using migrant labor comprised 58 percent of the total economic activity generated by the state's farm sector and related input supply industries. "Without migrant workers, some farmers would reduce output or leave the business," the report stated.[45]

Michigan growers describe the loss of foreign-born workers as a threat to their livelihoods. During a Senate Agricultural Committee Field Hearing held at Michigan State University in May 2011, Michigan Apple Association Chair Julia Rothwell said that if Michigan farmers do not have immigrants to harvest their crops, "we will cease to exist."[46]

This view is echoed by other Michigan fruit and vegetable growers, who are unequivocal about the importance of immigrant workers. "We're sweatin' bullets every day that they'll knock on the door and take our help away," said Charles Smith [a pseudonym], a third-generation specialty crop farmer. "We

Figure 3.4 Major Fresh Fruit and Vegetable Exports, 2009

Fresh fruits	Value ($ millions)
Apples	$753
Grapes	588
Oranges	345
Strawberries	325
Cherries	286
Grapefruit	185
Pears	153
Peaches	137
Lemons	110
Subtotal	$2,882

Fresh vegetables	
Lettuce & cabbage	$431
Tomatoes	179
Carrots	127
Onions	126
Potatoes	125
Broccoli	119
Subtotal	$1,107

Note: Includes only fresh fruits and vegetables with export value over $100 million in 2009.

Source: USDA, Economic Research Service.

rely on migrants. If they go away, we'll go back to growing soybeans. At that point, you are dealing with the same commodities they grow in Iowa ... with many thousands of acres when we have only hundreds of acres." When asked if he could switch to citizen workers instead of immigrants, Smith echoed other specialty crop growers around the country: "They won't do it." Frank Jones [also a pseudonym], a fourth-generation specialty crop farmer, relies on immigrant workers to grow strawberries, cantaloupes, cucumbers, and apples, among other crops, on his 1,200-acre farm. Jones said that if he lost access to his migrant workforce—about 200 seasonal workers—he'd switch to growing corn and soybeans. But even if he can make a go of it with new crops, the switch would harm his 12 full-time employees, all of whom are U.S. citizens that he employs to operate heavy machinery. "[They] will not have a job," said Jones.

According to farm worker advocates, small and medium-sized farmers like Smith and Jones are likely to treat their workers better than larger operations that employ farm workers. "[Problems are less common with] the family farms that have the same migrants coming back year after year ... they are good to their workers," said Theresa Hendricks, director of Michigan Migrant Legal Assistance.

Michigan farm worker Pasqual Hernandez said he earns $8 an hour and enjoys working in agriculture as his father did in Chiapas, Mexico. He sends some of his earnings to his family in Mexico for food and medicine, but he's unable to visit them. Like many immigrants, Hernandez planned to work in the United States for a couple of years, save up money, and return home. But the dangers of crossing the border have dissuaded him from going back, at least for now: "I changed opinions because I saw that a lot of people were going ... and there are some that do not return; they die in the desert."

Regardless of the quality of their relationships with their employers, the primary concern of most unauthorized farm laborers is their legal status. Among the states that employ large numbers of unauthorized farm workers, Michigan is one of the more hospitable, but the fear of being deported is pervasive here, too. "The biggest difficulty is the fear one has of being captured and being sent back to Mexico," Hernandez said.

Robert Sierra, a farm field manager, described the difference between being authorized and unauthorized to work in these terms: "Nothing is ever sure with the undocumented. You don't live peacefully; it's hard to sleep at night. You are fearful of investing in anything because if you are sent back to Mexico, all that you have saved for will stay here."

Research indicates that most workers stay in agriculture for 10 or fewer years. But some immigrant farm workers say that if the working conditions and pay are decent, they wouldn't want to do anything else. A much larger share of the population earns a living in agriculture in Mexico than in the United States—less than 2 percent of Americans work in agriculture. Many rural Mexicans, when they can't make ends meet, end up moving to Mexican cities. But some opt to leave the country for the United States, and they often end up living and working in rural America.[47]

Sierra, 40, said he began working in agriculture at age 12 in Querétaro, Mexico. He came to the United States because he couldn't make a living in rural Mexico. "I have always been used to working in the fields and it's what I know best," he said. "You become accustomed to it. You feel you have more freedom than in construction or warehouses."

Georgia

Agriculture (which includes fishing, forestry, and hunting) is a $3.9 billion industry in Georgia. In 2009, fruits, nuts, vegetables, and ornamental horticulture—all heavily dependent on immigrant workers—accounted for 27 percent of the state's total farm income.[48]

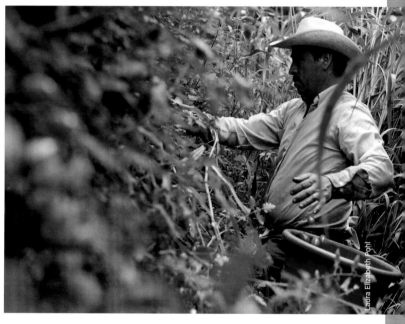

In April 2011, Georgia passed one of the most aggressive state immigration enforcement laws. The legislation may seem like a resounding victory to those opposed to the presence of unauthorized immigrants in the state, but Georgia farmers see things much differently. "The worker shortage really translates into a monetary loss," said Gary Butler [pseudonym], a fifth-generation Georgia farmer, "about a 15-20 percent loss of revenues [for my farm]."

"There's no question that we've seen a pretty severe shortage," said Bryan Tolar, president of the Georgia Agribusiness Council. "Fifty percent of the labor force that we've relied on ... to get those fresh fruits and vegetables to the market [has left]." Georgia's growers have a history of alarmist rhetoric on the subject of labor shortages. In this case, Latino advocates in the state agree that the law has deterred immigrants from passing through the state, and they agree with growers' view that the law has led to an exodus of immigrants.

Between 1989 and 2009, the value of U.S. agricultural exports increased by 250 percent, while exports of high-value agricultural products, including fruits and vegetables, more than tripled.

In June 2011, possibly realizing the risk that farmers would lose a large part of their labor force, Georgia Governor Nathan Deal called on the state's commissioners of labor, corrections, and agriculture to connect unemployed people on probation with farms seeking workers. "This points to a complete out-of-touch perspective that some ... of our leadership in this state have with regard to the current immigration crisis," said Jerry Gonzalez, executive director of the Georgia Association of Latino Elected Officials.[49]

Some Georgia farm worker advocates say that Deal's plan and grower claims of a labor shortage are phony, both part of a time-honored strategy to ensure an oversupply of cheap and pliable labor. "I think it's a lot of hot air," said attorney Greg Schell of Migrant Farmworker Justice. "If these guys were really desperate ... all they need to do is to put the word out [for workers]." Schell, who works with farm laborers in neighboring Florida, said that his state has many unemployed *legal* farm laborers looking for work, but growers prefer to continue hiring unauthorized laborers. Dawson Morton, a senior staff attorney for Georgia Legal Services, also said that growers' claim of a labor shortage was "a manufactured problem." "They could get H-2A workers," Morton said. "They just don't want to pay those wages."

Regardless of the ultimate impact of Georgia's new immigration law, the state's unauthorized farm laborers continue to work and live in limbo. Ernesto Alvarado, 40, has been a farm worker for 20 years, most of that time in Georgia. His family worked in agriculture in the Mexican state of Nuevo León before he came to the United States, and he's proud to do the work that most Americans refuse. "People who have papers don't want to work under the sun," Alvarado said. "We want to be strong in the heat, [strong] in our work."

But the emotional cost of living and working without legal authorization has been high. Alvarado said it's been 10 years since he's seen his parents in Mexico. Although Nuevo León borders Texas, Alvarado said the relatively short journey is too hazardous. "If I go over there, I can't come back," he said. "I don't care about the money, but you can die doing that trip."

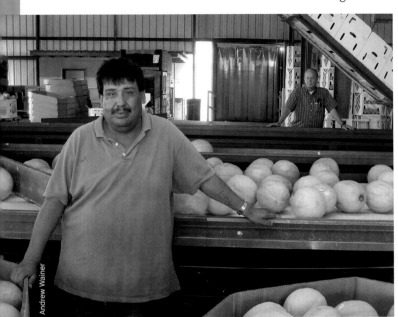

A worker at a packing warehouse in South Georgia.

AgJOBS: The Grand Compromise

In 2000, after decades of wrangling over the contours of an updated guest worker program, the Agricultural Job Opportunity, Benefits and Security bill (AgJOBS) was introduced in Congress. It has been periodically reviewed and debated—but it has not been enacted into law.[50]

Although the bill's details have changed—and are still being negotiated to reflect the changing political dynamics—AgJOBS reforms key parts of the agricultural labor system. The proposal is a compromise that follows years of negotiations between legislative adversaries—farm worker advocates and growers. Here we discuss two of the main components of AgJOBS:

Earned Legalization for Current Farm Workers

AgJOBS provides up to 1.5 million unauthorized farm workers with the opportunity to earn temporary legal immigration status—called a "Blue Card"—with the possibility of becoming permanent residents of the United States. In order to participate, workers must have two or more years of U.S. farm work experience before the passage of the bill. AgJOBS also offers workers an opportunity to legalize the status of family members.

Legalization would be contingent on workers' continuing to work in agriculture for three to five years (the requirement depends on how many days per year they are employed) after enactment of the bill. This part of the compromise would mainly affect unauthorized immigrants already living in the United States and working in agriculture—many of them for decades.

BOX 3.4   FARM WORK IS A SKILLED PROFESSION

by Ivone Guillen
Sojourners

At a July 2011 congressional hearing on "The Economic Imperative for Enacting Immigration Reform," Mayor Paul Bridges of Uvalda, GA, praised his state's farm workers. "The Georgia peaches, strawberries, blueberries, and many other fruits and vegetables they harvest end up on family dinner tables across the country. These crops are harvested by skilled migrant farm laborers who have harvesting down to a fine art."

The produce that most Americans find in their supermarkets looks fresh and tasty. Rarely do retailers sell fruit with bruises, even though bruises actually make no difference to the fruit's nutritional value. One reason much of the food Americans consume consistently looks so good is due to the skill of the farm workers who grade, pick, and package them.

The value-added to produce by farm workers comes in their skills in sowing, cultivating, and harvesting the crops. Techniques such as tree pruning and trimming require knowledge of how and when to use sharp tools like hand pruners to selectively remove parts of a plant or tree; done correctly, the techniques improve the plant's strength and health.

Different crops require a variety of techniques to be successful. For example, an orange orchard is maintained quite differently than a tomato field. When producing different crops, farm workers must understand how each is affected by soil quality, fertilizers, irrigation, and cultivating techniques.

The increasing use of machinery to improve productivity and efficiency requires additional skills. Farm workers operate machines that require agility, precision, and technical knowl-edge. During the processing and packing phase, farm workers must rapidly pack the fruits and vegetables to keep up with the conveyor belts and other equipment in the sorting facility.

Farm workers must regularly improve their skill set; agriculture is a competitive industry that requires workers' constant adaptation. There is no question: farm work is a skilled profession.

Ivone Guillen is the immigration campaigns fellow at Sojourners. She was an immigration policy fellow at Bread for the World Institute from September 2010 to September 2011.

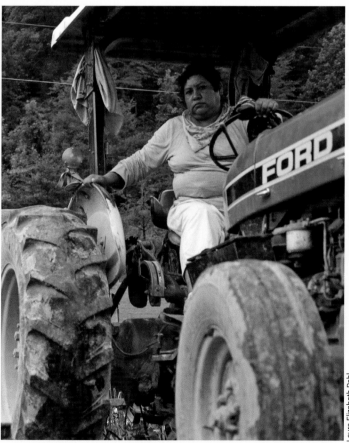

Laura Elizabeth Pohl

Earned legalization would require that workers pay a fine and any back income taxes they owe. While working to earn a long-term legal immigrant visa, farm workers would be eligible for unemployment insurance and the Earned Income Tax Credit, which makes a tax refund available to qualifying low-income workers, but they would not be eligible for means-tested federal benefits such as the Supplemental Nutrition Assistance Program (SNAP), formerly food stamps.[51]

H-2A Guest Worker Reform

The AgJOBS bill includes a reformed H-2A agricultural guest worker program that would reinforce the program's status as the nation's only legal source of agricultural labor. According to agricultural economist Philip Martin, about 100,000 (10 percent) of the total 1 million long-season farm jobs are now filled through the H-2A program, up from about 30,000 in the mid-1990s.[52]

Under the bill's provisions, employer "attestation" would replace "certification" in the H-2A program, reducing the Department of Labor's (DOL) involvement in confirming employers' need for guest workers. Employers would assure the DOL that they have vacant jobs available, are paying minimum wage, and are complying with other H-2A requirements. DOL would review and approve employer attestations within seven days.[53]

Under the current H-2A program, growers are required to provide free housing for workers. AgJOBS would allow employers the alternative of paying a housing allowance to workers, provided that the governor of the state where a farm is located agrees that sufficient rental housing is available. Experts say that this allowance would result in an increase in wages of about $200-$300 a month, depending on local rental costs.[54] A housing allowance would provide farm workers with more options as to where to live, but it could also mean they spend more of their own income on housing.

Under the current law, agricultural guest workers must be paid the "Adverse Effect Wage Rate" (AEWR), the state or federal minimum wage, or the local prevailing wage of their occupation, whichever of these is higher.[55]

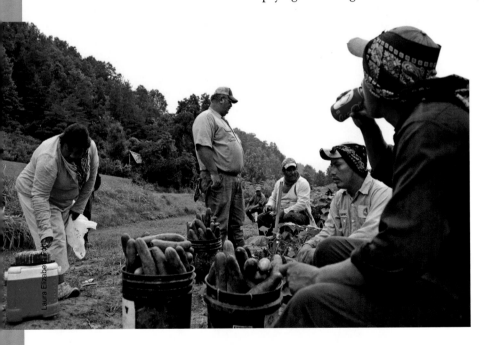

Migrant workers rest after picking cucumbers all morning.

The current AEWR ranges from about $9 to $11 an hour.[56] AgJOBS would roll back the AEWR by $1-$2 and subject it to studies by government and independent commissions. If Congress did not agree on a new wage rate within three years of the enactment of AgJOBS, future raises would be tied to the Consumer Price Index and could rise by as much as 4 percent per year.[57] If this happened it would increase the earnings of lower-paid farm workers, who are working at or near the minimum wage. The average wage rate of U.S. farm workers is $10.07 per hour.[58]

The Politics of AgJOBS

With both growers and farm workers on board for agricultural labor reform, the prospects for AgJOBS would seem good. At one time, the bill appeared to be headed straight for passage; a version of AgJOBS introduced in the Senate in 2000 had strong Republican support and was seen as the most likely immigration policy reform to pass.

But over the past decade, the opponents of immigration reform have blocked the enactment of AgJOBS. "Gradually the moderate Republicans that have supported AgJOBS have been weeded out of the Senate either by retirement or they've lost," says Rob Williams, project director of Migrant Farmworker Justice. "On the Republican side we had strong support ... [More recently] we haven't had a Republican [champion]."[59]

Another reason for delay is that AgJOBS has become part of a comprehensive immigration reform package, rather than remaining a standalone bill. Immigration reform components such as the DREAM Act and AgJOBS typically garner more public and political support than a broader comprehensive reform proposal because they focus on specific immigrant populations (youth and agricultural workers). "Ten years ago we were by ourselves [in advocating for AgJOBS] and then we became an element of comprehensive reform," said Williams.

The U.S. agricultural sector has a lot to lose from increasingly restrictive immigration legislation at the state and federal levels. Restarting immigration reform discussions in a sector where immigrants are most vital economically can provide a path forward for reform, so the AgJOBS bill would be a logical place to start the discussion. Both the dampening effect on immigration of the struggling economy and the reauthorization of the farm bill may provide added impetus for including immigrant farm labor in the broader discussion of agricultural policy.

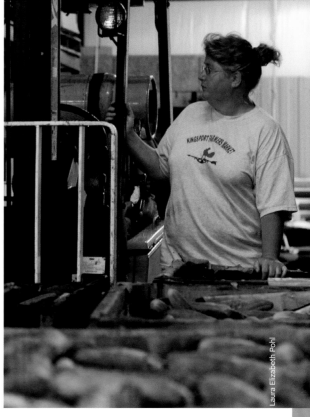

Sherilyn Shepard, a farmer in Blackwater, Virginia, drops off crates of freshly picked cucumbers to the Appalachian Harvest packing house in Duffield, Virginia.

The Other Side of the Border

While immigration reform, including passage of AgJOBS, is a long-term struggle, there is potential to improve the H-2A program more expeditiously, making it work better for growers, farm workers, and immigrant-sending communities in Latin America. "This is the only option that we are seeing to improve things right now on the ground," said Diego Reyes, executive board member of the Farm Labor Organizing Committee (FLOC), a union affiliated with the AFL-CIO.

In spite of the abuses associated with the H-2A program, legal guest worker permits are sought after in Mexico and would-be farm workers can easily go into debt to obtain them. Although the H-2A visa officially costs

$231, workers can end up paying $400-$600 or more with paperwork, transportation, and fees paid to recruiters. This is a significant sum of money for rural Mexicans. In some cases, potential guest workers obtain loans at high interest rates to pay for the opportunity to participate in the program. By the time they arrive in the United States for their $9 an hour jobs, they may already be deeply in debt.[60]

FLOC has pioneered a strategy to improve the H-2A program by creating a fairer recruitment process for workers in Mexico. On the U.S. side of the border, FLOC has established a framework that includes corporations, grower associations, and H-2A guest workers (represented by FLOC).

In 2004, FLOC used a corporate boycott to help get North Carolina growers who hire H-2A workers to agree to a contract that delineated workers' rights. It was the first-ever union contract for guest workers in the United States. After several more rounds of boycotts, the Mt. Olive Pickle Company and the North Carolina Growers Association (NCGA) also signed an agreement with FLOC. The NCGA hires Mexican H-2A

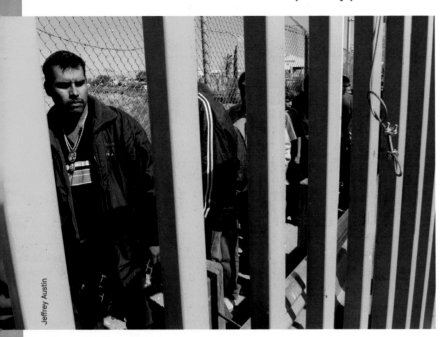

Deported immigrants are dropped off by U.S. officials along the Arizona-Mexico border.

workers, who are sent to the North Carolina farms that supply cucumbers to Mt. Olive.[61] When the contract was signed in 2004, the NCGA represented 1,000 farmers and 8,500 guest workers covered by the agreement.[62] The North Carolina agreement includes an arbitration process so that workers and growers can resolve disputes more efficiently.

The agreement goes beyond protecting the rights of H-2A workers in the United States: FLOC maintains a permanent office in Monterrey, Mexico, where it provides training and education for workers before they leave home. The program explains the rights and responsibilities of guest workers in the United States. FLOC's model is uncommon in its panoramic vision of addressing immigrant agricultural labor issues from both sides of the border.

Migration and Development

FLOC works on guest worker recruitment, education, and training issues on the Mexican side of the border—but it doesn't address the impact of the H-2A program on the Mexican communities that send these workers. In fact, this is one of the most under-analyzed parts of the H-2A program. It is rare for anyone, including the Mexican government, to raise the concerns of sending communities. The reasons Mexicans leave home to become farm workers in the United States are often not part of this or most other discussions of immigration reform.

But there are the beginnings of a framework that envisions the H-2A program as a way to benefit both growers in the United States and sending communities in Mexico. The bi-national Independent Agricultural Workers' Center (CITA by its Spanish acronym) is pioneering such a model; it plans to integrate the H-2A program with Mexican rural development efforts.

Farm worker advocate Chuck Barrett founded CITA along the Arizona-Mexico border in 2007 to serve as a "matchmaker" between prospective Mexican guest workers and U.S. growers. For the past several years, CITA has been focused on helping workers on both sides of the border: in Mexico with the recruitment process, and in the United States with disputes between workers and growers.

CITA helps growers recruit workers in Mexico and assists in getting growers' H-2A applications—which Barrett says are notoriously onerous—through the Department of Labor and other agencies. It also provides services to Mexican guest workers, including financial literacy information, low-interest loans to pay for guest worker visas, psychological counseling, and education on the guest worker system. In addition to the fees it earns from growers, CITA is supported by organizations such as Catholic Relief Services and the Howard Buffett Foundation.

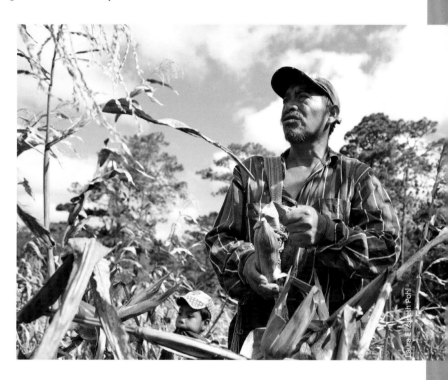

Barrett is hoping to expand the CITA model to become self-sustaining in rural communities throughout Mexico, saying that this expansion would help Mexican migrant-sending communities obtain "some beginning of control over migration, replacing illegal out-migration with legal migration." According to this model, communities would be trained to facilitate employer petitions, prescreen workers, and expedite the visa process—all tasks for which U.S. growers now pay CITA a fee. "Because they would be doing the training and passport process ... they [Mexican rural areas] will get a portion to be used by the community to fulfill their own development objectives," Barrett said.

Marvin Garcia Salas, a farmer in Chiapas, Mexico, twice migrated to the United States to do farm work before returning home for good.

While Barrett—like almost everyone else—said that the H-2A program is dysfunctional, he also believes that its use will increase. "Whether people like it or not ... H-2A is going to be a growing process," he said. "Every version of AgJOBS includes an expansion of H-2A. I see the next couple of years as a window of opportunity to find alternatives ... that are fairer for the workers and more effective for the employers, and also lend themselves ... to connecting the migration process to the development process."

CITA's concept of connecting its H-2A employer services to rural development in migrant-sending Mexican rural communities is still on the drawing board. But based on the relationships they've forged through their outreach to growers and services to workers, Barrett and CITA executive director Janine Duron said that the program can be extended to the source of the immigrant farm worker issue—the poor Mexican communities that provide U.S. growers

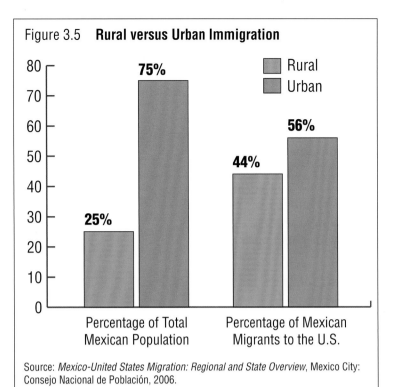

Figure 3.5 **Rural versus Urban Immigration**

Source: *Mexico-United States Migration: Regional and State Overview*, Mexico City: Consejo Nacional de Población, 2006.

with both unauthorized and H-2A farm workers. "It's an amazing relationship that can be built if you have reconciliation rather than adversity," said Duron.

Reducing migration pressures will require development and job creation throughout Mexico, but poverty and migration are particularly concentrated in the countryside. Although about a quarter of all Mexicans live in rural areas, 60 percent of Mexico's extremely poor people are rural, and 44 percent of Mexican immigrants come from rural communities (see Figure 3.5). Immigration reform and development assistance need to be linked, particularly for rural Mexico.

After decades of declining support, agriculture and rural development is now re-emerging as a vital development focus. The World Bank's 2008 World Development Report, *Agriculture for Development,* states, "Agriculture continues to be a fundamental instrument for sustainable development and poverty reduction."[63] Research has also found that agriculture is one of the best returns on investment in poverty-reduction spending.[64] Each 1 percent increase in crop productivity in Asia reduces the number of poor people by half a percent. This correlation also holds for middle-income countries such as Mexico.[65]

REGULARIZE AND RATIONALIZE FARM LABOR

by Philip Martin
University of California, Davis

It makes sense for farm policies to encourage more labor-saving mechanization—through research, for example—and to rationalize and regularize the farm-labor market. This would be in the best interest of everyone: farm workers and farmers, plus the rural areas of the United States and Mexico that farm workers have migrated to and from.

On a per-capita basis, nonmetro areas of the United States receive more government transfer payments than metro areas. In 2008, such payments made up 23 percent of nonmetro residents' incomes, versus 14 percent of metro income.[66] Unlike metro areas, which receive immigrants at both the top and the bottom of the education ladder, most of the newcomers in nonmetro areas have not finished high school. Immigrant parents hope their children will escape poverty in the United States, but the odds are not good.

If illegal migration were curbed and wages did not rise, more farmers might turn to the H-2A guest worker program, the only program currently available to hire legal foreign guest workers. Most farmers do not pay social security, Medicare, and federal unemployment insurance taxes on the earnings of H-2A guest workers—making guest workers up to 20 percent cheaper than U.S. workers. One way to rationalize and regularize the farm-labor market would be to levy payroll taxes on the earnings of guest workers.

The amount of money generated from payroll taxes on guest worker earnings would be significant—perhaps $1.2 billion a year. Half of this money could be used to support research on agricultural mechanization and the other half to support development of guest workers' areas of origin. This would have positive effects in both the rural United States and rural Mexico.

Research accelerated by additional resources from payroll taxes could promote rationalization and ensure

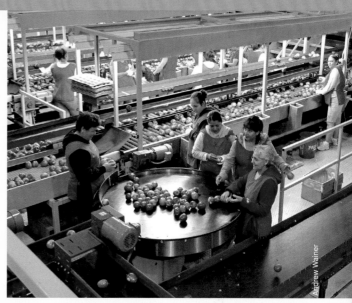

Immigrant workers sort apples at a warehouse in eastern Washington state.

that future guest workers have incentives to return to their areas of origin. This leaves the question—what should be done about the million or more unauthorized farm workers currently employed in U.S. agriculture?

There is no easy answer to this question of those now laboring in U.S. fields. The passage of the AgJOBS legislation would allow them and their families to become legal immigrants, meaning the United States would gain several million additional legal Mexican immigrants because families would be united here. AgJOBS would create a path to immigrant visas by requiring continued U.S. farm work, but this strategy goes against decades of experience that demonstrate that the best way to help farm workers increase their incomes is to get them out of agriculture.

AgJOBS would solve part of Mexico's rural poverty problem by transferring some poor people from rural Mexico to rural America. Given the failures of the Bracero program and 1986 immigration reforms, we need a new approach to immigration and agriculture.

Philip Martin is a professor of agricultural and resource economics at the University of California, Davis.

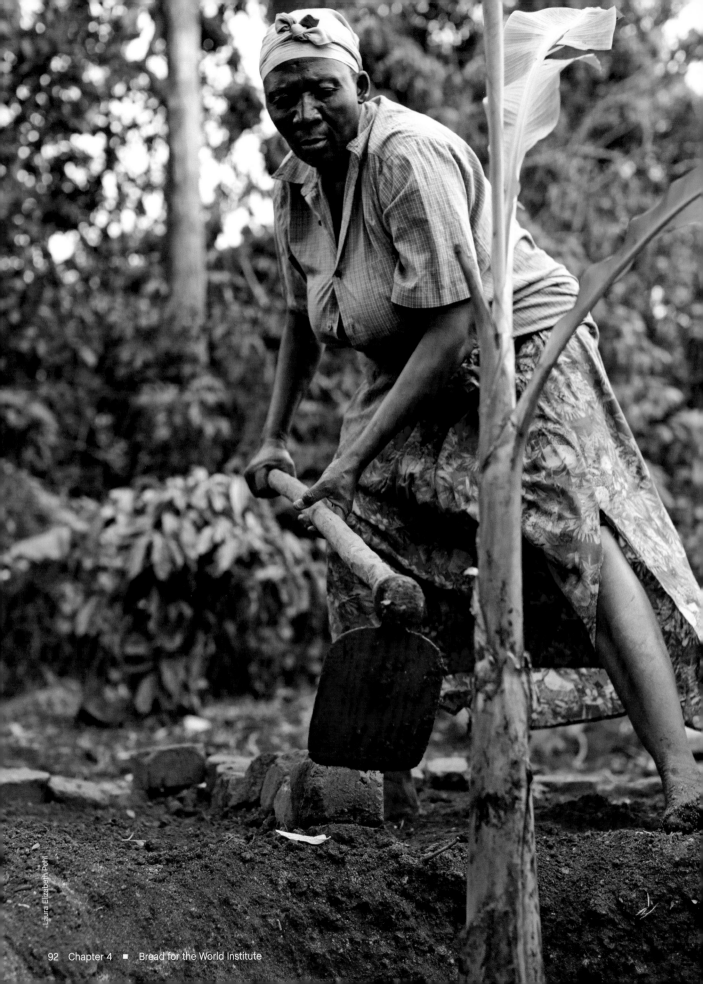

Rebalancing Globally

CHAPTER SUMMARY

The United States responds directly to hunger and malnutrition in the developing world with food aid and agricultural development assistance.

U.S. food aid programs and agricultural development assistance are increasingly focused on pregnant and lactating women and children younger than 2. Even brief episodes of hunger among people in these vulnerable groups are cause for alarm. A third of all child deaths are attributable to malnutrition, while survivors face lifelong physical and/or cognitive disabilities.

The United States should strengthen its traditional role as the largest provider of food aid, while also moving quickly to improve its nutritional quality. New mothers, young children, and other vulnerable people, such as those living with HIV/AIDS, can benefit from highly nutritious forms of food aid now available. These cost more than the foods normally included in U.S. food aid, but it is possible to reduce costs by purchasing in or near the countries where they are needed and by phasing out the inefficient practice of monetizing food aid to conduct development projects.

The United States should strengthen its commitment to Feed the Future, the innovative U.S. Global Hunger and Food Security Initiative critical to long-term progress against hunger and malnutrition. Feed the Future represents the U.S. government's strongest support in decades for agricultural development in poor countries. The focus on agriculture is especially valuable because the vast majority of poor people in developing countries earn their living by farming, and the majority of these farmers are women.

The United States must make larger investments in agricultural research to help meet the global need to produce crops that can feed a growing population, respond to shifts in dietary patterns, and adapt to changes in climate. Current funding for both U.S. research institutions and the international network of agricultural research centers is hardly adequate to meet these challenges.

All poverty-focused development assistance is instrumental in helping poor countries achieve the Millennium Development Goals. Cuts to U.S. foreign assistance, including USAID's operating budget, would harm efforts to make foreign assistance more effective, efficient, and sustainable.

Chapter 4

Recommendations

- The United States should strengthen its traditional role as the largest provider of food aid, while also moving quickly to improve its nutritional quality.

- The United States should strengthen its commitment to Feed the Future, the innovative Global Hunger and Food Security Initiative that is critical to sustainable progress against hunger and malnutrition.

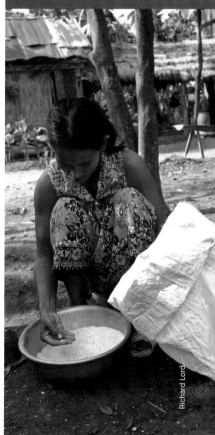

Richard Lord

1,000 Days

The U.N. Millennium Development Goals (MDGs) treat hunger and poverty as interdependent problems. The first MDG—dramatically reducing hunger and poverty—measures progress against hunger by gauging how many children remain chronically undernourished.

"Hunger" seems like a simpler concept than "undernutrition," but it's most accurate to say that it's the effects of undernutrition that kill children or limit their potential for the rest of their lives. Young children need calories to grow and gain weight, but vitamins and minerals matter every bit as much. In developing countries, one-third of all children are stunted or underweight as a result of undernutrition; it is the leading cause of child mortality. Reducing the high rate of undernutrition among children in the developing world is one of the greatest challenges in global health.

The most critical period in human development is the first 1,000 days of life, starting at pregnancy and lasting through a child's second year.[1] Healthy development, particularly brain development, depends on getting the right foods at this critical time in life. Hunger during this time is catastrophic, because the resulting physical and cognitive damage is lifelong and largely irreversible.

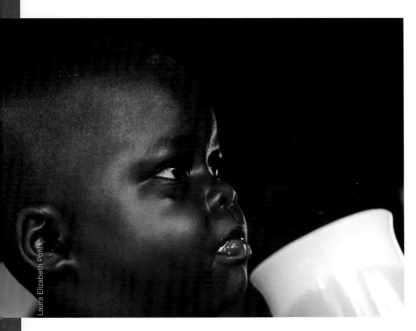

Healthy development, particularly brain development, depends on getting the right foods during the early years of life.

Early hunger and malnutrition is associated with later problems such as chronic illness and poor school attendance and learning. As adults, the survivors have lower productivity and lifetime incomes, which costs developing countries an estimated 2 to 3 percent of their economic output (Gross Domestic Product).[2]

Until recently, international development programs did not focus much attention on improving the nutritional status of young children. But that has changed since 2008, when a series of reports on early childhood appeared in the leading medical journal *The Lancet*. The series emphasized the connection between nutrition during the first 1,000 days and development outcomes, and showed how practical, inexpensive interventions during this "window of opportunity" can dramatically alter the arc of a person's life.

0.6%

of the federal budget is spent on poverty-focused development assistance.

The Food and Agriculture Organization of the United Nations (FAO) estimates that if women had the same access to productive resources as men, they could **increase yields** on their farms enough to **reduce the number of hungry people** in the world by **12–17%—up to 150 million people.**

The Lancet series appeared at the height of a global hunger crisis driven by dramatic spikes in the prices of staple foods, which forced an additional 100 million people into hunger and led to rioting in a number of countries. In the aftermath, the United Nations formed a High-Level Task Force on Global Food Security. In addition, representatives of the governments and civil societies of dozens of countries came together to prepare a framework for nutrition action based on *The Lancet* reports. From this effort came the Scaling Up Nutrition (SUN) movement to support the action plan.

During a U.N. summit on the MDGs in September 2010, Secretary of State Hillary Clinton and her Irish counterpart launched the "1,000 Days: Change a Life, Change the Future" initiative. 1,000 Days and SUN seek to make nutrition an integral component of development programs. SUN's plan for accomplishing this has been endorsed by national governments, multilateral institutions such as the World Bank and other international development banks, civil society organizations, development agencies, academics, and philanthropic bodies.[3] During the U.N. event, David Beckmann, president of Bread for the World, and Tom Arnold, CEO of Concern Worldwide, committed to convening a follow-up meeting of SUN. This meeting was held June 13, 2011, in Washington, DC, and drew government and civil society representatives from both SUN countries and developed countries. Bread for the World and Concern Worldwide continue to be instrumental in keeping policymakers focused on SUN and the critical importance of the first 1,000 days.

The United States has two development programs, Feed the Future and the Global Health Initiative, that put nutrition front and center. Bread for the World Institute's 2011 Hunger Report, *Our Common Interest: Ending Hunger and Malnutrition*, focused on Feed the Future, an agricultural development initiative designed to address the root causes of hunger in developing countries. Feed the Future is the first U.S. global food security program of this magnitude— and the only one to focus both on nutrition

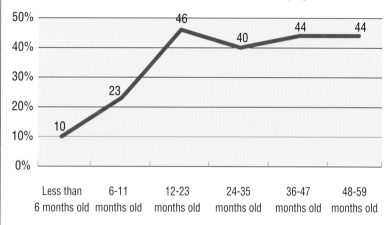

Figure 4.1   Stunting is Largely Irreversible after Age 2

Percentage of children 0-59 months old who are stunted, by age

Age	Percentage
Less than 6 months old	10
6-11 months old	23
12-23 months old	46
24-35 months old	40
36-47 months old	44
48-59 months old	44

Note: Analysis is based on data from 40 countries covering 56% of children under 5 years old in developing countries. Prevalence estimates are calculated according to the NCHS reference population, as there were insufficient data to calculate estimates according to WHO Child Growth Standards.

Source: DHS and National Family Health Survey, 2003-2009, with additional analysis by UNICEF.

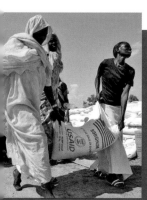

About $1.5 billion

The amount the United States spent in fiscal year 2010 on emergency food aid that reached about **46.5 million beneficiaries.**

1,000 days

From pregnancy to age 2 is the "window of opportunity" to prevent malnutrition from causing largely irreversible damage.

BOX 4.1 UNDERSTANDING MALNUTRITION AND RESPONDING EFFECTIVELY

by Rebecca J. Vander Meulen
Director of Community Development,
Anglican Diocese of Niassa, Mozambique

Children under the age of 5 are most at risk of death from malnutrition. As Figure 4.2 shows the odds of death from diarrhea, pneumonia, malaria, and measles are higher for children under 5 who are malnourished compared to those who are properly nourished.[4]

Children who lack adequate energy and protein suffer from what is known as "protein-energy malnutrition." Children suffering from chronic protein-energy malnutrition become "stunted"—shorter than they should be for their age. "Wasting" occurs when children suffer from acute food shortage (such as famine). Wasting is what we see in photographs of emaciated children, such as the shocking images from Somalia in 2011.

Severe malnutrition poses an immediate threat to a child's life, but more children die every year because of mild or moderate malnutrition.[5]

Humans also need micronutrients (vitamins and minerals) to lead a healthy and productive life. Micronutrient malnutrition may not always have obvious signs, but left untreated the consequences are serious. Zinc and Vitamin A deficiencies, for example, put children at increased risk of dying from diarrhea and malaria.[6]

Childhood death is not the only potential danger from malnutrition; multiple extended studies have shown that early childhood malnutrition also shapes lifelong development. Guatemalan adults who had been given a protein-enhanced nutrition supplement through age 2 were found to have better intellectual functioning than adults who had been given a sugar-sweetened nutrition supplement.[7] Improvements in nutritional status through age 2 have lifelong impacts: studies in Brazil, Guatemala, India, the Philippines, and South Africa found that healthy weight gain until age 2 was associated with more years of schooling and lower risk of failing a grade—yet improvements made in a child's nutritional status between ages 2 and 4 had little relationship to schooling outcomes.[8]

Maternal malnutrition also affects a child's nutrition and health. Women who are underweight before pregnancy and who gain little weight during pregnancy are particularly at risk of giving birth to babies of low birth weight. Even excluding those born prematurely, babies who are born at low birth weight are more likely to die as newborns than babies born at a healthy weight. Babies born between 4 pounds, 6 ounces and 5 pounds, 8 ounces are 2.8 times as likely to die as newborns than heavier babies. This figure rises to 8.1 times as likely for full-term babies born between 3 pounds, 5 ounces and 4 pounds, 6 ounces.[9]

Inadequate levels of maternal iodine during pregnancy can cause

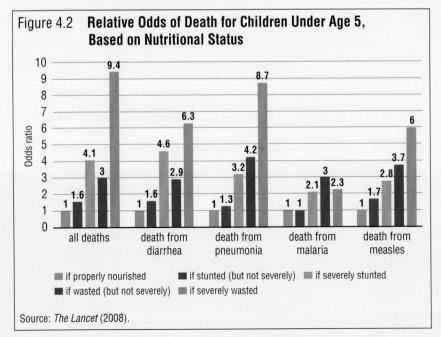

Figure 4.2 **Relative Odds of Death for Children Under Age 5, Based on Nutritional Status**

- if properly nourished
- if stunted (but not severely)
- if severely stunted
- if wasted (but not severely)
- if severely wasted

Source: *The Lancet* (2008).

brain damage in the child.[10] Populations with high rates of chronic iodine deficiency have dramatically lower IQ scores—an average of 14 points lower.[11]

A malnourished mother can produce breast milk containing all of the fat, protein, and carbohydrates (macronutrients) a baby needs. Only under famine or near-famine conditions would the macronutrient content of the milk be affected.[12] Babies given partial or no breastfeeding in the first few months of life are nearly 2.5 times as likely to die as babies who are breastfed exclusively.[13] However, if a mother experiences certain micronutrient deficiencies, she requires micronutrient supplements in order to pass these micronutrients on to her baby.

Nutrition is critical throughout life, but nutrition from pregnancy to age 2 has dramatic potential to shape the trajectory of a child's life. To reduce child mortality, interventions must cover all malnourished children, not simply those experiencing severe forms of malnutrition. Simple, cost-effective nutrition interventions would not only save millions of children from illness or death, it would also improve their health, intelligence, and productivity for the rest of their lives.

Because investing in the nutrition of children under age 2 has such a multiplier effect, agricultural development and food aid should focus particularly on targeting benefits to young children and pregnant mothers. Well-nourished young children become productive adults who have the potential to improve the outlook of entire nations.

Rebecca J. Vander Meulen is the director of community development for the Anglican Diocese of Niassa (Mozambique). From June 2011 to September 2011, she was a fellow in Bread for the World Institute.

outcomes and agricultural development, two issues that are inseparable.

Food aid is another tool the United States uses to respond to hunger crises. Most of this assistance is devoted to supplying food and other essentials directly to people trapped in humanitarian emergencies. Food aid is also used to improve food security in food-deficit countries where people are chronically hungry. While food aid is not a sustainable long-term solution to hunger and malnutrition, it can and should complement agriculture and food security programs such as Feed the Future.

Rural Mozambique: Constantia, Gustavo, and Their Neighbors

Mozambique is a southern African country of 23 million people, most of whom (81 percent) live below the international poverty threshold of $1.25 per day.[14] In the Mozambican village of Cobue, Constantia and her family farm a small plot of maize and cassava. They are subsistence farmers who eat what they grow themselves. Most rural Mozambican farmers have neither fertilizer nor formal training in agricultural techniques or management. A hoe and machete are the tools of their trade.

Constantia's experience with her firstborn child, Gustavo, is all too common here and in other villages around the world where a large share of people are hungry and poor. Gustavo developed normally until he was a year old, but then he contracted malaria. Constantia stopped breastfeeding him out of fear that her milk was contributing to his illness. But this weakened Gustavo's immune system and he developed other infections that stole his appetite.

As advised by her family and neighbors, Constantia fed him a thin porridge of maize flour and salt. The porridge kept Gustavo from becoming dehydrated, but it also worsened his malnutrition by filling his stomach without giving him the nutrients he needed. He had no appetite and began to refuse all food.

Gustavo then gained some weight back—but this was bad news because it meant his body was retaining water. At 18 months, Gustavo weighed only 17 pounds—including the water weight. His condition, known as edema, put him in mortal danger.

In addition to medical care, Gustavo needed food aid. Constantia brought him to a clinic, where she learned how to feed him a fortified milk formula with a syringe and then did so, every two to three hours around the

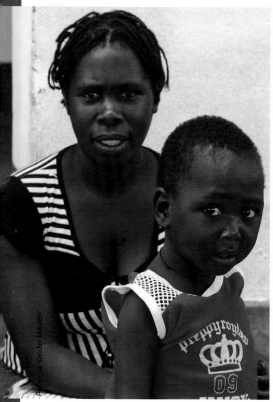

Only a year after Gustavo's brush with death, he is a healthy 2-year-old thanks to food aid. He is shown here with his mother, Constantia, whose persistent dedication to feeding him paid off.

clock. The formula was specially designed to maximize the toddler's absorption of energy, protein, and micronutrients.

Gustavo's appetite slowly returned and finally he could be coaxed into eating solid foods. He was given Plumpy'nut, a high-protein therapeutic food served as a paste. Though he rejected the other protein-rich foods he was offered, Gustavo found Plumpy'nut tasty and he ate it voluntarily.

Now, a year later, Gustavo is able to eat the same food as the rest of his family. Although his attending physician had suspected he would die, the little boy runs and plays with other children in the village. But the whole family still lives on the edge of hunger.

Quantity versus Quality: How Does Food Aid Do the Most Good?

For decades, the United States has been the world's leading provider of food aid to vulnerable and malnourished people. Under the International Food Aid Convention, the country agreed to provide a minimum of 2.5 million metric tons of food per year.[15] Over the years, the United States and other donor countries have delivered many millions of tons of food aid.

In theory, food aid is distributed according to the needs of a targeted population, but more often than not it is distributed according to what is available, which may not be appropriate nutritionally. Providing food aid is complex because it must respond to the complex, intertwined problems of famine, food insecurity, and malnutrition. Each year, tens of millions of people rely on food aid as their primary—sometimes their only—source of sustenance. This means that food aid donors must provide the right food—with the right nutrients.

No single food will meet the nutritional needs of all food aid recipients. In fact, studies show that a combination of different foods contributes more to overall nutrition than a combination of nutrients in a single food aid product.[16] Similarly, no single approach to providing food aid will work in all circumstances. Food aid may be provided at community feeding centers, as in Gustavo's case, or through home-based care programs or at health facilities.

Vulnerable groups, particularly severely malnourished children, need food aid that is specially designed to boost caloric intake and/or meet specific nutritional needs. This "targeted" food aid is usually intended for children younger than 5, women who are pregnant or lactating, or people living with HIV/AIDS or other chronic illnesses.

"Therapeutic feeding" is part of an emergency response to treat severely malnourished children; it includes foods high in fats, proteins, and vitamins and minerals (micronutrients). Milk-based therapeutic products, with formulas developed by UNICEF and the World Food Program, have been commonly used in therapeutic settings. Newer products have also become available that deliver precise, measurable quantities of nutrients to severely malnourished children.

Food aid for general distribution, provided to meet the needs of an entire population, is generally a dry commodity distributed in bulk. It can be fortified with micronutrients, either at the production plant or in the field, but usually whole grains (rice, corn, wheat, sorghum) are not fortified. Fifteen commodities account for the majority of food aid provided by the United States, although the list of approved products is much larger.[17] U.S. food aid is made up mostly of cereal-based products (see Figure 4.3). Corn Soy Blend (CSB) is made of cornmeal, soy flour, salt, and vegetable oil, fortified with micronutrients. Other formulations of CSB include powdered milk protein, which helps the body absorb nutrients. Some types of CSB include additional micronutrients, milk powder, de-hulled soybeans, vegetable oil, and/or sugar, giving them nutritional content similar to the newer lipid (fat)-based products. CSB is now sometimes available in the form of nutrition bars. The newest CSB products have not yet been tested with large numbers of at-risk people.

Clean water—whether from an improved water source, boiled, or treated—is a necessity anywhere cereal-based food aid is distributed, because these food products must be mixed with water. Food-borne and water-borne diseases, such as cholera and dysentery, are leading causes of illness and death in developing countries. The World Health Organization estimates that about 2.2 million people, most of them children, die from diarrhea each year.

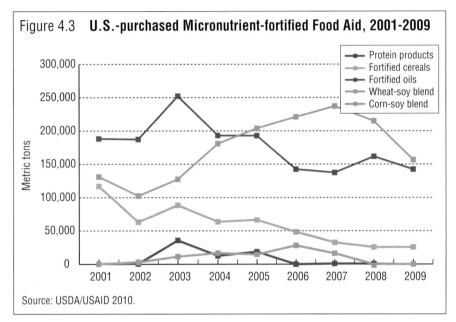

Figure 4.3 **U.S.-purchased Micronutrient-fortified Food Aid, 2001-2009**

Source: USDA/USAID 2010.

People who are malnourished or have weakened immune systems are more susceptible to contracting food-borne and water-borne diseases and more likely to die from them.

The general distribution food aid commodities fall short of meeting the nutrition needs of pregnant and lactating women, small children, and people with compromised health. This is especially true in chronic food shortage emergencies, where food aid is the main source of nutrition for more than a year. More than half the food aid provided by the United States is for multi-year programs (see Figure 4.4). According to the U.S. Government Accountability Office (GAO), 21 of the 30 countries that received U.S. emergency food aid in fiscal year (FY) 2010 had been receiving it for four or more years.

Developments in Food and Nutrition Science Focus Attention on Improving the Quality of Food Aid

New food aid products are improving the health of those suffering from both moderate and severe levels of malnutrition. Probably the best known is Plumpy'nut, developed by the French company Nutriset. Plumpy'nut has garnered a great deal of attention in the mainstream media; it's sometimes called a "miracle drug" for its ability to bring children wasted from malnutrition back from the brink of death. A recent study in Niger showed that feeding Plumpy'nut to severely malnourished children under age 2 was associated with a reduction in mortality of roughly 50 percent.[18]

Plumpy'nut and products like it are known as lipid-based nutritional supplements (LNS). Lipids are fats—key ingredients in food aid since they promote rapid weight gain, which is precisely what malnourished children need. LNS can be made from legumes (peas, lentils), peanuts, chickpeas, sesame seeds, maize, and/or soybeans.

LNS products have revolutionized the use of ready-to-use supplemental and therapeutic foods in treating malnutrition. They are also being tested as a complementary food for general distribution to food aid recipients. LNS are normally available in the form of a spreadable paste. In packaged form, they can be safely stored for extended periods, even in tropical climates, and children can eat them directly from the package with little assistance and no further preparation or cooking. LNS can also treat adults with chronic malnutrition, HIV/AIDS, and/or long-term illnesses. The packaging, storability, and design of LNS promote home-based therapy, which is less expensive since patients don't need to travel to feeding centers.

LNS can also be manufactured with simple technology available in developing countries. Dr. André Briend, the French pediatrician who invented Plumpy'nut, demonstrated by whipping up batches in a home blender.[19] There are still some quality and safety concerns about local production, mainly related to preventing bacterial contamination. For example, in-country testing must be done to ensure that the foods can be produced without being contaminated by aflatoxin, which can come from mold growth on peanuts and corn—particularly because exposure to aflatoxin causes malnutrition and suppresses the immune system.[20] But where solutions to such risks have been developed, local production and distribution of LNS can cut costs significantly.

Another group of nutritional supplements that show promise in treating moderate and severe malnutrition is micronutrient powders, which can be formulated to address specific micronutrient deficiencies and can be added as a complement to home meals or to other types of food aid to boost nutritional content. The World Food Program has successfully introduced micronutrient powders in South Asia but noted that packaging and labeling must make it clear that, for example, a supplement is for pregnant women or for babies and toddlers.[21] These supplements are low-cost and, as with lipid-based products, they can be produced locally.

The cost of different types of food aid varies widely. In 2011, the GAO determined the cost ranges of one day's worth or one dose of a product to be: grain-based food aid, 2-5 cents; micronutrient powders, 3-4 cents; corn-soy blend, 6-24 cents; and lipid-based, 12-41 cents.[22] Clearly, the cost determines the number of people who can be assisted for a given amount of money.

U.S. food aid fills many empty bellies, but it hasn't made nutrition the priority it should be. Policymakers should identify and implement the most

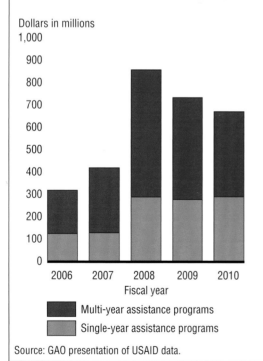

Figure 4.4   Emergency Food Aid Commodity Purchases, Multi-year and Single-year Assistance Programs, FY2006 through 2010

Dollars in millions

Multi-year assistance programs

Single-year assistance programs

Source: GAO presentation of USAID data.

effective and rapid ways to change the situation. One starting point: a review of the quality of U.S. food aid by researchers from Tufts University, commissioned by USAID, outlined ways to enhance its quality and effectiveness. The Tufts review affirmed the importance of nutrition during the first 1,000 days; identified how food aid can improve nutritional outcomes in older infants, young children, and pregnant and lactating women;[23] and recommended reformulating food aid products to take advantage of developments in nutrition science.

These new developments are, in fact, fueling discussions at both the policy and program levels about improving the quality of food aid.[24] Additional studies are needed to assess the effectiveness of new food aid products in actual field settings. In the absence of a substantive body of evidence on nutrition outcomes, cost considerations are likely to carry disproportionate weight. But it's quite clear that the nutritional quality of U.S. food aid can be improved by fortifying and targeting various types of foods and by including a wider range of foods.

Food Aid is Vital for People with HIV/AIDS

Veronica lives in the village of Ngofi in Mozambique, where families live on what they grow on their farms. She, her husband Marcos, and their four children had a herd of goats; they were wealthier than most of their neighbors since goats are worth 400 pounds of maize each.

Marcos fell ill and, on a visit to the hospital in neighboring Malawi, discovered that he had HIV. It's not necessary for everyone with HIV to begin treatment immediately after diagnosis, but Marcos needed to go on antiretro-

viral therapy right away. He had to make regular trips across Lake Niassa by ferry to get medical checkups and pick up medication. Each time, he had to pay for food and lodging in addition to the ferry fee, because the ferry ran only once a week. Veronica and Marcos had to sell a goat every couple of months to get the money.

Veronica and Marcos quickly depleted their resources, including the goats. The family went from being one of the wealthiest in their village to one of the poorest. After Marcos began treatment, Veronica was also diagnosed as HIV-positive, although she was not in immediate need of treatment. Both needed extra calories to help sustain their immune systems, working at full throttle against HIV. They also needed sufficient vitamins and minerals—important to the body's struggle against opportunistic infections—but normally their meals centered on cassava or maize, staple foods that filled them up and provided calories but had little nutritional value.

Their health deteriorated after they exhausted their resources. Production plummeted on the family farm because Marcos was too weak to work.

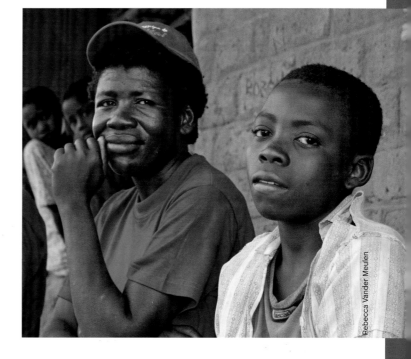

Thanks to HIV medication and food aid, Veronica is healthy and well-nourished. She is shown here with her son.

Veronica, though still physically able to work, spent much of her time and energy caring for her husband. Eventually Marcos died from an opportunistic illness and Veronica, much weaker by now, was left with the children and little food.

Just as she was selling the last of the goats, a medical facility opened closer to home, which made it possible for her to begin antiretroviral treatment. Veronica made the trip with fellow villagers who also needed HIV treatment. She received food aid along with her medication. The food she was given—flour, oil, and sugar—enabled her to make an enriched porridge and regain her strength. She added the oil and sugar to the porridge while it was cooking in order to increase its caloric density. The maize flour was fortified with protein and fat by the addition of ground beans and peanuts.

With the combination of HIV medication and food aid, Veronica recovered to the point where she could work on her farm and feed herself and the children. Other families in her village—including those not affected by HIV—also started to mix beans and peanuts into their porridge whenever possible.

Going the Distance: The Food Aid Supply Chain

U.S. food aid passes through three stages between farmers and food aid recipients.[25] Each offers opportunities to improve efficiency, thus enabling the program to provide higher-quality foods and/or serve more people.

- **Procurement.** The Office of Food for Peace at USAID and the Foreign Agricultural Service of USDA fill orders for food aid placed by the World Food Program and nongovernmental organizations such as World Vision, Catholic Relief Services, and Mercy Corps. The raw

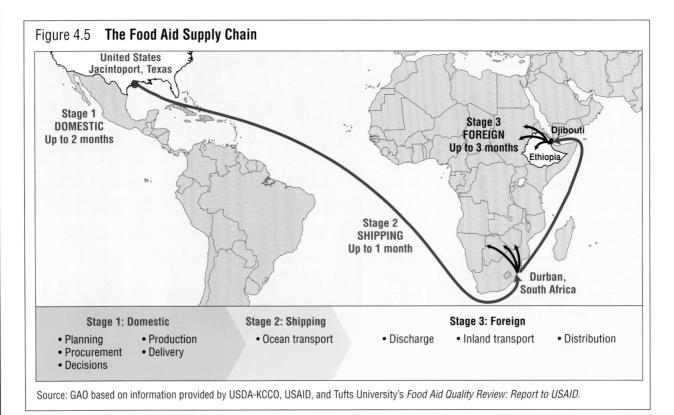

Figure 4.5 **The Food Aid Supply Chain**

Source: GAO based on information provided by USDA-KCCO, USAID, and Tufts University's *Food Aid Quality Review: Report to USAID*.

commodities are then sent for milling and fortification. There is a strict protocol for quality control, but a 2011 GAO report noted several concerns, including instances of failure to meet vitamin content specifications, the presence of salmonella and insects, rodent infestation, and poor data tracking through various stages of the supply chain.[26] To their credit, government offices in charge of quality control processes have taken steps to address problems. But they themselves admit that quality assurance would be jeopardized if funding cuts force the elimination of services.[27]

- **Transport.** U.S. policies require that 75 percent of food aid must be shipped on U.S.-flagged vessels,[28] so there is little room to economize under current law. However, shipping from the United States uses up as much as 50 percent of the total food aid budget[29] and takes four to six months.[30] Thus, no area presents a greater opportunity to save money than the reform of "cargo preference" laws.

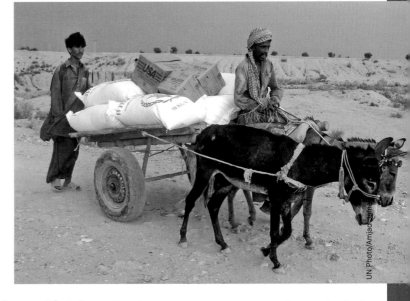

- **Distribution.** When the food aid arrives, the World Food Program or another implementing partner takes possession of it and distributes it to the recipients. This is the end of the supply chain, but it would improve the process if there were also an evaluation of nutritional outcomes. After all, improving people's nutritional status is the whole purpose of food aid, and no one can know whether the goal is being met without evaluation. Evaluation would also provide information to help identify problems at the end of the supply chain—for example, is food aid at risk of contamination from being mixed with unclean water?

Displaced Pakistanis pull a cartload of rations distributed by the U.N. World Food Program after massive floods in 2010.

Cost-Effective Improvements in the Quality of U.S. Food Aid

Improving the nutritional quality of U.S food aid is a daunting challenge in the context of a shrinking federal budget. Cost will significantly affect how quickly U.S. food aid can be changed to better meet the nutritional needs of the most vulnerable groups. Bulk commodities and unfortified cereal products cost less per ton than fortified or processed foods with enhanced nutritional value. Yet efforts to strengthen nutritional status, particularly those that supply people with more micronutrients,[31] yield an extraordinarily high return on investment: they enable people to live longer, more productive lives.

As a wider range of new and/or reformulated foods become available, understanding and evaluating the tradeoffs is increasingly complex. When food aid costs are calculated on a per ton basis, the real value of these new and improved products is not apparent. But considering the cost of each improvement in nutritional status is a different approach that leads to a different verdict. This is particularly true of food aid designed for very young children and pregnant women. As mentioned earlier, undernutrition before age 2 leads to irreversible damage to growth and brain development. It causes stunting and wasting.[32] Women who are malnourished during pregnancy face a greater risk of dying in childbirth and of giving birth to a low birth weight baby.

The U.S. government and implementing partners should begin taking steps immediately to move effective nutrition interventions "to scale" so they reach more of those who could benefit. Here are some ways to cut down on the cost of such initiatives:

1. *Adopt local and regional purchase (LRP).* Under this arrangement, implementing partners receive cash grants to purchase food aid commodities from nearby areas with surpluses rather than procuring them in the United States. This not only reduces transport fees but helps get food to people in need more quickly.

LRP is coming into widespread use. For fiscal year 2011, USDA has eight LRP projects and USAID's Food for Peace Office has 13, valued at $11.5 million and $98 million respectively. The World Food Program and other bilateral donors also purchase food aid locally and regionally. Of the 3.2 million tons of commodities that the World Food Program purchased in 2010, more than 78 percent came from developing countries.[33] Donor use of LRP increased from 13 percent of total food aid in 1994 to 50 percent in 2009.[34] LRP projects continue to evolve and yield additional information on reducing costs and working more efficiently.

2. *Preposition food aid closer to where it is most likely to be needed.* USAID has scaled up its efforts to do this; it now has six sites around the world where food aid is stockpiled.[35] The World Food Program also maintains advance-purchase facilities so that food aid is closer to areas that frequently face food shortages.

3. *Coordinate more effectively.* A Food Aid Consultative Group, consisting of multiple government agencies and stakeholders, should update policy recommendations for best practices and help offices coordinate with each other. Several offices in USDA, USAID, and the State Department develop and guide the implementation of U.S. food aid policy regulations. The current division of labor has USDA approving food aid commodities and arranging their purchase and delivery to port, after which USAID receives, transports, and distributes food aid in the field.

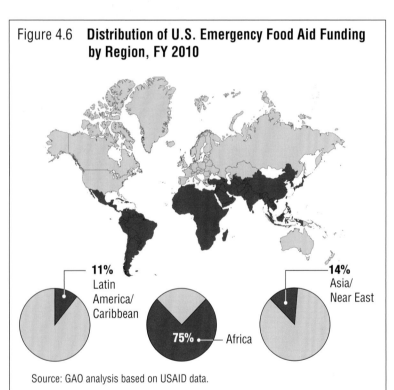

Figure 4.6 Distribution of U.S. Emergency Food Aid Funding by Region, FY 2010

11%
Latin America/ Caribbean

75% — Africa

14% Asia/ Near East

Source: GAO analysis based on USAID data.

4. *Report nutrition outcomes.* Current end-of-year reporting by implementing partners does not include reporting on nutrition.[36] A simplified Country Progress Report on nutrition outcomes will provide timely information on program successes and needed changes.

5. *Seek advice from experts.* Outside expertise on nutrition is widely available and should be weighed when the time comes to make decisions. In particular, the USDA/USAID food aid coordination group should consult with research institutions in the United States, such as Tufts University, as well as comparable institutions in developing countries.

6. *Reform the Food Aid Convention.*[37] The Food Aid Convention is a multilateral treaty set up to guarantee a minimum annual disbursement of food aid, thus enabling the international community to better respond to emergencies and build global food security. The United States, as the largest food aid donor, needs to lead an effort to reform the treaty. (See Box 4.2, next page.)

Phasing Out Monetization

Not all U.S. food aid is distributed directly to hungry people. Every year, hundreds of millions of dollars' worth of food aid is "monetized"—sold in recipient country markets for cash to pay for development projects. The practice started in the 1980s and has grown steadily. It has been used primarily to improve long-term food security—for example, providing technical training to farmers or improving the infrastructure farmers need to gain access to markets.[38]

Monetization has been widely criticized as an inefficient way of funding development projects. Research by the GAO in 2011 is one of many reports showing that monetization costs significant amounts of money that would otherwise go to programs for hungry and poor people. Of $722 million in food aid that was monetized between 2007 and 2009, $508 million was spent on development programs, while $219 million (30 percent) paid for freight charges to ship food aid commodities from the United States, transportation to bring the commodities to markets in the recipient countries, and other costs of monetization. U.S. cargo preference policies accounted for most of this lost funding.[39]

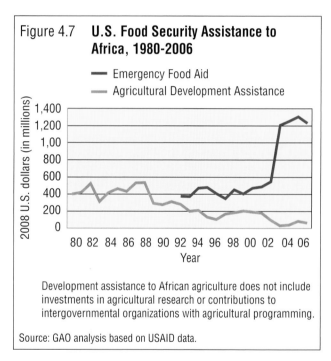

Figure 4.7 **U.S. Food Security Assistance to Africa, 1980-2006**

— Emergency Food Aid
— Agricultural Development Assistance

Development assistance to African agriculture does not include investments in agricultural research or contributions to intergovernmental organizations with agricultural programming.

Source: GAO analysis based on USAID data.

In addition to being inefficient, as the GAO report notes, monetization can also displace or crowd out of the market the products of domestic farmers. Ironically, flooding the market with food aid hurts the sales of the same people the commodities were intended to help—the smallholder farmers who count on domestic markets for their livelihoods.

There's a general consensus that long-term food security depends on new investments in agricultural development.[40] But for too long, the principal source of U.S. assistance for agricultural development was—in another striking irony—food aid. For most of the last 30 years, there has been little interest in agriculture's role in development. (See Figure 4.7.) U.S. agricultural assistance plummeted from $400 million in the 1980s to $60 million by 2006,[41] while World Bank lending for agricultural assistance fell from 30 percent of all loans to 8 percent over the same timeframe. Governments of aid-recipient countries followed the international community and slashed their own support for agriculture.

With donors slashing agricultural assistance and using food aid as their preferred mode of conducting food security policy, monetizing food aid kind of made sense: otherwise, development organizations simply had no resources to support smallholder farmers. But this is no longer the case. In 2009, the U.S. government launched Feed the Future, a new agricultural development program, starting with 20 countries, and President Obama pledged $3.5 billion over three years to support agricultural development initiatives. The United States also called on other developed countries to prioritize agriculture, and several donors pledged resources at the 2009 G-8 meeting in L'Aquila, Italy.

Although no one can promise that funding for Feed the Future—or any government program—will be allo-cated in coming years, its establishment signals a major shift in U.S. government policy on global food security. Feed the Future is the first initiative of its kind to explicitly focus on overcoming long-term food security challenges. It should mean that it is no longer necessary to monetize food aid to obtain resources for long-term food security programs. Food aid is still a valuable tool, but now there's a division of labor: food aid can be used for humanitarian emergencies and protracted food shortages while Feed the Future promotes longer-term food security.

The need to improve the nutritional quality of food aid, discussed earlier, is one major reason to reassess U.S. food aid policy. Another is the need to phase out the practice of monetization as Feed the Future and multilateral initiatives make more resources available for agricultural development. The two areas of change dovetail quite well: saving hundreds of millions of dollars per year in monetization costs would make it possible to fund significant efforts to improve the nutritional quality of food aid.

BOX 4.2   A MOMENT OF UNCERTAINTY ON FOOD AID

by Trans Atlantic Food Assistance Dialogue (TAFAD)

The Food Aid Convention (FAC) was established in 1967 as a multilateral instrument under the International Grains Agreement. Every year member states commit to provide a minimum flow of food and food-related resources to recipient countries. Since the last renegotiation in 1999, the FAC has guaranteed 5 million tons per year of food assistance.

As yet, there has been no discussion of a new commitment on guaranteed tonnage in the ongoing FAC negotiations scheduled to be completed in December 2011. Overall assistance will likely be the sum of individual member pledges in whatever form is convenient (in tonnage or in cash). The risk of the absence of a collective commitment is that governments will have no binding target to reach, thereby making food assistance to recipient countries less predictable.

Abandoning the tenet of a guaranteed floor on food assistance would greatly undermine the value of the treaty. The FAC should not become another donor coordination mechanism. The treaty must continue to guarantee an adequate and predictable minimum amount of food assistance. This assistance is vital in responding to food emergencies such as the current East African Food Crisis and supporting food safety net programming.

Many countries and observers have called for the new FAC to be needs-based rather than resource-based. A real needs-based convention should therefore ensure a collective commitment every year. There should be a way to reconcile cash and food commitments in a common unit. If the collective commitment were lost in the current negotiations, the FAC would be a weaker instrument of food assistance and therefore less useful as an element of a global food security strategy.

TAFAD is a coalition of 11 major food aid programming NGOs from Europe, Canada, and the United States.

Aligning Food Aid and Feed the Future

"We will design and implement programs that enable the rural poor to participate in and contribute to food security," reads the Feed the Future Guide, the initiative's official implementation strategy.[42] The guide describes Feed the Future's goals; what stands out are the "two key objectives of accelerating inclusive agriculture sector growth and improving nutritional status."[43]

Directly linking improvements in nutrition with agriculture-led growth makes Feed the Future more sophisticated than previous U.S. approaches to food security. Similarly, an approach that recognizes that progress against hunger and poverty requires full partnership with poor people themselves is much more likely to be successful. The governments of developing countries are also essential partners. Sustainable progress requires taking ownership of development initiatives. An encouraging sign in Africa, for example, is the formation of the Comprehensive Africa Agriculture Development Program (CAADP), which brings together leaders from a number of African countries who have pledged to increase their funding for agriculture and to improve regional integration of their agricultural sectors.

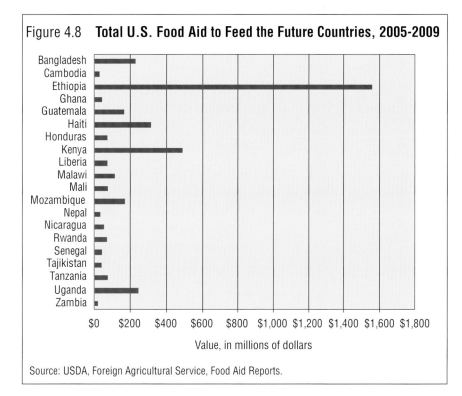

Figure 4.8 **Total U.S. Food Aid to Feed the Future Countries, 2005-2009**

Value, in millions of dollars

Source: USDA, Foreign Agricultural Service, Food Aid Reports.

In theory, food aid comes first, development later. In practice, the two frequently co-exist, which is why food aid programs and Feed the Future need to be coordinated. Of Feed the Future's initial 20 partner countries, some are beginning to realize steady growth in their agricultural sectors, while others are major recipients of U.S. food aid. (See Figure 4.8.) One way to coordinate the two is through local and regional purchase (LRP) of food aid commodities.

Sadly, it is unlikely that humanitarian emergencies in poor countries—whether caused by war, drought, floods, or one-off natural disasters such as earthquakes—will abruptly cease. Food aid will continue to be essential. One possible silver lining is an increased demand for local crops from LRP of food aid commodities. In this way, farmers in the country or region where food aid is needed will benefit from supplying it. Enabling farmers to sell more of their crops in markets will, in turn, help build stronger local economies—precisely the point of Feed the Future's focus on agriculture-led growth as a way to build resiliency among rural poor people.

In a comprehensive analysis of LRP programs around the world, most of them operated by the World Food Program, GAO concluded, "While the pri-

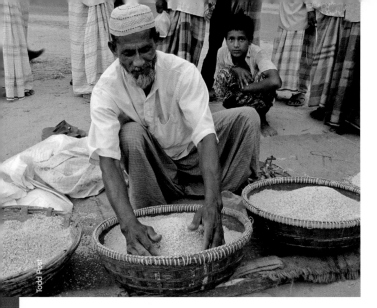

Smallholder farmers carry out most of their trade in village markets, such as the one shown here in Bangladesh. U.S. agricultural development assistance helps farmers gain greater access to markets.

mary purpose of LRP is to provide food assistance in humanitarian emergencies in a timely and efficient manner, a potential secondary benefit is contributing to the development of the local economies from which food is purchased. This can be accomplished by increasing the demand for agricultural commodities, thereby increasing support for all levels of the commodity value chain."[44]

GAO found reasons why in some countries LRP might not be an efficient alternative to shipping food aid commodities from the United States—for example, a shortage of reliable suppliers, poor infrastructure, or the inability of processors to meet food safety requirements. However, Feed the Future is oriented toward resolving such problems. In 2010, at the International Food Aid and Development Conference in Kansas City, MO, Ann Tutwiler, then USDA's coordinator of Feed the Future, used similar terms to describe the initiative as GAO had used for LRP: "Feed the Future seeks to develop the entire value chain: production, storage and handling, transport and rural infrastructure, and finally increasing market access."[45]

In spite of its potentially significant benefits, LRP does not enjoy universal support among people involved in U.S. food aid. A report by the Congressional Research Service summarizes two objections: "Critics... maintain that allowing non-U.S. commodities to be purchased would undermine the coalition of agribusinesses, private voluntary organizations, and shippers that participate in and support the U.S. food aid program, and would reduce the volume of U.S. commodities provided as aid."[46]

It is often very difficult to change the status quo, even in a representative democracy. But policymakers should focus on outcomes and efficiency. Sustainable solutions to hunger depend on the capacity of countries to meet their own food security challenges. Feed the Future can help countries build their capacity, while food aid policies such as local and regional purchase can support the infrastructure necessary to respond more quickly to humanitarian crises.

Feed the Future in Mozambique

Mozambique, like other Feed the Future countries, is poor but committed to taking ownership of its own development. As mentioned earlier, four of every five people live in poverty and spend a large portion of their incomes on food; soaring food prices led to riots in the capital city of Maputo in fall 2010. The country's turbulent past includes a 16-year civil war that ended in 1992.

U.S. food aid and development assistance work well together in Mozambique, as Ambassador Amelia Matos Sumbana explained to participants in the 2011 International Food Aid and Development conference in Kansas City, MO: "In the 1990s, in the aftermath of 16 years of armed conflict, [U.S. food aid programs] helped our country recover and transition to a more stable and inclusive democracy. Food distribution helped meet immediate needs, and in a short period of time the program shifted to a developmental focus."[47] Mozambique continues to rely on U.S. food aid but is also well on its way to self-sustaining agricultural production. It works with both Feed the Future and the U.S. Millennium Challenge Corporation (through a five-year development compact signed in 2007).

With a resource base of rich soil, abundant water, relatively low population density, and a smallholder-dominated farm sector, the agriculture sector would seem to have great potential to jump-start the nation's economy and drive it into rapid development. Mozambique is also in a key regional trade location—on the Atlantic coast and bordering five southern African countries.

Feed the Future supports partnerships that provide Mozambican farmers with technical assistance. For example, Ikuru is the country's largest farmer-owned business, with more than 22,000 members. It's in Nampula Province in the north, one of the poorest regions of the country, where 43 percent of children are stunted and 51 percent are underweight. Ikuru's main crop and source of income is groundnuts (peanuts). In 2004, group members sold just 300 metric tons of groundnuts. Production began to rise once the farmers were receiving technical support from USAID and its implementing partners, primarily Michigan State University and the Cooperative League of the USA. By 2009, the volume of nuts sold had reached 2,250 metric tons—an increase of more than 700 percent in just five years. Feed the Future hopes to cultivate more of these types of partnerships in Mozambique.[48]

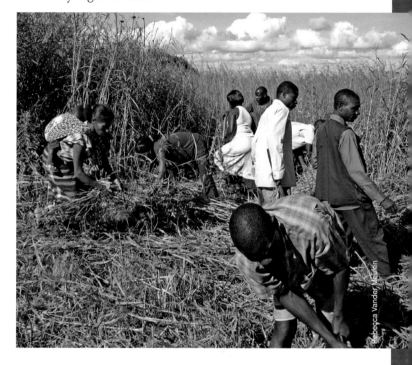

Mozambican farmers clear land by hand. Most Mozambican farmers grow food without mechanical tractors or animal traction.

The technical support available to U.S. agriculture is one of the reasons it is so productive. Much of it is offered to farmers through USDA's cooperative extension service. Such technical support is much less common in developing countries. Through partnerships with U.S. land grant universities and the private sector, USAID has been able to offer extension services in Mozambique and other developing countries. Ikuru is just one of the farmers' groups that have made substantial gains in productivity in a short time.

Although Feed the Future supports research and technology innovation, many of the solutions to the problems that limit agricultural production do not require sophisticated technology. In another of Mozambique's poorest regions, Zambezia, 61 percent of smallholders harvest mangos, but only 5 percent are able to market them. Fruit production in Mozambique is marred by post-harvest loss—25-40 percent of production[49]—because most of the country's farmers lack access to basic storage facilities that protect their fruit from bugs and rodents.

In Chapter 1, we were introduced to Arlyn Schipper, an Iowa corn and soybean farmer, who has visited developing countries with other U.S. farmers to offer his assistance to smallholders. U.S. farmers would be providing more help to smallholder farmers by sharing what they know about farming than by selling a small fraction of their own harvests to U.S. food aid programs. Knowledge-sharing trips are also an important way to build public understanding in the United States of the conditions and struggles of smallholder farmers overseas and of what U.S. development assistance tries to achieve. But opportunities for U.S. farmers to do this are scarce.

Farmers in developing countries do need access to better technologies, but even more important are effective policies and strong support from their governments, and commitment and true partnership from donor countries. Continued U.S. support for Feed the Future is a vital part of what will help them build stronger local economies and stronger families.

Protecting Today's Investments, Looking Toward Tomorrow

The world is not producing enough food to keep pace with increasing demand.[50] There is no doubt that this is everyone's problem: the consequences of failing to solve it will affect us all. Nothing fuels global instability like hungry people taking their frustration to the streets of capital cities, as we've seen in recent years when food prices spiked.

It will take a concerted effort by governments and the private sector to turn the situation around so that global food production is on track to meet human needs. Developed countries have more influence over the outcome than others. They must come forward and lead because they have the greater share of resources to bring to bear on the problem.

The agricultural challenge is exacerbated by the effects of climate change. The most recent news is quite alarming: if climate change continues at its current rate, child malnutrition rates will increase by 20 percent by 2050.[51] This forecast is based on existing data and scientific models which extrapolate from that data. For example, the model combines data on the increasing severity of droughts with research from West Africa showing that children born during drought years are 72 percent more likely to be stunted.[52] Adapting to climate change would be hard enough with a set population, but in fact, world population increases every day. By the end of the century, the number of mouths to feed is expected to reach 10 billion. Agricultural productivity must be increased quickly enough to stay ahead of climate change and population growth combined.

Developing countries are experiencing the destructive effects of climate change now—before many of the developed countries have truly mobilized to help slow the changes. Most developing countries are in southern latitudes whose higher temperatures create environments that are inherently difficult for agricultural production. In parts of sub-Saharan Africa, where rain-fed agriculture employs 70 percent of the population, drier conditions are producing smaller harvests or none at all, posing a grave threat to already-fragile food security

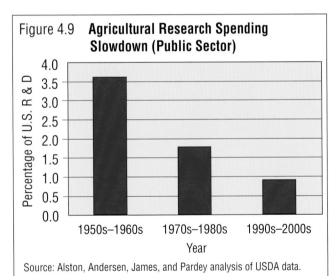

Figure 4.9 **Agricultural Research Spending Slowdown (Public Sector)**

Percentage of U.S. R & D

Year

Source: Alston, Andersen, James, and Pardey analysis of USDA data.

BOX 4.3   A U.S. – UGANDAN RESEARCH PARTNERSHIP

by Laura Elizabeth Pohl
Bread for the World

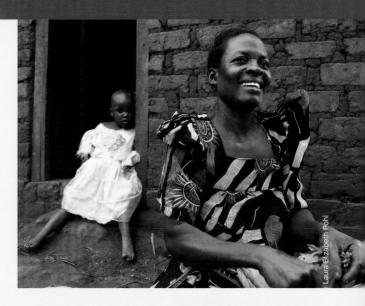

The hoe falls in a rhythmic "thud, thud, thud" as Jane Sabbi and her sister-in-law hack at the undergrowth on Sabbi's shaded, fertile vegetable farm. The sun is still rising in Kamuli, Uganda, and Sabbi has already cooked breakfast, washed the dishes, cleaned the goat and pig pens, and laid out several pounds of beans to dry. Still ahead: pounding amaranth, harvesting bananas, shelling beans, feeding the animals, and cooking lunch for her husband and seven children.

"I want to work hard, get enough money to educate the children to the university level and attain degrees," said Sabbi. "That's my hope and desire in life."

Back in 2004, Sabbi was like many other farmers in Uganda: working hard, subsisting on her harvests, and generating a small income. Then she joined Volunteer Efforts for Development Concerns (VEDCO), a Ugandan civil society group. She learned updated farming methods and began planting more nutritious crops, such as beans.

In a country where, according to USAID, one in five people is undernourished and two in five children are malnourished, helping farmers like Sabbi improve food and nutrition security is crucial to a healthy future. That's why, at about the same time Sabbi joined, VEDCO began a partnership with Makerere University—Uganda's top college—and Iowa State University. VEDCO benefits from research and development, as well as on-the-ground training, conducted by the two universities. In turn, the universities benefit from VEDCO's cadre of members willing and eager to improve their agricultural practices and to test different approaches to sustainable development.

"If you say, 'We're going to dictate the terms of this,' then that doesn't work," said Professor Robert Mazur, associate director of Iowa State's Center for Sustainable Rural Livelihoods. "But if you're learning together and raising questions together, I think you not only have a better chance of being able to introduce change but to make change."

Although women do the majority of the agricultural work in many countries, they often face higher rates of malnutrition than men, due partly to their lower social status. So in 2008, VEDCO, Makerere, and Iowa State launched a four-year nutrition project focused on helping women grow high-quality beans for both consumption and sale.

So far, the project has field-tested various beans to determine which are hardiest, improved market access for the bean growers, and developed fast-cooking bean flour.

Jane Sabbi used to grow beans only for cooking as a sauce and mixing with other foods. Now she harvests high-quality beans for the market. She earns 2,500 shillings (about $1) per kilo for her improved beans, versus 800 shillings per kilo for regular beans.

"Sometimes I go to the farms and I ask about the production system, 'Who clears the land?' 'The women.' 'Who plants the seeds?' 'The women.' 'Who does the weeding?' 'The women.' 'Who does the harvesting?' 'The women,'" said Dr. Dorothy Nakimbugwe, a food technology and nutrition professor at Makerere who develops bean-related food products. "So, women actually do the majority of the work of farm production and ensure food security for their families."

Laura Elizabeth Pohl is a writer and multimedia manager at Bread for the World. She visited Uganda and this project in May 2011.

situations.[53] In coastal regions, climate change is producing more frequent and severe cyclones, leading to flooding and outbreaks of disease.

Some of the countries facing the most alarming climate change impacts are partners in the U.S. Feed the Future initiative. Mozambique's National Disaster Management Institute reports, "The exposure to natural disaster risk will increase significantly over the coming 20 years and beyond," as more severe cyclones hit the coast.[54] Even Mozambique's "normal" exposure to natural disaster risk can bring significant damage; for example, severe flooding in 2000 cost the country $550 million and lowered the national GDP by 1.5 percent.[55] In our era of rapid change, building the resilience of families and communities is arguably the best way to help them. Feed the Future investments are focused on improving food security and reducing poverty; families with greater access to resources will be better able to help themselves adapt to climate change.

Climate change is no longer avoidable. The only questions are how soon, and by how much, we allow it to happen. The last decade was the hottest on record; the one before that was the second-hottest. Residents of developed countries have more choice than others about when and how to get serious about containing the damage caused by climate change. The surest way to slow climate change is to reduce greenhouse gas emissions. Because agriculture itself contributes one-third of all greenhouse gas emissions, the agricultural sector must become more sustainable while simultaneously becoming more productive.

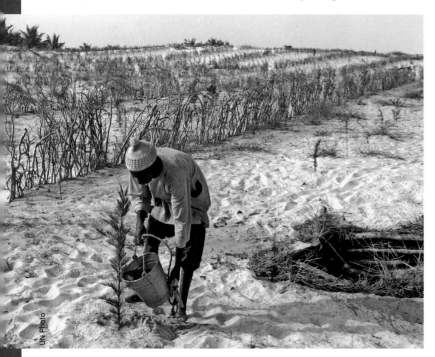

Climate change poses a serious threat to food production in sub-Saharan Africa. The region experiences the highest risk of drought of anywhere in the world.

The United States has tools to raise productivity in sustainable ways that poor countries don't. One of these is a sophisticated research and development (R&D) sector. Historically, U.S. public investments in agricultural R&D have paid off handsomely, with cost-benefit ratios of 20:1 or even higher.[56] The United States also contributes to global agricultural R&D, primarily through the Consultative Group on International Agricultural Research (CGIAR). Established in 1971, CGIAR is a network of research centers around the globe, all focused on innovations to support poor farmers in developing countries—something that the private sector tends to neglect. Investments in CGIAR have a comparable track record, with a rate of return on investments estimated up to 17:1.[57]

U.S. support to CGIAR peaked in the early 1980s and then declined steadily for more than two decades. One reason for this, according to The Chicago Council on Global Affairs, was "the erroneous impression that the world's food problems had been solved. It seemed to some that support for more productivity was no longer needed; food problems came to be understood in some circles as only problems of distribution."[58] 2008 brought a rude awakening as food prices surged and a global hunger crisis ensued. At the height of the crisis, U.S. support to CGIAR was only a quarter of what it had been in the early 1980s.[59]

In 2011, when CGIAR turned 40, the global agricultural system appeared eerily similar to the way it had looked in 1971 when the center was founded. At the time, Malthusian predictions of a world growing too fast to keep up with the demand for food were influential. The Green Revolution that spread across Asia and Latin America stilled those voices for a time. But, as described earlier, global leaders became complacent, and investments in both agriculture and agricultural R&D fell off.

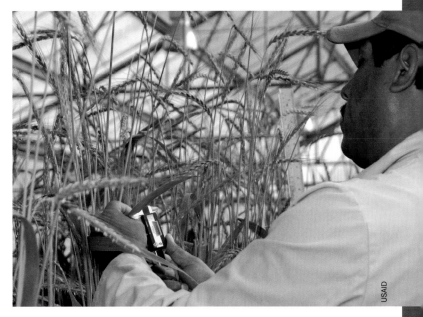

This chapter raises many questions that cannot be answered without additional agricultural research and development, and therefore more funding for it. Just one example: How can agriculture most effectively improve nutrition in countries with high malnutrition rates? Agricultural R&D questions are not academic, but immediately relevant to human problems. In the past decade, the magnitude of the threat that climate change poses to agricultural productivity has become much clearer to researchers and policymakers. We also know more now about the importance of delivering the right nutrition at the right time in life, and about effective ways to do this. All of this is knowledge gained because of investments in R&D.

USAID has supported various agricultural research programs to improve crop production and incomes for farmers in Mexico.

R&D rarely pays off quickly; it usually takes more than a decade to realize returns on investment. But the results are well worth waiting for, as many examples show.[60] Instead of restricting R&D funding, we must urge policymakers and the private sector to stay focused on making the investments that are necessary to solve the urgent problems of global hunger and poverty.

SAFE-FARMING: CROP INSURANCE FOR SMALLHOLDERS

by Stephanie Hanson
Director of Policy and Outreach, One Acre Fund

Trophus Nyaga is a smallholder farmer in Kamwana, a village in eastern Kenya. He has two acres of land, where he plants maize, beans, millet, and sorghum. He also has avocado trees. Last year, Trophus planted maize for the short planting season, and the rains failed. He harvested less than one bag of maize, not even enough to pay for seed and fertilizer for the next planting season.

But Trophus had purchased crop insurance for the first time that season, and in March 2011, he received a payout. He immediately used that money to purchase maize seeds for the long planting season, which began in March.

Unfortunately, the rains for the long planting season were irregular, and Trophus' germination rate was disappointing. When I met him, at the end of June, he was surprisingly sanguine. "If I do not harvest maize, I will get money for replacing the seeds," he told me.

Trophus had only been an insurance customer for a year, but he was fully convinced of its benefits, as are many of the farmers in his area that have purchased the

One Acre Fund

same insurance, a product called Kilimo Salama, which means safe farming in Swahili.

Nancy Njeii said that she tripled the quantity of maize seed that she planted because she was confident that she would receive compensation if the rains failed. Before the insurance, she would only plant part of her land, in an attempt to minimize her potential loss.

"There is a hope," a farmer named Enos Ngondi told me. "Either you will be paid if the rains fail, or you will have a good harvest."

Kenyan smallholder farmers are not used to having the kind of hope that crop insurance brings. Though the majority of farmers in Kenya, and across sub-Saharan Africa, depend on rain-fed agriculture, if the rains fail, they traditionally have no way to recover from the loss. They bear 100 percent of the risk.

Farmers in the United States also must contend with the vagaries of the weather. In America, however, crop insurance is universally adopted. Every farmer has it. In fact, the U.S. government highly subsidizes the cost of crop insurance for farmers. It is one of the few agriculture subsidies that the World Trade Organization permits.

But insuring an American farmer with thousands of acres of land is much easier than insuring an African farmer with two acres of land. There is an abundance of historical weather data available in the United States, which makes it possible to calculate risk, and transaction costs are manageable for large farmers. Until recently, these two challenges prevented the spread of crop insurance in sub-Saharan Africa.

Kilimo Salama, the insurance product that Trophus, Nancy, and Enos all purchased, is showing that it is possible to measure risk and administer insurance at a reasonable cost for smallholder farmers.

The product's cost is kept low by technology. Farmers can purchase the insurance at a local agrodealer when

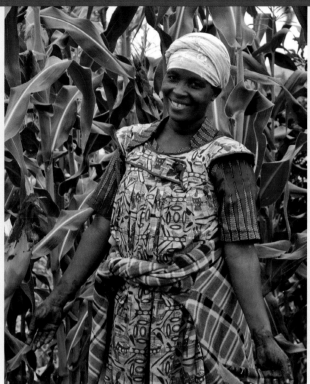

One Acre Fund

they purchase their seed and fertilizer. They receive the insurance policy by text message. Over the course of the agriculture season, Kilimo Salama uses solar-powered weather stations to measure rainfall levels and determine whether the farmers in a particular district should receive a payout. If rainfall levels are either too low or too high during certain critical periods of the growing season, the insurer automatically disburses a payout to every insured farmer in the district. There is no need to check each farmer's fields, or even to write a check to each farmer; the payout is distributed by mobile phone.

Kilimo Salama was developed by the Syngenta Foundation for Sustainable Agriculture in 2009 and was piloted with 200 farmers. In 2011, it is insuring over 21,000 smallholder farmers in Kenya (with plans to reach 50,000 in 2012), in partnership with the Kenyan insurance company UAP. The foundation is looking at offering crop insurance products in other African countries.

One Acre Fund, the agriculture organization that I work for, partners with Syngenta to offer Kilimo Salama to all of our farmers in Kenya who live in districts with its weather stations. We offer the crop insurance as part of our financing package—farmers receive inputs on credit, and the cost of crop insurance is included in the cost of the loan. Because farmers have never had access to crop insurance before, we make it incredibly easy for them to adopt; it is packaged with their loans.

Expanding crop insurance across the continent is particularly important as global food prices rise ever higher. Africa's smallholder farmers have the potential to significantly increase their agriculture production, but without a tool for mitigating risk, most farmers won't be willing to invest in improved seed and fertilizer. Increasing their own production will protect these farmers against further food price increases, but it will also help stabilize global food prices by increasing the overall supply of food. There are roughly 500 million smallholder farmers in the world; in sub-Saharan Africa and southeast Asia, they produce 80 percent of food.

If more of the world's smallholder farmers had crop insurance, they would feel more confident trying new agriculture techniques to improve their productivity. Some of the farmers insured by Kilimo Salama are already doing this. Now that Trophus has crop insurance, he wants to plant different crops and see if he can increase the profitability of his land. "I want to try new things and then I will see the outcome," he said.

Stephanie Hanson is director of policy and outreach at One Acre Fund, an agriculture organization that serves over 55,000 smallholder farmers in East Africa through a complete service model that includes farm inputs, financing, training, and market facilitation. In 2010 and 2011, One Acre Fund won the Financial Times/IFC Sustainable Finance Award for Achievement in Basic Needs Financing.

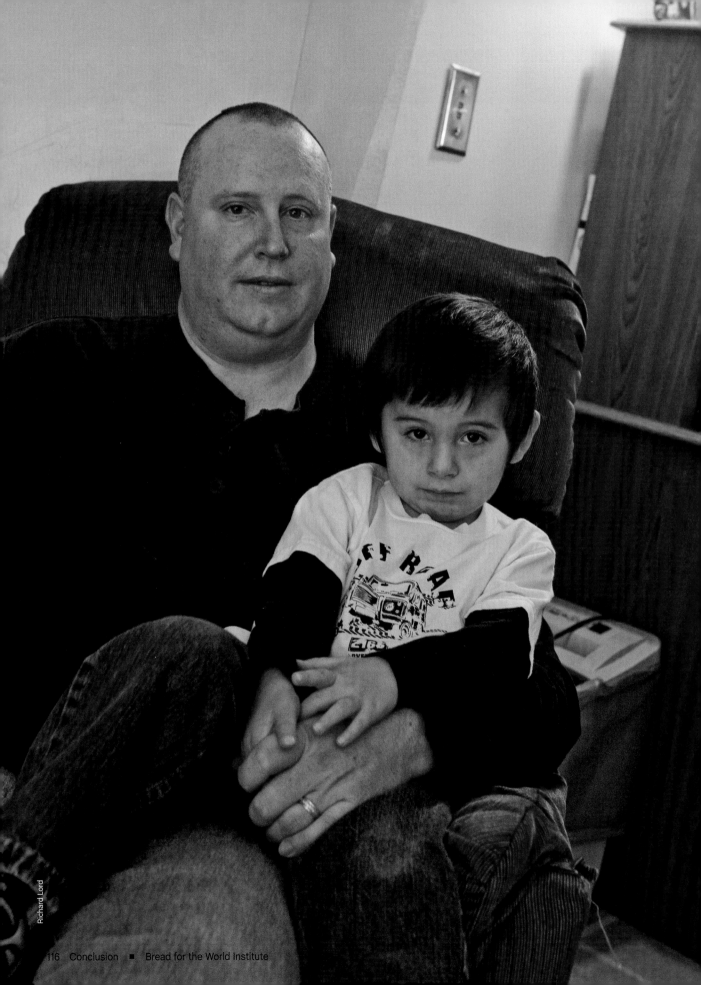

The Hidden Faces of Hunger

Kate Hagen
Bread for the World Institute

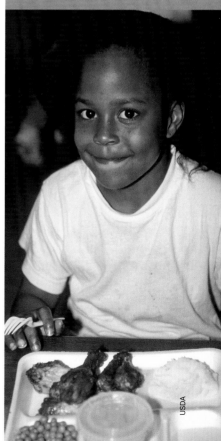

Conclusion

❝Everything we have achieved for hungry and poor people in the last 35 years is under severe threat of budget cuts—nutrition programs such as the Special Supplemental Nutrition Program for Women, Infants and Children (WIC), and SNAP (formerly food stamps), as well as poverty-focused development assistance."

– Rev. David Beckmann, president of Bread for the World and Bread for the World Institute

After college I served in South Africa for a year through the Evangelical Lutheran Church in America. Following a year of enriching experiences, I had to decide whether to stay in sub-Saharan Africa or return to the United States. I thought I could make more of a difference back home, working in Washington, DC, where the U.S. government makes decisions every day that affect the lives of millions of hungry and poor people around the world.

When I applied for an internship in Bread for the World Institute, the editor of the Hunger Report asked if I knew anything about the farm bill. In my head I saw tractors. He explained that the farm bill should be called the food bill because two-thirds of its funding goes to national nutrition programs. I was still concerned that my focus would be on rows of corn in the Midwest and not on people struggling for food.

During my first week in the Institute, one of Bread for the World's field organizers asked for information about the national nutrition programs. With many new members of Congress calling for steep cuts in government spending, voters in these districts were asking why should the government feed hungry people in the United States. Couldn't the churches do the job?

Because a voter in Kansas asked this question, my first project was to compile information on public and private sources of food assistance in Kansas. In 2009, the year we had the most consistent data, one in seven people in the United States was receiving Supplemental Nutrition Assistance Program (SNAP) benefits. In Kansas, it was one in 13 people, mostly because half the people who were eligible did not enroll. How can it be that one in seven people in the country use SNAP to help meet their nutritional needs and I can't name seven people in the program? Where are all of these hungry people and why does the problem of hunger in the United States seem so invisible?

Figure c.1

Private and Public Sector Sources of Food Assistance in Kansas, 2009

6%

94%

◼ Private sector sources of food assistance

☐ Public sector sources of food assistance

Sources: USDA, Food and Nutrition Service; Private—Kansas Food Bank, Harvester: The Community Food Network, Second Harvest Community Food Bank.

The task of identifying all the sources of food assistance for hungry people in Kansas overwhelmed me. Thankfully, information about public sector food assistance is easy enough to find on the U.S. Department of Agriculture's website. Where do people find private sector food? I didn't know how private food systems work. I soon learned that soup kitchens and pantries, like the Salvation Army chapter that I had volunteered for in my hometown, often get their food through a food bank. Food banks receive donations from businesses and individuals, as well as commodities provided by the U.S. government. Most of these food banks are members of Feeding America, an umbrella organization of more than 200 food banks around the country.

It's not possible to account for every dollar of food from every private source. All the organizations I contacted—the Salvation Army in Kansas, the United Way in Kansas, Feeding America's three food banks in the state, Feeding America's main office in Chicago, and the Food Research and Action Center in Washington, DC—told me the largest sources of private sector food donations are delivered through the food banks.

The Kansas food banks provided me with extensive information. In Kansas, it turns out that only 6 percent of food assistance comes from the private sector. It was astonishing to realize that 94 percent of food assistance is delivered through the public sector.

In most states, government distributes the vast majority of food assistance. As I learned about how many people in the United States receive food through government programs, I called the Salvation Army chapter where I had volunteered in high school. Pat, the social services director, talked with me about the value of food assistance that comes from private sources. Volunteers help to strengthen connections between hungry and non-hungry people who live in the same community. Pat believes the advantage of the public sector is the financial power it can bring to bear on the problem.

When I worked as a volunteer in my community, serving in a soup kitchen, collecting trailers full of food for food drives, it seemed like we were providing so much food. Without seeing and recognizing the faces of hungry people there, I would not be working in Bread for the World Institute today. But if I had known what I know now, I would've included a letter-writing campaign to members of Congress—asking them to support SNAP and other nutrition programs—as part of every canned food drive I helped run at my church and high school.

In 2010, the share of the population in deep poverty (below half of the poverty line) hit a record high of **6.7%**

312 out of 435 congressional districts have at least 1 in 5 households with children struggling with food hardship, according to an August 2011 Gallup poll.

Please do not misunderstand me: churches, communities, organizations, and individuals should do their best to help support people in need. Public and private assistance are both essential. Sadly, even with the public and private sectors trying to make food available, together they still don't provide for everyone in need. But the notion that the private sector, much less churches alone, can make up for the difference in cuts to public sector funding now seems dangerously ignorant to me. Unfortunately, most people don't grasp the extent of the government's contribution to fighting hunger.

In 2011, David Beckmann, Tony Hall, and tens of thousands of people around the country fasted to ask God for guidance and to raise awareness about the importance of nutrition programs. This fast has turned into the campaign called the "circle of protection," declaring that Congress and the administration must not balance the budget on the backs of poor people. I joined the fast by not eating for the first 30 hours. The experience reminded me how food is a gift from God, and this gift should not be denied to anyone.

Kate Hagen is the project assistant on the 2012 Hunger Report.

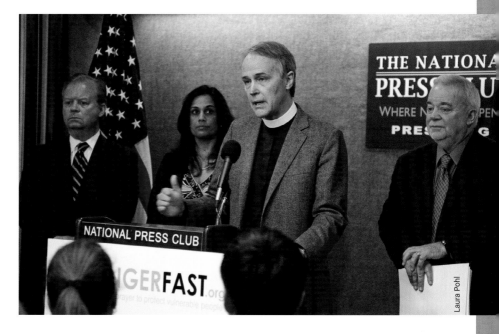

David Beckmann, Bread for the World president (at lectern), is joined by (from left) Ambassador Tony Hall, executive director of the Alliance to End Hunger; Ritu Sharma, president and co-founder of Women Thrive Worldwide; and Jim Wallis, president and CEO of Sojourners, as they launch a fast to form a circle of protection around U.S. government programs that help hungry and poor people at home and abroad.

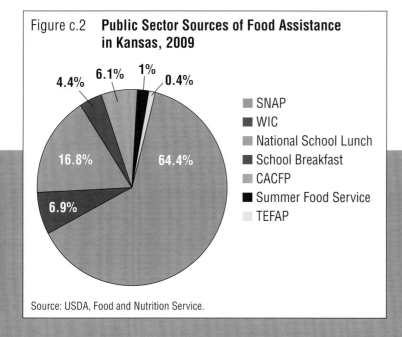

Figure c.2 **Public Sector Sources of Food Assistance in Kansas, 2009**

- SNAP
- WIC
- National School Lunch
- School Breakfast
- CACFP
- Summer Food Service
- TEFAP

4.4% 6.1% 1% 0.4%
16.8% 64.4%
6.9%

Source: USDA, Food and Nutrition Service.

62

The number of religious leaders, denominations, and organizations who have joined the circle of protection.

Study Guide Contents and General Process Suggestions

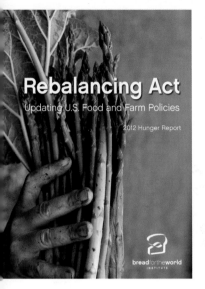

1. The 2012 Christian Study Guide includes six small-group sessions rooted in the content of the 2012 Hunger Report, Rebalancing Act: Updating U.S. Food and Farm Policies. Session 1 sets the context, while the following five sessions develop particular themes emphasized in the Hunger Report. If your group cannot do all the sessions, we recommend that you do Session 1 before any others.

2. We anticipate that each session will have a facilitator, but the leader needs no specific expertise on the report's content to facilitate the session.

3. The study guide is designed for Christians of many theological and political viewpoints. You should feel free to adapt the guide to enhance the experience for your group. The section below, Preparation Notes for Group Leaders, steers your group to websites relating social policies to different Christian traditions.

4. The activities will direct participants to read relevant sections of the report during the sessions. However, *Rebalancing Act* is filled with detailed analysis, statistics, and stories, so additional reading will enrich your conversation, but it is not required.

5. Each session includes:

- Biblical reflection materials and questions.
- A summary of the theme as presented in the Hunger Report, along with reflection questions.
- Activities to engage group members in analyzing current realities, using content from the Hunger Report and their life experiences.
- An invitation to pray and act in light of the discussion.

6. The sessions as written may take an hour to 90 minutes each, but should be adapted to meet the scheduling needs of the group.

Preparation Notes for Group Leaders

1. At least one Bible is required for each session. Participants could be encouraged to bring additional translations.

2. It will be helpful to have a copy of the session materials for each participant.

3. After you familiarize yourself with the outline of the session, you may adapt the activities to best serve the needs of your group.

4. To learn more about social policy in your own Christian tradition, you should visit the website of your denomination or national group. Sometimes these include a discussion of social policies. You might also visit:

National Association of Evangelicals
www.nae.net/government-affairs

U.S. Conference of Catholic Bishops
www.usccb.org/sdwp/projects/socialteaching

The National Council of Churches
www.ncccusa.org/NCCpolicies

5. Most sessions include activities using newsprint, a flip-chart, or a white board.

Group Leaders

For notes about specific sessions, see
www.bread.org/go/hunger2012

Ideas for Action

Each session of the Study Guide invites participants to consider how they might take action in response to the issues discussed. Here are suggestions for activities to engage your whole group. The size and nature of your group may require you to adapt the activities, but the descriptions below provide a template.

1. Learn from firsthand experience

Find a way for your group to spend time with someone whose life experience has given him or her personal knowledge of hunger, farming, and/or U.S. development assistance.

2. Write about your concerns

a. *Bread for the World's Offering of Letters*

Each year, Bread for the World invites churches and campus groups across the country to take up a nationwide Offering of Letters to Congress on an issue that is important to hungry and poor people. The Offering of Letters enables individuals to see their concerns translated into policies that help hungry and poor people improve their lives. To learn more about Bread for the World's Offering of Letters this year, visit www.bread.org/OL2012

b. *Write to your state or local representative*

Write letters to your representative in the city council, state assembly, or Congress to share your thoughts and concerns about food and farm policy.

Learn what your denomination or national association is doing related to food and farm policy.

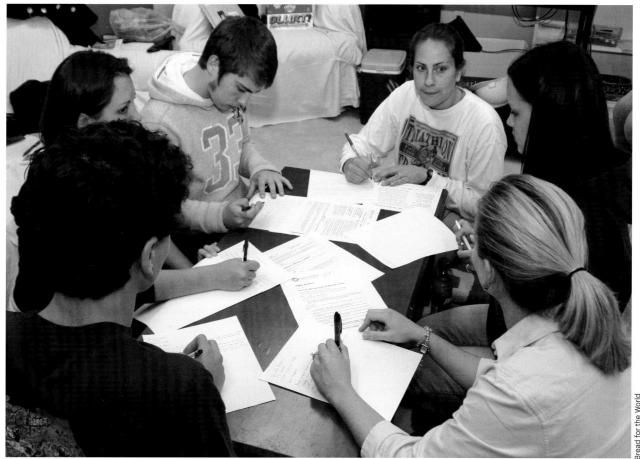

Bread for the World

SESSION 1: OUR BROKEN FOOD SYSTEM CAN BE TRANSFORMED

Biblical Reflection

Read Micah 3:9-12 and 4:1-4

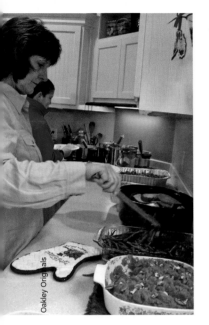
Oakley Originals

The prophesy of the book of Micah addresses both Israel and Judah. The prophet is critical of the leadership in these two kingdoms. In verse 3:11, he says that the leaders give judgment for a bribe, the priests teach for hire, and the prophets make predictions for money. Vulnerable people are being exploited.

Today in our nation, various special interests work to influence government decisions, often without regard to the needs of hungry and poor people. At times of economic crisis, we see cuts to vital safety net programs that help people stay out of poverty. Just like in Israel and Judah, the systems that support vulnerable people are broken.

Micah, like many other prophets, warns Israel and Judah that they will suffer consequences if they do not change their ways. In chapter four, after three chapters describing how the people will suffer, Micah offers a vision of a world transformed. All people will come to the Lord and "walk in his paths" (4:2). Nations will no longer fight each other, and their weapons will be turned into tools for agriculture. All people will sit under their own vine and fig tree without fear.

It is our responsibility as people of faith to share God's vision of transformation with the world. It is a vision of a world where everyone has enough to eat, where everyone has a safe place to sleep, and where everyone can live at peace with one another. We are called to be God's voice today. Like the biblical prophets of ancient times, we are called to be advocates who urge our leaders to do right and to act with justice.

Reflection Questions

1. Describe what the world could look like if God's justice reigned. What's present? What's absent?

2. How does our current world compare to the world you just described? What's broken and not working for vulnerable people?

3. In what ways do groups and individuals have power to change these patterns of brokenness? In what ways should God's vision influence our advocacy?

Hunger Report Theme Summary

Our food system is broken, but it can be transformed! Many objectives shape our systems of agriculture, trade, energy, and immigration through what are sometimes conflicting and inconsistent policies. U.S. laws subsidize an approach to crop production that rewards quantity much more than nutritional value. These policies subsidize products people can't eat, such as cotton and ethanol, in addition to encouraging the consumption of less nutritious foods.

Meanwhile, other policies undercut small scale farmers globally, while also making it difficult for low-income families in the United States to access healthy food. A desire for cheap food contributes to a demand for cheap farm labor. Farmers and farm workers need U.S. policy to provide a safety net and to support dignified, sustainable livelihoods. Policy options based around nutritious food and decent livelihoods would offer transformation. The Hunger Report shares some ways to get there.

Discussion Questions

1. What, in your opinion, currently works well in our food and agriculture system? What isn't working well, particularly for poor and vulnerable people? What improvements could make the system work better?

2. In the process of transforming our food system, which people could be perceived as losers? How can we help ensure that they don't lose their livelihoods?

Activities

1. Review "A World of Change since the Farm Bill" (Box i.2, page 17). Have members of your group restate these trends in their own words. Then, on newsprint or a flip-chart sheet, make three columns labeled "helpful," "neutral," and "unhelpful." Put each trend in a column based on how helpful it is for hungry and poor people. Draw lines to connect items that seem to be related to each other. What could be done to reverse trends that are unhelpful for hungry and poor people?

2. Read "U.S. Agriculture Has to Become More Productive and Sustainable" (Box 1.1, page 26). Imagine your group has been tasked with identifying top concerns in the food and farm system. Name as many challenges as you can (even beyond what you read in the article). Discuss how you would prioritize which issues to address first. How might you group the various concerns? What further plans would you want to make to begin to work toward transformation? How might your group remain hopeful about the transformations that are possible, even while grappling with the enormity of this broken system?

3. As you conclude, pray for efforts to transform our nation's food and farm system, and consider if there is something God might be calling you to do as a result of this conversation.

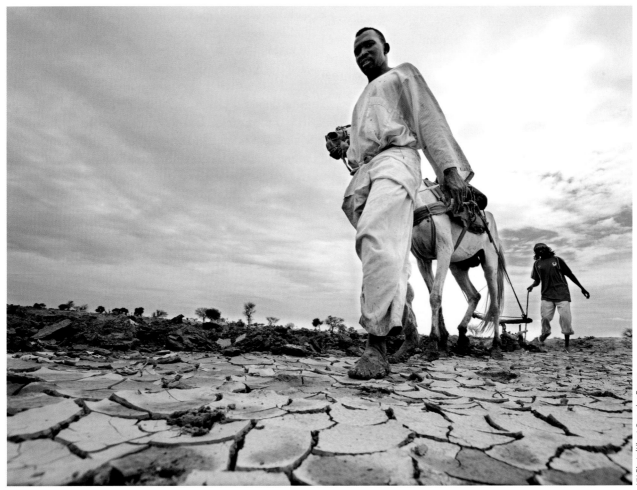

UN Photo/Albert Gonzalez Farran

Biblical Reflection

Read Deuteronomy 30:11-20

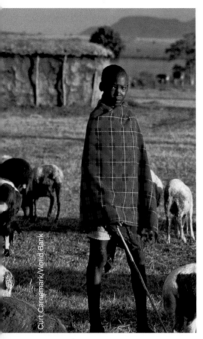

Curt Carnemark/World Bank

"Choose life," exhorts the Deuteronomy passage! In English we have only one word to describe "life," but in many other languages there are multiple concepts or aspects of "life" that each get their own word. Biblical Hebrew is one such language. The Hebrew word in this passage is "hayim" חַיִּים, meaning life in its fullness, health, well-being, and wholeness. "Hayim" is also the word used in connection to the "tree of life" in Genesis.

In the Kiswahili translation of Deuteronomy 30, the word is "uzima," which means wholeness, well-being, and abundance. "Uzima" to the Maasai people of Tanzania is beyond breathing, and it's more than mere survival. It includes good health, healthy animals, having enough to live sufficiently, and even abundantly, but not excessively. It includes spiritual health, mental health, emotional health, and physical health. Maasai Christians understand that being faithful to God does not guarantee that life will be easy or prosperous in the material sense. But their faith grasps a vision of the well-being that God wants for all people, the wholeness God wants for the world.

Jesus says, "I have come that they may have life (uzima), and have it to the full" (John 10:10). Let us choose life, abundant and full, for all our neighbors in God's world!

Reflection Questions

1. What is needed for abundant life, wholeness, and well-being? What does this imply for both spiritual and physical well-being? What does it mean in situations of hunger or malnutrition?

2. What do you see in today's world that is life-giving or life-taking? What must change to bring "uzima" or "hayim"?

Hunger Report Theme Summary

Malnutrition, which simply means a "lack of proper nutrition," has serious long-term consequences at both the individual and societal levels. In the 2012 Hunger Report we read that malnutrition in the first 1,000 days (from pregnancy through 2 years of age) is associated with low birth weights, stunting, poor school attendance and learning, chronic illness, and lifelong reductions in economic activity. The physical and cognitive damage from malnutrition during this period is largely irreversible. Recent studies have also shown a 2-3 percent loss in gross domestic product (GDP) in countries where malnutrition is common. U.S. food aid policy has largely overlooked the unique dietary needs of populations such as young children, pregnant women, and nursing mothers. Here in the United States, our food policy contributes to malnutrition, often in the form of obesity. This has long-term individual and societal consequences, including potentially serious health complications.

Discussion Questions

1. Many international and domestic anti-hunger programs have focused more on caloric intake than on nutrition. What are some of the consequences of that?

2. What attitudes and policies need to change so that our food system pays as much attention to the quality of food as it does to quantity? What are the domestic and international implications?

Activities

1. Look at "The Cycle of Food Insecurity and Chronic Disease" (Figure i.2, page 12). Consider how obesity, hypertension, and diabetes are indirectly caused by food insecurity. Now redraw the cycle with "Food Security" at the top. Replace the rest of the content accordingly, so it becomes a positive, life-giving cycle. Consider the effects of food security, healthy food options, etc. What are the practical challenges to transforming the cycle?

2. Read "Understanding Malnutrition and Responding Effectively" (Box 4.1, page 96). On newsprint, make three columns. In the first column, list actions households can take to improve the nutrition of women and children. In the second column, list ways the community can support better nutrition. And in the third, list ways governments must be involved. What are your key observations, learnings, and surprises?

3. As you conclude, pray for efforts to transform our nation's food and farm system, and consider if there is something God might be calling you to do as a result of this conversation.

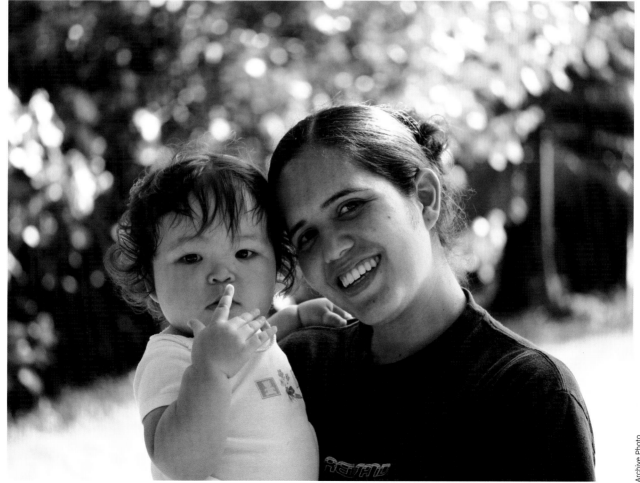

Archive Photo

Biblical Reflection

Read James 2:1-7 and 1 Corinthians 12:12-26

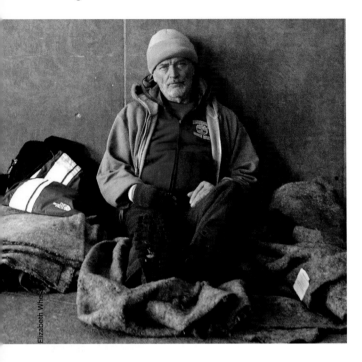

Elizabeth Whelan

The biblical vision of community and nation lifts up the voices of those who are vulnerable and marginalized. Even within big systems and structures, those who are marginalized need to have a voice.

Using the metaphor of the body, the Corinthians passage says that all parts have a unique purpose and that each part should be honored. In fact, greater honor should go to those parts that lack it. The James passage warns against giving special treatment based on wealth and appearance. Those who are poor and marginalized should be honored and respected because God has chosen them to be "rich in faith and heirs to the kingdom which God has promised to those who love him."

These admonitions are directed to the Christian community, but their truth also applies to the broader relationships of communities and nations. God calls us to raise up the voices of those who are marginalized and vulnerable and to lift up the plight of those who do not have powerful lobbyists and financial resources on their side.

Reflection Questions

1. How do we honor the voices of vulnerable and marginalized people in our communities?

2. In a society where money and powerful interests play such influential roles, how can we work to ensure that the voices of marginalized people are included in institutional decision-making processes?

Hunger Report Theme Summary

The Hunger Report shows that U.S. farm policy, with its system of commodity payments, favors large-scale farms over smaller farms. While all farmers need some protections from the risks associated with farming, the current system undermines farmers in the developing world and does not adequately support smaller farms in the United States.

Policy reform could include 1) helping farmers transition from traditional commodity crops, 2) offering better support to fruit and vegetable farmers, and 3) assisting small scale farmers in developing countries to be more productive. This means not undercutting small scale farmers in other countries by keeping traditional commodity prices artificially low or by monetizing food aid. On the positive side, it means targeting poverty-focused development assistance to better address farmers' needs through a new program called Feed the Future. For terms that are unfamiliar, please see the Glossary on pages 144-147.

Discussion Questions

1. How does government's disproportionate support for commodity crops impact what we eat and the nutritional composition of our food system? [Leader: Help the group think back to issues raised by the Hunger Report Theme Summary in Session 1 on page 122.]

2. Recent budget debates have included calls for dramatic cuts to foreign aid, including food aid and development aid. A troubling underlying tension in these debates is the question of whether U.S. taxpayers should continue to provide assistance overseas and at what levels. How can we move beyond an "us"

versus "them" mentality and focus the conversation on how we can all benefit?

Activities

1. Read pages 33-34, beginning with the paragraph on Recommended Daily Allowances (RDAs). Examine Figure 1.8. Imagine that you work for the U.S. Department of Agriculture. Divide group members into the following roles: 1) liaisons to program crop farmers, 2) nutritionists or those working to improve diets, 3) liaisons to fruit, vegetable, and organic producers, 4) liaisons to farmers in conservation programs, 5) liaisons to ethanol producers, and 6) those working with nutrition programs, such as SNAP, WIC, and school lunches. Depending on the size of the group, make sure that roles 1 and 6 get greater representation.

   Within each role, take a moment to identify the interests you want to protect and write them on newsprint. Note why those interests are important. Retain your small group roles as you rejoin the full group. What joint recommendations can you propose to Congress that advance the interests of the people you serve, but also improve the food system? The goal is nutritious food, grown in sustainable ways, adequate

livelihoods for the producers, and adequate access to nutrition, especially for low-income families.

Debrief: How difficult is it to bring so many different interests to the table? What are the implications of supporting the production of more nutritious food? What does this mean for policies, for farmers hoping to transition, for public health? Who are the perceived losers in the process? Are there ways to help everyone feel like a winner?

2. Read "Phasing out Monetization" (pages 105-106). Map out the relationships between U.S. farmers, the U.S. government, development organizations, and smallholder farmers in developing countries. Trace the movement of money and crops. Add dollar signs for the movement of money and corn ears for the movement of agricultural products. Notice what happens to the U.S. crops. Notice what happens to the small farmers' crops in Africa. Who benefits and how?

3. As you conclude, pray for efforts to transform our nation's food and farm system, and consider if there is something God might be calling you to do as a result of this conversation.

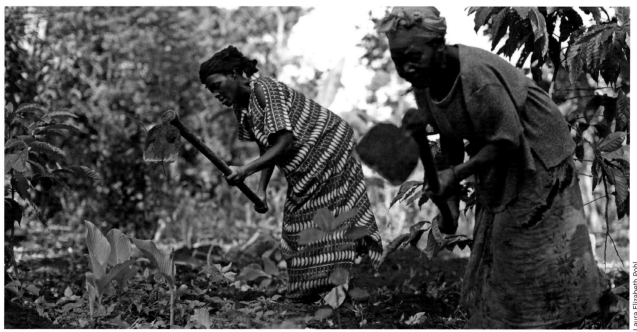

Laura Elizabeth Pohl

Biblical Reflection

Read Psalm 72

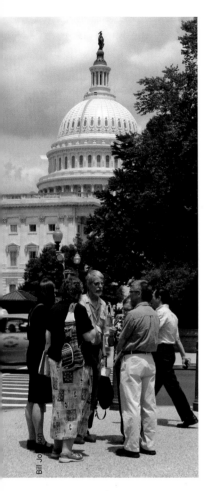

Bill Jo...

What an amazing vision of an earthly kingdom and its king functioning as God desires! Although we are unaccustomed to life under a king's rule, we can read Psalm 72 in light of our present reality and discern the characteristics of godly leadership. One clear characteristic is the protection of poor and vulnerable people. In verse 4 the good king is called to "defend the cause of the poor of the people," and in verses 12-14 he "delivers the needy when he calls" and saves them "from oppression and violence." Protection of those who are weak is an integral part of the grand kingdom vision. Justice for the poor goes hand-in-hand with the kingdom's prosperity and abundance (v. 3 and 16), the king's dominion over his enemies (v. 8-9), and his long life and enduring fame (v. 15 and 17).

In the world of Psalm 72, the king was the government. It was his decision whether to defend the poor and deliver the needy of his land. While our present government bears little resemblance to a king, it still decides whether to save those who are weak from oppression and violence. And in a representative democracy such as ours in the United States, a government "of the people, by the people, for the people," we have a voice in these decisions. We are collectively in our country what the king of Psalm 72 was in his. And although the forms of government may change and have changed, God's desired characteristics have not.

When Israel's leaders did not uphold God's kingdom vision, the role of the prophet was to call them to account. In God's eyes, the leaders were not free to rule their nation as they desired. When poor and vulnerable people were not protected, when weak and needy people in the land were oppressed and exploited, God spoke through the prophets to the rulers of the land. From Isaiah to Jeremiah to Amos to Micah, God's message through the prophets was clear: Leaders are not living according to God's vision when they fail to protect those who are needy and vulnerable. Societies are not in right relationship to God as long as there is injustice in the land. The outward symptom of disregard for the poor betrays an inner disregard for God. Disaster awaited if Israel did not change its course and restore justice to the land.

Reflection Questions

1. Given what God teaches us, what should the role of government be in protecting poor and vulnerable people today?

2. How does our government here in the United States currently align with God's vision for a just society? In what ways are we living up to God's vision? In what ways are we falling short?

Hunger Report Theme Summary

In 2011, rising food prices have again drawn attention to the plight of poor people around the world. The 2012 Hunger Report argues that poor and vulnerable people should be protected as governments seek to fix the broken food system. Even as our nation struggles to address budget deficits, our food and farm policies should strengthen the food and nutrition safety net for people in the United States and around the world. This includes improvements in food aid and support for sustainable agriculture, as well as food and nutrition programs such as SNAP, WIC, and school meals. See the Glossary on pages 144-147 for unfamiliar terms.

Discussion Questions

1. How does society benefit when people are well-nourished?

2. How do U.S. safety net programs benefit society as a whole? How does poverty-focused development assistance to poor countries benefit more than just the recipients of that aid?

Activities

1. "Starvation in the Horn of Africa" (Box i.1, page 16) notes that "food shortages may be triggered by drought, but famine is not the inevitable result." Make a list of actions that could protect poor and vulnerable people from starvation in a future drought. Circle the items on your list that could be influenced by U.S. foreign assistance. Are there other ways the United States might help prevent famine overseas?

2. Identify the people in your group who do the most grocery shopping for their households. How much do they spend for each person for each meal? Consider that with SNAP benefits (formerly food stamps), a family of four receives $4.50 per person per day for food. Now plan a grocery list for one month with this figure in mind. What foods did you include? What foods did you exclude? How is this similar to or different from your diet? Will you make it through the end of the month? What will you do if you can't? Look at Figure 1.2 (page 25). Notice how variations in food prices affect household budgets.

3. As you conclude, pray for efforts to transform our nation's food and farm system, and consider if there is something God might be calling you to do as a result of this conversation.

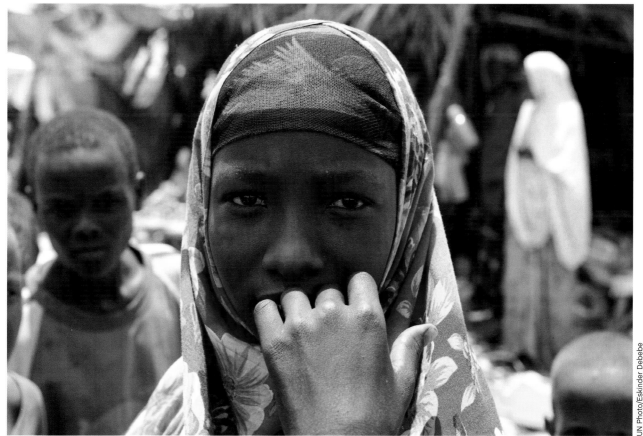

UN Photo/Eskinder Debebe

Biblical Reflection

Read Proverbs 13:23 and 1 Corinthians 9:7-11

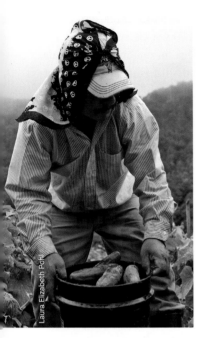

There are various passages in the Bible that call for decent and fair treatment of workers, acting justly toward them and not exploiting their labor. Proverbs 13:23 suggests that injustice makes it difficult for poor farmers to benefit from what their fields produce. In the 1 Corinthians passage, Paul reaffirms the biblical principle that workers should earn an adequate livelihood from their labor. He states this within the context of addressing the care and livelihood of those called to be apostles.

Throughout the Bible, calls for justice reflect a basic understanding that within the community, honest work deserves a decent livelihood. It is basic to how people should live in relationship with one another in God's world.

Read Leviticus 19:33-37

Immigrants (also referred to as strangers, aliens, or sojourners) are recognized in the Bible as one of the most vulnerable populations. For this reason, they are lifted up time and again for special care and consideration along with the other most vulnerable groups, the widows and the orphans. Throughout the Old Testament law, there is provision for the immigrants, in leaving gleanings for them, allowing them Sabbath rest, protecting their rights in legal disputes, paying them a fair wage, and not exploiting their labor. The people of Israel were constantly reminded by God that they had been slaves and immigrants, and should therefore care for and protect this vulnerable class of people in the land. Interestingly, many prominent people in the Bible were also immigrants or foreigners. How many can you name? (See Leader's Notes at www.bread.org/go/hunger2012 for a list.) Clearly, immigrants are near and dear to the heart of God!

Reflection Questions

1. Decent wages and protections for workers, native-born or immigrant, is important within the biblical vision of justice and right relationship among people. What might that mean for us today within our society?

2. Unauthorized immigrant workers are among the most marginalized and vulnerable populations in the United States, due primarily to their legal status. How does a biblical vision of justice instruct our perception and treatment of unauthorized immigrants? How might such a vision guide us to respond to the legalization debates in our country?

Hunger Report Theme Summary

One of the values this Hunger Report lifts up is the need for a food system that supports sustainable livelihoods for all farmers and farm workers. For farmers, the report lifts up revenue insurance as an important way to manage the risks of farming. Since specialty crops are heavily dependent on immigrant labor and many of the workers are unauthorized to work in the United States, an important policy change would be for Congress to legalize immigrant workers, giving them greater protection under the law. Reforming our agricultural guest worker program so that it benefits U.S. growers *and* poor small farmers in Mexico is also an important part of making our agricultural labor system beneficial to farm communities on both sides of the border.

Discussion Questions

1. How should those who work the land (farmers, farmworkers, migrant laborers) be protected from having the fruit of their labor "swept away by injustice"?

2. How would you define a sustainable livelihood for farmers and farm workers?

Activities

1. On newsprint, make a list of potential risks that a farmer might face. Now look for the article on risk management (pages 41-45). Read the introductory paragraphs, the first two paragraphs in the section titled "Revenue Insurance for the Whole Farm," and the first two paragraphs under the section called "Shared Responsibility and Fairness." Also, review the definition for "commodity payments" in the Glossary on page 144.

   Discuss the following questions in small groups. How will revenue insurance create some protections in the face of these risks? Evaluate revenue insurance and commodity payments in light of the principles of sustainable livelihoods for farmers and fairness overall. How do they compare?

2. Read "Maria's Story" (page 72). On newsprint, make two lists. In the first, note the factors contributing to Maria's coming to the United States. In the second, note both the challenges she faces here and the reasons she stays. Read the two sections under the AgJOBS heading (pages 84 and 86). How might Maria's life improve and become more sustainable through the AgJOBS legislation? What challenges would not be addressed by AgJOBS?

3. Review Figure 3.2 (page 76). In small groups, create a budget based on the crop farm worker wage. Make sure to include rent, utilities, transportation, groceries, insurance, toiletries, cleaning supplies, entertainment, and clothing, etc. In the full group, discuss the following questions: What was the most difficult thing to give up? What was essential? How did you prioritize the essentials?

4. As you conclude, pray for efforts to transform our nation's food and farm system, and consider if there is something God might be calling you to do as a result of this conversation.

For an additional activity, see
www.bread.org/go/hunger 2012

The AgJOBS Bill: A Step in the Right Direction

One of the most promising options for Congress to better support all farmers and farmworkers is the Agricultural Job Opportunity, Benefits and Security bill (AgJOBS). The bill contains two main components: The first would provide a path to earned legalization for unauthorized farm workers. This part of the bill addresses agricultural workers already living and working in the United States. The second part addresses the future flow of farm workers by reforming the H-2A agricultural guest worker program. This part of the bill makes it easier for farmers to recruit agricultural guest workers and provides the workers with additional protections.

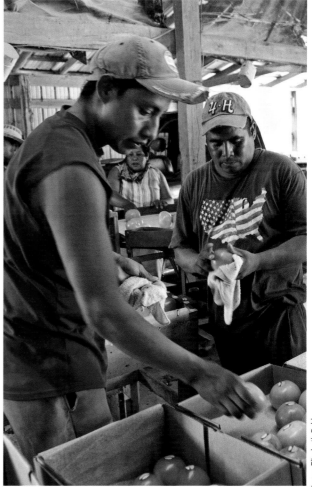

Laura Elizabeth Pohl

Biblical Reflection

Read Mark 2:1-5 and Luke 5:17-20

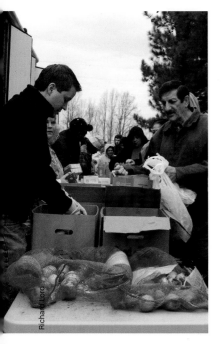

Both versions of this gospel story offer a vivid image of a group working together for a positive goal. God calls us into such community. Genesis makes it clear from the beginning of creation that God intends for us to have helpers. God says of Adam, "it is not good that the man should be alone" (Genesis 2:18). The biblical story continues as a description of the relationship between God and the people of God. It is a community, not an individual, called to the Promised Land. And God blesses community. In Matthew, Jesus promises the disciples, "Where two or three are gathered in my name, there am I in the midst of them."

In the community described in our passage, a collection of individuals combined their resources and skills to get the paralytic to the place where he could receive what he needed. Note the differences and similarities in these two versions of the story. (See Leader's Notes at www. bread.org/go/hunger2012 for ideas on the similarities and differences.) Consider the many gifts that people in the story likely offered: resources such as a ladder and tools to get through the roof, creativity, strength to carry the man, and even the willingness of the homeowner to have a hole put in the roof. After the group achieved its goal, Jesus recognized their faith, not simply the faith of the paralytic.

Reflection Questions

1. What struggles might this group have faced as they saw the challenge ahead? What might have helped and hindered their efforts?

2. How are these same dynamics in play as communities face the challenge of ensuring everyone is fed?

Hunger Report Theme Summary

It will take a variety of efforts to change the food system. Many communities around the country (and world) are taking important steps to promote the distribution of and access to nutritious food. Throughout the report you will find stories about communities that are harnessing their own resources to improve their lives.

There are stories of farmers working domestically and internationally with local school systems to provide food for healthy meals. There are communities organizing to bring supermarkets to their neighborhoods in order to improve access to a wider variety of fresh foods. Former tobacco farmers in Virginia have come together to learn more about organic and sustainable practices to produce healthier food, and they have partnered in distribution to gain access to wider markets. They are

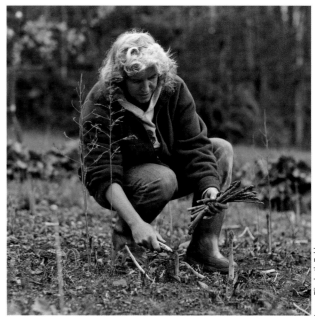

getting educated, getting organized, and improving the reach of healthy foods to communities in need. The positive impacts of these efforts can be multiplied if supported by better food policy.

Discussion Questions

1. What efforts are happening in your community to promote the growing and processing of nutritious food?

2. Where have you seen unlikely collaborations between individuals and groups to improve the availability and quality of food?

Activities

1. Read "Eat Well and Create Jobs" (Box 1.3, page 40) and "Closing the Healthy Food Gap in Rural Oregon" (Box 2.2, pages 56-57). In the middle of a piece of flip-chart paper, draw stick figures representing a household with small children that decides to start eating more fresh fruits and vegetables. Around the figures, draw (or list) in a different color marker all the people and groups you can think of who will be affected by the family's choice. Using a third color marker, add the names of all the people or groups who can make it easier for the household to eat more fresh fruits and vegetables. What connections do you see among these groups?

2. Read "An Appetite for Sustainably Produced Food Creates New Opportunities for Farmers" (pages 34-36). How did this community come together to make the transition from tobacco farming? What community resources did they tap? Break into pairs and see which pair can come up with the best idea for a similar transformation from program crops (rice, corn, soy, cotton, wheat) and commodity programs in your community.

3. Read "Farm-to-School Programs Help Kids Eat Better and Benefit Local Farmers and Communities" (Box 2.3, page 64). Now find your state on the tables for youth fruit and vegetable consumption at www. fruitsandveggiesmatter.gov/health_professionals/

maps_youth.html. In no state are adults or youth eating the recommended amounts of fresh fruits and vegetables. What do you make of your state's results? How can this story serve as inspiration for what might happen in your community or state? Now find your state on the chart of "Policy and Environmental Indicators" at www.fruitsandveggiesmatter.gov/health_professionals/statereport.html. Using the data you find, list ways you believe people could increase the fruit and vegetable consumption in your state.

4. As you conclude, pray for efforts to transform our nation's food and farm system, and consider if there is something God might be calling you to do as a result of this conversation.

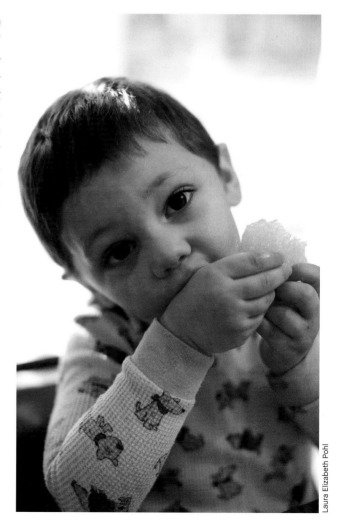

Laura Elizabeth Pohl

Endnotes

Introduction

1   CDC Online Newsroom, Centers for Disease Control and Prevention, U.S. Department of Health and Human Services (July 27, 2009), "Study Estimates Medical Cost of Obesity May be as High as $147 Billion Annually," press release.

2   Larry Brown and others (June 5, 2007) *The Economic Cost of Domestic Hunger: Estimated Annual Burden to the United States*, see "Table 4," Sodexho Foundation.

3   Sarah Treuhaft and Allison Karpyn (2010), *The Grocery Gap: Who Has Access to Healthy Food and Why it Matters*, PolicyLink and The Food Trust.

4   White House Task Force on Childhood Obesity (May 2010), *Solving the Problem of Childhood Obesity Within a Generation*, Report to the President.

5   Marcus Noland (interviewee) (Fall 2005), "Asia's Post-War Economic Growth," *Education About Asia*, Vol. 10, No. 2.

6   William Masters (lead evaluator) (2011), *2011 Progress Report on U.S. Leadership in Global Agricultural Development*, Global Agriculture and Development Initiative, The Chicago Council on Global Affairs.

7   U.S. Government Accountability Office (May 2011), *International Food Assistance: Better Nutrition and Quality Control Can Further Improve U.S. Food Aid*, Report to Congressional Requesters.

8   1,000 Days (September 2010), *Scaling Up Nutrition: A Framework for Action*, policy brief.

9   Jean-Claude Maswana (2006), "Economic Development Patterns and Outcomes in Africa and Asia," working paper, *Congo Economic Review*.

10 Stephen Censky (April 7, 2011), "Statement by Stephen Censky, Chief Executive Officer, American Soybean Association," before the Rural Development, Research, Biotechnology, and Foreign Agriculture Subcommittee, Agriculture Committee, U.S. House of Representatives.

11 U.S. Agency for International Development (September 8, 2011), "Horn of Africa – Drought," Fact Sheet, No. 11.

12 Poverty Reduction and Equity Group, The World Bank (August 2011), "Food Price Watch,"

13 John Norris and Bronwyn Bruton (September 2011), *Twenty Years of Collapse and Counting: The Cost of Failure in Somalia*, Center for American Progress and One Earth Future Foundation.

Chapter 1

1   Timothy Park and others (December 2010), *Agricultural Income and Finance Outlook*, Economic Research Service, U.S. Department of Agriculture.

2   Economic Research Service, U.S. Department of Agriculture (accessed on June 9, 2011), "Foreign Agricultural Trade of the United States (FATUS): Monthly Summary."

3   Interagency Agricultural Projections Committee, U.S. Department of Agriculture (February 2011), *USDA Agricultural Projections to 2020*.

4   Economic Research Service, U.S. Department of Agriculture, op. cit.

5   Joseph W. Glauber (February 24, 2011), "Prospects for the U.S. Farm Economy in 2011," U.S. Department of Agriculture.

6   Economic Research Service, U.S. Department of Agriculture (March 2009), "U.S. Agricultural Trade."

7   Stephen Censky (April 7, 2011), "Statement by Stephen Censky, Chief Executive Officer, American Soybean Association," before the Rural Development, Research, Biotechnology, and Foreign Agriculture Subcommittee, Agriculture Committee, U.S. House of Representatives.

8   Economic Research Service, U.S. Department of Agriculture (May 19, 2011), "State Fact Sheets: United States," source: *2007 Census of Agriculture*.

9   Zachary Cain and Stephen Lovejoy (4th Quarter 2004), "History and Outlook for Farm Bill Conservation Programs," *Choices: The Magazine of Food, Farm, and Resource Issues*, Agricultural and Applied Economics Association.

10 Lawrence C. Hamilton and others (2008), *Place Matters: Challenges and Opportunities in Four Rural Americas, Reports on Rural America*, Vol. 1, No. 4, Carsey Institute, University of New Hampshire.

11 Economic Research Service, U.S. Department of Agriculture (accessed on February 14, 2011), "2010 Farm Income Forecast."

12 GPS.gov, National Coordination Office for Space-Based Positioning, Navigation, and Timing and Civil GPS Service Interface Committee, U.S. Department of Homeland Security (April 29, 2011), "Agriculture."

13 Intel Corporations, "Intriguing Applications: Robot Tractors Roll."

14 Carolyn Dimitri, Anne Effland, and Neilson Conklin (June 2005), *The 20th Century Transformation of U.S. Agriculture and Farm Policy*, Economic Information Bulletin, No. 3, Economic Research Service, U.S. Department of Agriculture.

15 The Voice of Agriculture, American Farm Bureau Federation, "Food and Farm Facts."

16 Michael Duffy (January 2011), "Estimated Costs of Crop Production in Iowa – 2011," *Ag Decision Maker*, University Extension, Iowa State University.

17 Ken Anderson (April 29, 2011), "Northeast Iowa Farmland Hits $10,000/Acre," Brownfield.

18 Michael Duffy (2nd Quarter 2011), "The Current Situation on Farmland Values and Ownership," *Choices: The Magazine of Food, Farm, and Resource Issues,* Agricultural and Applied Economics Association.

19 Federal Deposit Insurance Corporation (March 2011), "Don't Bet the Farm: Assessing the Boom in U.S. Farmland Prices."

20 Center for Rural Affairs, "Beginning Farmer Financing Programs."

21 Val Dolcini (April 14, 2011), "State-

ment by Val Dolcini, Acting Administrator, Farm Service Agency, U.S. Department of Agriculture," before the Conservation, Credit, Energy, and Research Subcommittee, Agriculture Committee, U.S. House of Representatives.

22 U.S. Department of Agriculture (2009), "Table 49: Selected Operator Characteristics for Principal, Second, and Third Operator: 2007," in *2007 Census of Agriculture*.

23 Justin Gillis and Celia W. Dugger (May 3, 2011), "UN Forecasts 10.1 Billion People by Century's End," *The New York Times*.

24 Food and Agriculture Organization, United Nations (September 23, 2009), "2050: A third more mouths to feed," press release.

25 Thomas R. Karl, Jerry M. Melillo, and Thomas C. Peterson (editors) (2009), *Global Climate Change Impacts in the United States*, U.S. Global Change Research Program.

26 David Pimentel (August 2006), "Impacts of Organic Farming on the Efficiency of Energy Use in Agriculture," An Organic Center State of Science Review, The Organic Center.

27 Susan S. Lang (March 20, 2006), "'Slow, insidious' soil erosion threatens human health and welfare as well as the environment, Cornell study asserts," *Chronicle Online*, Cornell University.

28 Natural Resources Conservation Service, U.S. Department of Agriculture (December 2009), *Summary Report: 2007 National Resources Inventory*.

29 Marc Ribaudo and Robert Johansson (2006), "AREI Chapter 2.2: Water Quality – Impacts of Agriculture," *Agricultural Resources and Environmental Indicators*, Economic Research Service, United States Department of Agriculture.

30 U.S. Environmental Protection Agency (March 2007), Nitrous Oxide: Sources and Emissions.

31 U.S. Environmental Protection Agency (June 2010), Nitrous Oxide: Science.

32 Economic Research Service, U.S.

Department of Agriculture (March 2009), "Environmental Interactions with Agriculture: Background."

33 Arthur Grube and others (February 2011), *Pesticides Industry Sales and Usage: 2006-2007 Market Estimates*, Biological and Economic Analysis Division, Office of Chemical Safety and Pollution Prevention, U.S. Environmental Protection Agency.

34 Helena Bottemiller (June 20, 2011), "Senate Bill Addresses Antibiotics in Animal Feed," *Food Safety News*.

35 James Pease, David Schweikhardt, and Andrew Seidl (3rd Quarter 2008), "Conservation Provisions of the Food Conservation and Energy Act of 2008: Evolutionary Changes and Challenges," *Choices: The Magazine of Food, Farm, and Resource Issues*, Vol. 23, No. 3, Agricultural and Applied Economics Association.

36 Andrew Hug (April 27, 2011), "Keeping Secrets Down on the Farm," *AgMag*, Environmental Working Group.

37 Timothy A. Wise (March 2011), "Still Waiting for the Farm Boom: Family Farmers Worse Off Despite High Prices," policy brief, Global Development and Environment Institute, Tufts University.

38 Catherine Greene, Edward Slattery, and William D. McBride (June 2010), "America's Organic Farmers Face Issues and Opportunities," *Amber Waves*, Economic Research Service, U.S. Department of Agriculture.

39 Dallas Tonsager (February 2011), "Value-Added Producer Grant Program," *Federal Register*, Vol. 76, No. 36, Rural Business-Cooperative Service and Rural Utilities Service, U.S. Department of Agriculture.

40 Committee on Twenty-First Century Systems Agriculture and National Research Council (2010), *Toward Sustainable Agricultural Systems in the 21st Century*, The National Academies Press.

41 Patrick Canning (February 2011), *A Revised and Expanded Food Dollar Series: A Better Understanding of Our Food Costs*, Economic Research Report, No. 114, Economic Research

Service, U.S. Department of Agriculture.

42 Christopher R. Knittel (2011), *Corn Belt Moonshine: The Costs and Benefits of U.S. Ethanol Subsidies*, American Boondoggle, American Enterprise Institute.

43 Gregory Meyer (July 12, 2011), "U.S. ethanol refiners use more corn than farmers," *Financial Times*.

44 International Energy Agency (2011), *Technology Roadmaps: Biofuels for Transport*.

45 Niketa Kumar (April 13, 2011), "Study: Algae Could Replace 17% of U.S. Oil Imports," Office of Public Affairs, U.S. Department of Energy.

46 Thomas W. Hertel and Jayson Beckman (revised on February 12, 2011), "Commodity Price Volatility in the Biofuel Era: An Examination of the Linkage between Energy and Agricultural Markets," paper prepared for the NBER Agricultural Economics Conference, National Bureau of Economic Research, March 4-5, 2010, Cambridge, Massachusetts.

47 Office of Transportation and Air Quality, U.S. Environmental Protection Agency (February 2010), "EPA Finalizes Regulations for the National Renewable Fuel Standard Program for 2010 and Beyond," regulatory announcement.

48 Christopher R. Knittel, op. cit.

49 Growth Energy (April 13, 2011), "Food vs. Fuel Fallacies."

50 David Dawe and Ali Doroudian (January 2011), "A Simple Price Monitoring Tool to Assess Monthly Changes in Food Prices," Agricultural Development Economics Division, Food and Agriculture Organization, United Nations.

51 Environmental Working Group (2011), "Note," 2011 Farm Subsidy Database.

52 Ibid.

53 Environmental Working Group (2010), "Rice Subsidies in Woodruff County, Arkansas totaled $192 million from 1995-2010," 2011 Farm Subsidy Database, source: U.S. Department of Agriculture; Small Area Estimates Branch, U.S. Census

Bureau; U.S. Department of Labor.

54 World Trade Organization (2010), "United States – Subsidies on Upland Cotton," Dispute Settlement: Dispute DS267.

55 Pascal Lamy, World Trade Organization (January 31, 2011), "The Man-Made Causes of Price Volatility," speech at the Global Commodities Forum, United Nations Conference on Trade and Development.

56 Centers for Disease Control and Prevention, U.S. Department of Health and Human Services (2008), "National Diabetes Fact Sheet, 2007."

57 Boyd A. Swinburn and others (May 2009), "Estimating the Changes in Energy Flux that Characterize the Rise in Obesity Prevalence," *American Journal of Clinical Nutrition*, Vol. 89, No. 6.

58 Supplemental Nutrition Assistance Program, U.S. Department of Agriculture (April 2011), "Healthy Incentives Pilot (HIP) - Basic Facts."

59 Julian M. Alston and Philip G. Pardey (August 2008), "Public Funding for Research into Specialty Crops," *HortScience*, Vol. 43, No. 5.

60 Food Consumer (July 7, 2010), "The United States Needs 13 Million More Acres of Fruits and Vegetables to Meet the RDA," press release.

61 Jill E. Krueger, Karen R. Krub, and Lynn A. Hayes (February 2010), *Planting the Seeds for Public Health: How the Farm Bill Can Help Farmers to Produce and Distribute Healthy Foods*, Farmers' Legal Action Group, Inc.

62 Informa Economics, Inc. (February 2007), *An Analysis of the Effect of Removing the Planting Restrictions on Program Crop Base*.

63 Jill E. Krueger, Karen R. Krub, and Lynn A. Hayes, op. cit., Chapter 2: Commodity Payments.

64 Sara Sciammacco (June 23, 2011), "City Slickers Continue to Rake in Farm Payments," Environmental Working Group.

65 Barry Krissoff and others (February 2011), *Fruit and Vegetable Planting Restrictions: Analyzing the Processing Cucumber Market*, Economic Research Service, U.S. Department of Agriculture.

66 Specialty Crop Farm Bill Alliance (March 2, 2007), "Specialty Crop Coalition Releases Comprehensive Planting Flexibility Study," news release.

67 Centers for Disease Control and Prevention, U.S. Department of Health and Human Services (September 2010), "Trends in Current Cigarette Smoking Among High School Students and Adults, United States, 1965-2009," National Health Interview Survey.

68 American Medical Association (October 2007), *AMA Policy Compendium on Issues Relating to Minority Health and Minority Physicians*, see "H-150.944 Combating Obesity and Health Disparities."

69 Steve Martinez and others (May 2010), "Local Food Systems: Concepts, Impacts, and Issues," Economic Research Report, No. 97, Economic Research Service, U.S. Department of Agriculture.

70 Matthew Wheeland (October 14, 2010), "Walmart Sows Major Sustainable Ag Commitment," GreenBiz.com.

71 J.P. Reganold and others (May 6, 2011), "Transforming U.S. Agriculture," *Science*, Vol. 332.

72 *Choices: The Magazine of Food, Farm, and Resource Issues* dedicates an entire issue to the subject of the local food movement. See Vol. 25, No. 1 (1st Quarter 2010).

73 Office of Communications, U.S. Department of Agriculture (September 15, 2009), "USDA Launches 'Know Your Farmer, Know Your Food' Initiative to Connect Consumers with Local Producers to Create New Economic Opportunities for Communities," news release.

74 Suzanne Briggs and others (June 2010), *Real Food, Real Choice: Connecting SNAP Recipients with Farmers Markets*, Community Food Security Coalition and Farmers Market Coalition.

75 Tom Philpott (April 29, 2011), "Is Walmart our best hope for food policy reform?," *Grist*.

76 Office of Research and Analysis, Food and Nutrition Service, U.S. Department of Agriculture (February 2011), "Benefit Redemption Patterns in the Supplemental Nutrition Assistance Program."

77 Office of Research and Analysis, Food and Nutrition Service, U.S. Department of Agriculture (March 2011), "Analysis of Verification Summary Data, School Year 2008-2009."

78 Katherine Ralston and others (July 2008), *The National School Lunch Program: Background, Trends, and Issues*, Economic Research Report, No. 61, Economic Research Service, U.S. Department of Agriculture.

79 David Wallinga (March 2010), "Agricultural Policy and Childhood Obesity: A Food Systems and Public Health Commentary," *Health Affairs*, Vol. 29, No. 3.

80 Ibid.

81 U.S. Census Bureau (2011), Table 857: Fresh Fruits and Vegetables-Supply and Use: 2000-2009, in "Section 17: Agriculture," *Statistical Abstract of the United States: 2011*.

82 Virginia A. Stallings and Christine L. Taylor (editors) (2008), *Nutrition Standards and Meal Requirements for National School Lunch and Breakfast Programs: Phase 1. Proposed Approach for Recommending Revisions*, Committee on Nutrition Standards for National School Lunch and Breakfast Programs, Institute of Medicine.

83 Office of Communications, Food and Nutrition Service, U.S. Department of Agriculture (April 26, 2011), "New USDA Rule Encourages the Purchase of Local Agricultural Products for Critical Nutrition Assistance Programs," press release.

84 Shermain D. Hardesty (1st Quarter 2010), "Do Government Policies Grow Local Food?," *Choices: The Magazine of Food, Farm, and Resource Issues*, Agricultural and Applied Economics Association.

85 Business Leaders for Michigan (June 2010), "Michigan Turnaround Plan."

86 Debbie Stabenow, Chairwoman (May 31, 2011), "Opening state-

ment," at Opportunities for Growth: Michigan and the 2012 Farm Bill field hearing, Agriculture, Nutrition, and Forestry Committee, U.S. Senate, Michigan State University.

[87] *The New York Times* (June 3, 2011), "Bigger Losses in Rural Areas," sources: Census Bureau; Economic Research Service, U.S. Department of Agriculture.

[88] Rick Snyder (January 19, 2011), "Michigan State of the State Address 2011," *Stateline*, transcript from the *Detroit Free Press*.

[89] Agriculture, Nutrition, and Forestry Committee, U.S. Senate (May 31, 2011), "Chairwoman Stabenow and Ranking Member Roberts Hold First Field Hearing in East Lansing, Discuss Opportunities for Economic Growth, Job Creation," press release.

[90] Ibid.

[91] Val Osowski (Winter/Spring 2010), "Research to Energize Michigan's Economic Development," *Futures*, Vol. 27, No. 4/Vol. 28, No. 1.

[92] Economic Research Service, U.S. Department of Agriculture (August 2009), "Farm Risk Management: Government Programs and Risk."

[93] Sherrod Brown and others (September 2011), "Aggregate Risk and Revenue Management (ARRM) Program," proposal.

[94] Robert Dismukes and Ron Durst (June 2006), "Whole-Farm Approaches to a Safety Net," Economic Information Bulletin, No. 15, Economic Research Service, U.S. Department Agriculture.

[95] Sherrod Brown and others, op. cit.

Chapter 2

[1] Food Research and Action Center (August 1, 2011), "Supplemental Nutrition Assistance Program: Number of Persons Participating – 1 Month (April 2011-May 2011)."

[2] Food Research and Action Center (September 1, 2011), "Supplemental Nutrition Assistance Program: Number of Persons Participating – 1 Month (May 2011 – June 2011)."

[3] Office of Communications, Food and Nutrition Service, U.S. Department of Agriculture (March 16, 2011), "Agriculture Secretary Joins Nutrition Partners to Launch Childhood Hunger Campaign," press release.

[4] Katherine Ralston and others (July 2008), *The National School Lunch Program: Background, Trends, and Issues*, Economic Research Report, No. 61, Economic Research Service, U.S. Department of Agriculture.

[5] Mission: Readiness (21 September 2010), Letter to Speaker Pelosi, Representative Boehner, and Senators Reid and McConnell.

[6] Ibid.

[7] Alfred Lubrano (October 29, 2010), "Food that's as poor as the family," *The Philadelphia Inquirer*.

[8] Gopal K. Singh, Mohammad Siahpush, and Michael D. Kogan (March 2010), "Neighborhood Socioeconomic Conditions, Built Environments, and Childhood Obesity," *Health Affairs*, Vol. 29, No. 3.

[9] Food and Nutrition Service, U.S. Department of Agriculture (September 29, 2011), "Supplemental Nutrition Assistance Program: Average Monthly Participation (Households)."

[10] Michele Ver Ploeg and others (June 2009), "Food Access and Its Relationship to Food Choice," Chapter 5 of *Access to Affordable and Nutritious Food: Measuring and Understanding Food Deserts and Their Consequences*, Economic Research Service, U.S. Department of Agriculture.

[11] Ibid.

[12] Nicole I. Larsen, Mary T. Story, and Melissa C. Nelson (2009), "Neighborhood Environments: Disparities in Access to Healthy Foods in the U.S.," *American Journal of Preventive Medicine*, Vol. 36, No. 1.

[13] Paula Tarnapol Whitacre, Peggy Tsai, and Janet Mulligan (rapporteurs) (2009), *The Public Health Effects of Food Deserts: Workshop Summary*, Institute of Medicine and the National Research Council of the National Academies, The National Academies Press.

[14] Mark Winne (2008), *Closing the Food Gap: Resetting the Table in the Land of Plenty*, Beacon Press.

[15] Community Alliance for Research and Engagement (2010), Documenting the Health of our Neighborhoods: West River and Dwight.

[16] Bread for the World Institute (December 14, 2010), interview with Linda Thompson-Maier.

[17] Ibid.

[18] Mark Winne, op. cit.

[19] Mary E. O'Leary (February 2, 2011), "Stop and Shop to Open on Whalley Ave. in New Haven (video)," *New Haven Register*.

[20] Children's HealthWatch, Witnesses to Hunger.

[21] A.D.A.M. Medical Encyclopedia (reviewed on August 2, 2009), definition of "Failure to Thrive," PubMed Health.

[22] Bread for the World Institute (February 17, 2011), interview with Marianna Chilton.

[23] Children's HealthWatch and Medical-Legal Partnership (December 2009), "Rx for Hunger: Affordable Housing."

[24] Lisa M. Troy, Emily Ann Miller, and Steve Olson (rapporteurs) (2011), *Hunger and Obesity: Understanding a Food Insecurity Paradigm: Workshop Summary*, Food and Nutrition Board, Institute of Medicine of the National Academies.

[25] Deborah A. Frank and others (May 1, 2010), "Cumulative Hardship and Wellness of Low-Income, Young Children: Multisite Surveillance Study," *Pediatrics*, Vol. 125, No. 5.

[26] Arloc Sherman (July 6, 2009), "Safety Net Effective at Fighting Poverty But Has Weakened for the Very Poorest," Center on Budget and Policy Priorities.

[27] Mark R. Rank and Thomas A. Hirschl (November 2009), "Estimating the Risk of Food Stamp Use and Impoverishment During Childhood," *Archives of Pediatric and Adolescent Medicine*, Vol. 163, No. 11.

[28] Mark Nord, Margaret Andrews, and Steven Carlson (November 2009), *Household Food Security in the United States: 2008*, Economic Re-

search Report, No. 83, Economic Research Service, U.S. Department of Agriculture.

29 Food and Nutrition Service, U.S. Department of Agriculture (September 29, 2011), "Supplemental Nutrition Assistance Program Participation and Costs."

30 Food and Nutrition Service, U.S. Department of Agriculture (June 23, 2010), "Supplemental Nutrition Assistance Program: American Recovery and Reinvestment Act Plan Update."; Food and Nutrition Service, U.S. Department of Agriculture (2009), "Supplemental Nutrition Assistance Program: American Recovery and Reinvestment Act of 2009."

31 Mark Nord and Mark Prell (April 2011), *Food Security Improved Following the 2009 ARRA Increase in SNAP Benefits*, Economic Research Report, No. 116, Economic Research Service, U.S. Department of Agriculture.

32 Office of Analysis, Nutrition, and Evaluation, Food and Nutrition Service, U.S. Department of Agriculture (June 2006), "An Analysis of Food Stamp Benefit Redemption Patterns."

33 Abdul G. Dulloo, Jean Jacquet, and Lucien Girardier (1997), "Poststarvation Hyperphagia and Body Fat Overshooting in Humans: A Role for Feedback Signals from Lean and Fat Tissues," *The American Journal of Clinical Nutrition*, Vol. 65, No. 3.

34 FRAC Action Council, Food Research and Action Center (August 10, 2010), "FRAC Statement: Time to Stop Raiding SNAP Benefits."

35 Food and Nutrition Service, U.S. Department of Agriculture (June 23, 2010), op. cit.

36 Jackie Calmes and Michael Cooper (November 20, 2009), "New Consensus Sees Stimulus Package as Worthy Step," *The New York Times*.

37 FRAC Action Council, Food Research and Action Center, op. cit.

38 Food Research and Action Center (August 2010), "Don't Cut SNAP to Pay For Other Priorities."

39 Food Research and Action Center (September 2009), Child Nutrition Fact Sheet: Women, Infants and Children (WIC).

40 Maureen M. Black and others (July 2004), "Special Supplemental Nutrition Program for Women, Infants and, Children Participation and Infants' Growth and Health: A Multisite Surveillance Study," *Pediatrics*, Vol. 114, No. 1.

41 Geri Henchy (2005), "WIC in the States: Thirty-One Years of Building a Healthier America," Food Research and Action Center.

42 Peter D. Hart Research Associates and McLaughlin & Associates (October 21, 2010), "Updated Review of Public Opinion Research on Nutrition and Hunger," memorandum to Food Research and Action Center.

43 John Cook and Karen Jeng (2009), *Child Food Insecurity: The Economic Impact on Our Nation*, Feeding America.

44 Anemona Hartocollis (October 6, 2010), "New York Asks to Bar Use of Food Stamps to Buy Sodas," *The New York Times*.

45 Chronic Disease Prevention and Health Promotion, U.S. Department of Health and Human Services (May 26, 2011), "Obesity: Halting the Epidemic by Making Health Easier at a Glance 2011."

46 Eric A. Finkelstein and others (September-October 2009), "Annual Medical Spending Attributable to Obesity: Payer-And Service-Specific Estimates," *Health Affairs*, Vol. 28, No. 5.

47 Lenny R. Vartanian, Marlene B. Schwartz, and Kelly D. Brownell (April 2007), "Effects of Soft Drink Consumption on Nutrition and Health: A Systematic Review and Meta-Analysis," *American Journal of Public Health*, Vol. 97, No. 4.

48 Anemona Hartocollis (October 7, 2010), "Plan to Ban Food Stamps for Sodas has Hurdles," *The New York Times*.; Ollice C. Holden, Regional Administrator (May 4, 2004), Letter to Ms. Maria Gomez, Supplemental Nutrition Assistance Program, U.S. Department of Agriculture.

49 Helen H. Jensen and Parke E. Wilde (3rd Quarter 2010), "More Than Just Food: The Diverse Effects of Food Assistance Programs," *Choices: The Magazine of Food, Farm, and Resource Issues*, Vol. 25, No. 3, Agricultural and Applied Economics Association.

50 Michele Ver Ploeg, Lisa Mancino, and Biing-Hwan Lin (February 2006), "Food Stamps and Obesity: Ironic Twist or Complex Puzzle?," *Amber Waves*, Vol. 4, Issue 1.

51 Lisa M. Troy, Emily Ann Miller, and Steve Olson (rapporteurs), op. cit.

52 Bread for the World Institute (February 17, 2011), interview with Witnesses to Hunger.

53 Jessica E. Todd and Chen Zhen (3rd Quarter 2010), "Can Taxes on Calorically Sweetened Beverages Reduce Obesity?" *Choices: The Magazine of Food, Farm, and Resource Issues*, Vol. 25, No. 3, Agricultural and Applied Economics Association.

54 Federal Trade Commission (July 2008), *Marketing Food to Children and Adolescents: A Review of Industry Expenditures, Activities, and Self-Regulation*, Report to Congress.

55 Federal Trade Commission, op. cit.

56 Tatiana Andreyeva, Frank J. Chaloupka, and Kelly D. Brownell (June 2011), "Estimating the Potential of Taxes on Sugar-Sweetened Beverages to Reduce Consumption and Generate Revenue," *Preventative Medicine*, Vol. 52, No. 6.

57 Minh Wendt and Jessica E. Todd (June 2011), "The Effect of Food and Beverage Prices on Children's Weights," Economic Research Report, No. 118, Economic Research Service, U.S. Department of Agriculture.

58 Office of Communications, Food and Nutrition Service, U.S. Department of Agriculture (August 19, 2010), "USDA Selects Massachusetts to Test Ground-Breaking Nutrition Pilot Program: SNAP Recipients to Receive Incentives for Healthy Eating," press release.

59 Ibid.

60 Economic Research Service, U.S. Department of Agriculture, Your Food Environment Atlas: Download the Food Environment Atlas Data.

61 Patrick G. Lee (August 19, 2010), "Food stamp discount for buying produce," *The Boston Globe*.

62 Adam Drewnowski and S.E. Specter (January 2004), "Poverty and Obesity: The Role of Energy Density and Energy Costs," *American Journal of Clinical Nutrition*, Vol. 79, No.1.

63 Office of Research and Analysis, Food and Nutrition Service, U.S. Department of Agriculture (September 2011), "Characteristics of Supplemental Nutrition Assistance Program (SNAP) Households: Fiscal Year 2010."

64 Bread for the World Institute calculation based on: U.S. Department of Health and Human Services (August 2010), "The HHS Poverty Guidelines for the Remainder of 2010 (August 2010)."

65 Bread for the World Institute (February 17, 2011), interview with Sara Cardinale.

66 Suzanne Briggs and others (June 2010), "Real Food, Real Choice: Connecting SNAP Recipients with Farmers Markets," Community Food Security Coalition and Farmers Market Coalition.

67 National Institute of Food and Agriculture, U.S. Department of Agriculture (revised February 2011), "2010 Impacts: The Expanded Food and Nutrition Education Program (EFNEP)."

68 Bread for the World Institute calculation based on: Food and Nutrition Service, United States Department of Agriculture (September 29, 2011), "Annual Summary of Food and Nutrition Service Programs."

69 Food Research and Action Center (2011), "Fresh Fruit and Vegetable Program."

70 Farm to School, Food and Nutrition Service, U.S. Department of Agriculture (accessed on May 27, 2011), USDA Farm to School Team Site Visit: Burlington School District in Burlington, Vermont.

71 Bread for the World Institute (June 15, 2011), interview with Doug Davis.

72 Mary Story and others (2008), "Creating Healthy Food and Eating Environments: Policy and Environ-

mental Approaches," *Annual Review of Public Health*, Vol. 29, University of Wisconsin.

73 Joel Kimmons and others (January 2009), "Fruit and Vegetable Intake Among Adolescents and Adults in the United States: Percentage Meeting Individualized Recommendations," *The Medscape Journal of Medicine*, Vol. 11, No. 1.

74 Ed Bruske (November 18, 2010), "White House to put 6,000 salad bars in schools," *Grist*.

75 School Nutrition Association (March 29, 2011), "SNA Submits Comments on Proposed School Meal Standards," press release.

76 Melissa D. Ho and Geoffrey S. Becker (January 12, 2010), *Farm and Food Support Under USDA's Section 32 Program*, Report for Congress, Congressional Research Service.

77 Food and Nutrition Service, U.S. Department of Agriculture (2011), "Food and Nutrition Service: 2012 Explanatory Notes."

78 Kari Hamerschlag (June 9, 2011), "Improving School Food: Do it Now or Pay the Price Later," Agriculture, Environmental Working Group.

79 Diane Conners (February 3, 2011), "For Some Kids, Farm to School a Health Lifeline," *Great Lakes Bulletin News Service*, Michigan Land Use Institute.

Chapter 3

1 Employment and Training Administration, Department of Labor (accessed September 9, 2011), The National Agricultural Workers Survey: Public Access Data.

2 Philip Martin, Michael Fix, and J. Edward Taylor (2006), *The New Rural Poverty: Agriculture and Immigration in California*, Urban Institute Press.

3 Philip Martin, Michael Fix, and J. Edward Taylor, op. cit.

4 Philip Martin (2009), *Importing Poverty?: Immigration and the Changing Face of Rural America*, Yale University Press.; Bread for the World Institute (July 2011), correspondence with Philip Martin.

5 Deborah Waller Meyers (January 2006), "Temporary Worker Programs: A Patchwork Policy Response," *Insight: Independent Task Force on Immigration and America's Future*, No. 12, Migration Policy Institute.; Philip Martin (2009), op. cit.; Bread for the World Institute (July 2011), correspondence with Philip Martin.

6 Marshall Ganz (April 2009), *Why David Sometimes Wins: Leadership, Organization, and Strategy in the California Farm Worker Movement*, Oxford University Press.

7 Vernon M. Briggs Jr., Cornell University (February 12, 2004), "Guestworker Programs for Low-Skilled Workers: Lessons from the Past and Warnings for the Future," testimony before the Immigration and Border Security Subcommittee, Judiciary Committee, U.S. Senate.

8 Philip Martin (2009), op. cit.

9 Ibid.

10 Ibid.

11 Philip Martin (April 30, 2011), "California Hired Farm Labor 1960-2010: Change and Continuity."

12 Philip Martin and Linda Calvin (2010), "Immigration Reform: What Does It Mean for Agriculture and Rural America?," *Applied Economic Perspectives and Policy*, Vol. 32, No. 2.

13 Daniel Carroll, Annie Georges, and Russell Saltz (May 12, 2011), "Changing Characteristics of U.S. Farm Workers: 21 Years of Findings from the National Agricultural Workers Survey," presentation for the Immigration Reform and Agriculture Conference: Implications for Farmers, Farm Workers, and Communities, University of California.

14 Employment and Training Administration, Department of Labor, op. cit.

15 Philip Martin and Linda Calvin, op. cit.

16 Economic Research Service, U.S. Department of Agriculture (accessed on June 24, 2011), "Rural Labor and Education: Farm Labor."; Philip Martin and Linda Calvin, op. cit.

17 William Kandel (July 2008), "Profile of Hired Farm Workers: A 2008 Up-

date," *Economic Research Report*, No. 60, Economic Research Service, U.S. Department of Agriculture.

18 Ibid.; Daniel Carroll, Annie Georges, and Russell Saltz, op. cit.

19 Katherine L. Cason, Anastasia Snyder, and Leif Jensen (November 2004), *The Health and Nutrition of Hispanic Migrant and Seasonal Farm Workers*, The Center for Rural Pennsylvania.

20 Manuel Valdes (August 14, 2008), "State farmworkers face low quality of life, study finds," *The Associated Press.*

21 John Thomas Rosen-Molina and Daniel A. Sumner (November 2009), "Agricultural Workforce," in *AIC White Papers on California Agricultural Issues*, University of California Agricultural Issues Center.

22 Sara A. Quandt and others (November-December 2004), "Household Food Security Among Migrant and Seasonal Latino Farmworkers in North Carolina," *Public Health Reports*, Vol. 119.

23 Kimberly Greder and others (June 2007), "Latino Immigrants: Food and Housing Insecurity," University Extension, Iowa State University.

24 Philip Martin (March 21, 2011), "Farm Exports and Farm Labor: Would a Raise for Fruit and Vegetable Workers Diminish the Competitiveness of U.S. Agriculture?," Briefing Paper, No. 295, Economic Policy Institute.; Philip Martin, Michael Fix, and J. Edward Taylor, op. cit.

25 Daniel Carroll, Annie Georges, and Russell Saltz, op. cit.

26 Katherine L. Cason, Anastasia Snyder, and Leif Jensen, op. cit.

27 Bureau of Labor Statistics, U.S. Department of Labor (August 25, 2011), "National Census of Fatal Occupational Injuries in 2010 (Preliminary Results)," news release.

28 United Farm Workers and Bon Appétit Management Company Foundation (March 2011), *Inventory of Farmworker Issues and Protections in the United States.*; Bread for the World Institute (July 2011), correspondence with Philip Martin.

29 Bread for the World Institute (April 26, 2011), interview with Nancy Foster.

30 Phil Glaize, Glaize Orchards (September 24, 2010), "Protecting America's Harvest," testimony before the Immigration, Refugees, and Border Security Subcommittee, Judiciary Committee, U.S. House of Representatives.

31 Phil Glaize, op. cit.

32 Human Smuggling and Trafficking Center (December 2008), *Domestic Human Trafficking: An Internal Issue.*

33 Terence Coonan and others (October 2010), *Florida Strategic Plan on Human Trafficking*, Center for the Advancement of Human Rights, Florida State University.

34 U.S. Citizenship and Immigration Services, U.S. Department of Homeland Security (June 24, 2011), "History and Milestones."

35 Ibid.

36 National Immigration Law Center (September 2011), Legal Workforce Act of 2011 (HR 2885).

37 David Harrison (May 2011), "Rep. Smith's E-Verify Measure Gets Mixed Reception from Industry Concerns," *CQ Today.*

38 National Immigration Law Center, op. cit."

39 Philip Martin (March 21, 2011), op. cit.

40 Ibid.

41 Gary Lucier and others (April 2006), *Fruit and Vegetable Backgrounder*, Electric Outlook Report, Economic Research Service, U.S. Department of Agriculture.

42 National Association of State Departments of Agriculture (2008), "Michigan Department of Agriculture and Rural Development."

43 Dinesh Ramde (November 15, 2010), "Food Production a Rare Growth Industry in Gloomy Economy," HuffPost Food, *Huffington Post.*

44 A. G. Sulzberger (June 2, 2011), "Rural Legislators' Power Ebbs as Populations Shift," *The New York Times.*; Economic Research Service, U.S. Department of Agriculture (September 2011), "State Fact Sheets: Michigan."

45 William A. Knudson (July 2006), "The Impact of Migrant Farm Workers on Michigan Agriculture," Product Center for Agriculture and Natural Resources, Michigan State University.

46 Julia Rothwell, U.S. Apple Association (May 31, 2011), "Panel 2: Michigan Agricultural Production and Farm Bill Principles," testimony at Opportunities for Growth: Michigan and the 2012 Farm Bill field hearing, Agriculture, Nutrition, and Forestry Committee, U.S. Senate, Michigan State University.

47 Philip Martin, Michael Fix, and J. Edward Taylor, op. cit.; John Burstein (April 13, 2007), "U.S.-Mexico Agricultural Trade and Rural Poverty in Mexico," report from a task force convened by the Woodrow Wilson Center's Mexico Institute and Fundación IDEA.

48 Bread for the World Institute (July 14, 2011), correspondence with Tom Hertz, U.S. Department of Agriculture.; Susan R. Boatright and John C. McKissick (compiled by) (May 2010), "2009 Georgia Farm Gate Value Report," Center for Agribusiness and Economic Development, College of Agricultural and Environmental Science, The University of Georgia.

49 Reid J. Epstein (June 14, 2011), "Georgia sends criminals to replace undocumented immigrants," *Politico.*

50 Philip Martin, Michael Fix, and J. Edward Taylor, op. cit.

51 Ibid.

52 Philip Martin (June 23, 2011), "Immigration Reform: Implications for Farmers, Farm Workers, and Communities."; Philip Martin (July 2011), "H-2A: AEWR, Global; H-2B," *Rural Migration News*, Vol. 17, No. 3.

53 Philip Martin (June 11, 2010), op. cit.

54 Philip Martin, Michael Fix, and J. Edward Taylor, op. cit.

55 William G. Whittaker (March 26, 2008), "Farm Labor: The Adverse Effect Wage Rate (AEWR)," Report for Congress, Congressional Research Service.

56 Employment and Training Administration, U.S. Department of Labor (March 1, 2011), "Adverse Effect Wage Rates – Year 2011," *Federal Register*, Vol. 76, No. 40.

57 Philip Martin (June 11, 2010), op. cit.

58 Ibid.

59 Bread for the World Institute (January 2011), interview with Rob Williams.

60 Bread for the World Institute (July 2011), interview with David Reyes, Farm Labor Organizing Committee Executive Board Member.

61 Philip Martin (July 2010), "Florida and NC: FLOC and CIW Boycotts," *Rural Migration News*, Vol. 16, No. 3.

62 Steven Greenhouse (September 17, 2004), "North Carolina Growers' Group Signs Union Contract for Mexican Workers," *The New York Times*.

63 World Bank (October 2007), World Development Report 2008: *Agriculture for Development*.

64 Prabhu Pingali (2010), "Agriculture Renaissance: Making 'Agriculture for Development' Work in the 21st Century," *Handbook of Agricultural Economics*, Vol. 4, Chapter 74.

65 Ibid.

66 Economic Research Service, U.S. Department of Agriculture (September 2010), "Rural Income, Poverty, and Welfare: Transfer Payments."

Chapter 4

1 1,000 Days (September 2010), *Scaling Up Nutrition: A Framework for Action,* policy brief.

2 Susan Horton and others (2006), *Scaling Up Nutrition: What Will It Cost?*, The World Bank.

3 1,000 Days, op. cit.

4 Robert E. Black and others (January 2008), "Maternal and Child Undernutrition: Global and Regional Exposures and Health Consequences," *The Lancet*, Vol. 371, Issue 9608.

5 D.L. Pelletier and others (1995), "The Effects of Malnutrition on Child Mortality in Developing Countries," *Bulletin of the World Health Organization*, Vol. 73, No.

4, World Health Organization, United Nations.; David L. Pelletier and others (1994), "A Methodology for Estimating the Contribution of Malnutrition to Child Mortality in Developing Countries," *The Journal of Nutrition*, Vol. 124, No. 10.

6 Robert E. Black and others, op. cit.

7 Aryeh D. Stein and others (2008), "Nutritional Supplementation in Early Childhood, Schooling, and Intellectual Functioning in Adulthood: A Prospective Study in Guatemala," *Archives of Pediatrics and Adolescent Medicine*, Vol. 162, No. 7.

8 Reynaldo Martorell and others (2010), "Weight Gain in the First Two Years of Life Is an Important Predictor of Schooling Outcomes in Pooled Analysis from Five Birth Cohorts from Low- and Middle-Income Countries," *The Journal of Nutrition*, Vol. 140, No 2.

9 Robert E. Black and others, op. cit.

10 Daniel Gilnoer and François Delange (October 2000), "The Potential Repercussions of Maternal, Fetal, and Neonatal Hypothyroxinemia on the Progeny," *Thyroid*, Vol. 10, No. 10.

11 Ming Qian and others (2005), "The Effect of Iodine on Intelligence in Children: a Meta-Analysis of Studies Conducted in China," *Asia Pacific Journal of Clinical Nutrition*, Vol. 14, No. 1.

12 Robert E. Black and others, op. cit.

13 Shams Arifeen and others (October 2001), "Exclusive Breastfeeding Reduces Acute Respiratory Infection and Diarrhea Deaths Among Infants in Dhaka Slums," *Pediatrics*, Vol. 108, No. 4.

14 World Bank (July 28, 2011), "Population 2010" World Development Indicators database; Bread for the World Institute (2010), 2011 Hunger Report: *Our Common Interest: Ending Hunger and Malnutrition*, see "Table 2: Millennium Development Goals."

15 U.S. Food Aid and Security, "Food Aid and Hunger Fast Facts," see "Fact 7."

16 Patrick Webb and others (April 2011), *Delivering Improved Nutrition:*

Recommendations for Changes to U.S. Food Aid Products and Programs, Food Aid Quality Review Report to the U.S. Agency for International Development, Tufts University.

17 Food for Peace Office, U.S. Agency for International Development (2009), "Annex H: Food Aid Commodities Availability List," in *Fiscal Year 2010: Title II Proposal Guidance and Program Policies*.

18 Medecins Sans Frontieres/Doctors without Borders (May 2011), *Reducing Childhood Mortality in Niger: The Role of Nutritious Foods*.

19 Andrew Rice (September 2, 2010), "The Peanut Solution," *The New York Times*.

20 Jonathan H. Williams and others (November 2004), "Human Aflatoxicosis in Developing Countries: A Review of Toxicology, Exposure, Potential Health Consequences, and Interventions," *American Journal of Clinical Nutrition*, Vol. 80, No. 5.

21 World Food Program, *2009 Food Aid Flows*.

22 U.S. Government Accountability Office (May 2011), *International Food Assistance: Better Nutrition and Quality Control Can Further Improve U.S. Food Aid*, Report to Congressional Requesters.

23 Patrick Webb and others, op. cit.

24 Ibid.

25 U.S. Government Accountability Office, op. cit.

26 Ibid.

27 Ibid.

28 U.S. Agency for International Development (February 19, 2009), "ADS Chapter 315: Cargo Preference," in *Functional Series 300: Acquisition and Assistance*.

29 Elizabeth R. Bageant, Christopher B. Barrett, and Erin C. Lentz (2010), "Food Aid and Agricultural Cargo Preference," paper presented at the 2010 Meeting of the Agricultural and Applied Economics Association, July 25-27, Denver, CO.

30 U.S. Government Accountability Office (April 2007), *Foreign Assistance: Various Challenges Impede the Efficiency and Effectiveness of U.S.*

Food Aid, Report to the Agriculture, Nutrition, and Forestry Committee, U.S. Senate.

31 The World Bank (2006), *Repositioning Nutrition as Central to Development: A Strategy for Large-Scale Action*.

32 Patrick Webb and others, op. cit.

33 Catherine Feeney, World Food Program, United Nations (June 2011), "USAID and USDA LRP Support to WFP," presentation at the International Food Aid and Development Conference, June 27-29, 2011, Kansas City, Missouri, see presentations under "Local Regional Procurement: USAID and USDA Initiatives."

34 Christopher B. Barrett and others (June 2011), "Misconceptions About Food Assistance," policy brief, Global Public Policy Institute and Cornell University.

35 Rajiv Shah, USAID (June 28, 2011), Remarks at the International Food Aid and Development Conference, Kansas City, Missouri.

36 Jeff Borns (July 30, 2009), "Food for Peace Information Bulletin: Memorandum for All Food for Peace Officers and Awardees," Food for Peace Office, U.S. Agency for International Development.

37 C. Stuart Clark (2010), "Food Aid Convention: Contributing to Global Food Security," in Bread for the World Institute's 2011 Hunger Report: *Our Common Interest: Ending Hunger and Malnutrition*.

38 Emmy Simmons (June 2009), *Monetization of Food Aid: Reconsidering U.S. Policy and Practice*, Partnership to Cut Hunger and Poverty in Africa.

39 U.S. Government Accountability Office (June 2011), *International Food Assistance: Funding Development Projects through the Purchase, Shipment, and Sale of U.S. Commodities is Inefficient and Can Cause Adverse Market Impacts*, Report to Congressional Requesters.

40 David Nabarro (2011), "Action Plan on Food Price Volatility and Agriculture," The Secretary-General's High-Level Task Force on the Global Food Security Crisis, United Nations.

41 Robert Paarlberg (August 2, 2011), "Famine in Somalia: What Can the World Do About It?," *The Atlantic*.

42 U.S. Government (May 2010), *Feed the Future Guide*.

43 Ibid.

44 U.S. Government Accountability Office (May 2009), *Local and Regional Procurement Can Enhance the Efficiency of U.S. Food Aid, but Challenges May Constrain Its Implementation*, Report to the Chairman, Africa and Global Health Subcommittee, Foreign Affairs Committee, U.S. House of Representatives.

45 Ann Tutwiler, Global Food Security Initiative (August 4, 2010), "Feed the Future Update from the International Food Aid and Development Conference," USDA Blog, U.S. Department of Agriculture.

46 Charles E. Hanrahan (January 26, 2010), "Local and Regional Procurement for U.S. International Emergency Food Aid," Congressional Research Service.

47 Amelia Matos Sumbana, Ambassador of Mozambique to the U.S. (June 29, 2011), Speech, at the International Food Aid and Development Conference, Kansas City, Missouri.

48 U.S. Agency for International Development (March 25, 2011), Mozambique: Strategic Review: Feed the Future.

49 Ibid.

50 Food and Agriculture Organization, United Nations (2009), *How to Feed the World in 2050*.

51 Gerald C. Nelson and others (updated October 2009), *Climate Change: Impact on Agriculture and the Costs of Adaptation*, Food Policy Report, International Food Policy Research Institute.

52 United Nations Development Program, United Nations (2007), Human Development Report 2007-2008: *Fighting Climate Change: Human Solidarity in a Divided World*.

53 Kavita Watsa (editor) (2009), Africa's Development in a Changing Climate, The International Bank for Reconstruction and Development, The World Bank.

54 Integrated Regional Information Networks (May 28, 2009), "Mozambique: Climate change adaptation can't wait," UN Office for the Coordination of Humanitarian Affairs, United Nations.

55 Ibid.

56 Philip G. Pardey and Julian M. Alston (July 2011), "For Want of a Nail: The Case for Increased Agricultural R&D Spending," American Boondoggle, American Enterprise Institute.

57 Science Council, Consultative Group on International Agricultural Research (December 2005), "Research Benefits Heavily Outweigh Costs," Science Council Brief, No. 1.

58 Independent Leaders Group on Global Agricultural Development (2009), *Renewing American Leadership in the Fight Against Global Hunger and Poverty*, The Chicago Council of Global Affairs.

59 Ibid.

60 Joachim von Braun and others (2008), *What to Expect from Scaling Up CGIAR Investments and "Best Bet" Programs*, Consultative Group on International Agricultural Research and International Food Policy Research Institute.

Sources for data strips on pages 4-5, 10-11, 22-23, 48-49, 72-73, 94-95, 118-119

Alliance to End Hunger
Bread for the World
Bread for the World Institute
Carnegie Endowment for International Peace
Center on Budget and Policy Priorities
U.N. Food and Agriculture Organization
Pew Hispanic Center
The Lancet
USDA, Economic Research Service
USDA, Food and Nutrition Service
U.S. Department of Labor, National Agricultural Workers Survey

Acronyms

ADHD	Attention-deficit hyperactivity disorder
AEWR	Adverse Effect Wage Rate
AgJOBS	Agricultural Job Opportunity, Benefits and Security bill
ARRA	American Recovery and Reinvestment Act
ARRM	Aggregate Risk and Revenue Management Act of 2011
ASD	Appalachian Sustainable Development
CAADP	Comprehensive Africa Agriculture Development Program
CACFP	Child and Adult Care Feeding Program
CGIAR	Consultative Group on International Agricultural Research
CITA	Independent Agricultural Workers' Center (Centro Independiente de Trabajadores Agrícolas)
CIW	Coalition of Immokalee Workers
CSB	Corn Soy Blend
CSBs	Calorically sweetened beverages
CSFP	Commodity Supplemental Food Program
DOL	U.S. Department of Labor
EBT	Electronic benefit transfer
EFNEP	Expanded Food and Nutrition Education Program
EITC	Earned Income Tax Credit
EPA	Environmental Protection Agency
FAC	Food Aid Convention
FAO	United Nations Food and Agriculture Organization
FLOC	Farm Labor Organizing Committee
FSA	Farm Service Agency
GAO	U.S. Government Accountability Office
GDP	Gross Domestic Product
GHGs	Greenhouse gases
GPS	Global positioning system
GWDC	Greater Dwight Development Corporation

HIP	Healthy Incentives Pilot
ICE	Immigration, Customs and Enforcement
LNS	Lipid-based nutritional supplements
LRP	Local and regional purchase
MDGs	Millennium Development Goals
NCGA	North Carolina Growers Association
NGO	Nongovernmental Organization
NSLP	National School Lunch Program
RDAs	Recommended daily allowances
SFSP	Summer Food Service Program
SNAP	Supplemental Nutrition Assistance Program
SUN	Scaling Up Nutrition
TAFAD	Trans Atlantic Food Assistance Dialogue
TANF	Temporary Assistance for Needy Families
TEFAP	The Emergency Food Assistance Program
USDA	U.S. Department of Agriculture
VEDCO	Volunteer Efforts for Development Concerns
WIC	Special Supplemental Nutrition Program for Women, Infants and Children
WTO	World Trade Organization

Glossary

1,000 Days: A public-private partnership promoting targeted action and investment to improve nutrition for mothers and children in the 1,000 day period from pregnancy to age two when better nutrition can have a life-changing impact on a child's future.

American Recovery and Reinvestment Act (ARRA): A $787 billion economic recovery plan enacted in February 2009 with provisions for federal tax cuts and incentives, an expansion of unemployment benefits and other social entitlement programs. In addition, 28 federal agencies received Recovery funds to finance contracts, grants, and loans around the country.

Biofuels: Fuels made from any organic matter that is available on a renewable or recurring basis. Ethanol made from sugarcane or corn would be an example of biofuels.

Budget deficit: The amount by which the federal government's total outlays exceed its total revenues in a given period, typically a fiscal year.

Cargo preference: Whenever the federal government pays for equipment, material, or commodities shipped to other countries, a minimum percentage of the gross tonnage shipped by sea must go by U.S.-flag vessels.

Circle of Protection: An initiative launched in 2011 by a broad coalition of Christian groups to oppose budget cuts to programs that would slash or eliminate programs that provide essential services for poor and vulnerable populations in the United States and abroad.

Civil society: The sphere of civic action outside of the government comprised of citizens' groups, nongovernmental organizations, religious congregations, labor unions and foundations.

Clean Air Act: The law that establishes the basic structure for government regulation of the nation's air quality and the stratospheric ozone layer.

Clean Water Act: The law that establishes the basic structure for regulating discharges of pollutants into the waters of the United States and regulating quality standards for surface waters.

Climate change: Climate change refers to a change in the state of the climate that can be identified (e.g., by using statistical tests) and that persists for an extended period, typically decades or longer.

Commodity payments: The U.S. government provides commodity payments for a select group of crops. The largest recipients are corn, soybeans, wheat, cotton and rice. Farmers who grow these can receive payments for losses in income due to low yields or low market prices. Other payments have nothing to do with market price or yield—farmers (or landowners) receive a payment by virtue of holding land with a history of raising one of the commodity crops.

Conservation: Activities, systems, practices, or management measures designed to address a resource concern. Structural, vegetative, and land management measures (including agricultural drainage management systems), and planning needed to address a resource concern are included.

Consultative Group on International Agricultural Research (CGIAR): A strategic partnership of diverse donors that support 15 international research centers, working in collaboration with many hundreds of government and civil society organizations as well as private businesses around the world.

Decoupled support: When commodity program payments are tied to current production or net returns, they can introduce market distortions by influencing planting decisions, overall production, and market prices. In contrast to such "coupled" programs, benefits from "decoupled" programs do not depend on the farmer's production choices, output levels, or market conditions.

Developed countries: An alternate way of describing highly industrialized nations such as the United States, Great Britain, France, Germany and Japan.

Developing countries: Countries with low per capita income. Terms such as less developed country, least developed country, underdeveloped country, poor, southern or Third World have also been used to describe developing countries.

Development assistance: Grants and loans to developing countries by donors to spur economic development and poverty reduction.

Direct payments: Fixed payments for eligible historic production of wheat, corn, barley, grain sorghum, oats, upland cotton, long and medium grain rice, soybeans, other oilseeds, and peanuts.

Doha Development Round: The name given to the current round of multilateral trade negotiations under the auspices of the World Trade Organization (see below).

Earned Income Tax Credit (EITC): A federal government program that provides a cash benefit to many low-income working people by refunding a portion of their income taxes.

Electronic benefit transfer (EBT) systems: Supplemental Nutrition Assistance Program (SNAP) benefits are provided through EBT systems under which recipients use an EBT card (similar to a debit card) to access their food stamp benefit "account" (replenished monthly) to buy food items.

Emergency food aid: Food aid provided to victims of natural or man-made disasters. It is freely distributed to targeted beneficiary groups and is usually provided on a grant basis.

Family farm: USDA defines a "family farm" as any farm organized as a sole proprietorship, partnership, or family corporation. Family farms exclude farms organized as nonfamily corporations or cooperatives, as well as farms with hired managers. Family farms are closely held (legally controlled) by their operator and the operator's household.

Famine: An extreme collapse in local availability and access to food that causes a widespread rise in deaths from outright starvation or hunger-related illnesses.

Farm bill: A multi-year, omnibus law that contains federal commodity and farm support policies, as well as other farm-related provisions, such as rural development, conservation, agricultural research, food aid and nutrition programs.

Farm programs: Generally meant to include the commodity programs administered by the Farm Service Agency, as well as the other U.S. Department of Agriculture (USDA) programs that directly benefit farmers.

Farm-to-school: Sourcing foods served in school meal programs (K-12) from local farms with the objectives of serving healthy meals and supporting local and regional farmers.

Farmer's markets: Farmer's markets are venues where agricultural and food producers sell directly to consumers.

Farmland: Land used for agricultural purposes. The United States has had roughly 1 billion acres of farmland.

Feed the Future: A new U.S. foreign assistance program that supports agricultural development initiatives. The U.S. Agency for International Development (USAID) launched the program in 2009, pledging $3.5 billion over three years to 20 targeted countries.

Food bank: A charitable organization that solicits, receives, inventories, stores and distributes food and grocery products from various sources to other charitable organizations.

Food insecurity: Uncertain availability or inability to acquire safe, nutritious food in socially acceptable ways.

Food security: Assured access to enough nutritious food to sustain an active and healthy life with dignity.

Fruit and vegetable planting restrictions: Planting for harvest of fruits, vegetables, and wild rice is prohibited on base acres of commodity program participants, except in certain situations specified in farm legislation.

Greenhouse gases (GHG): Gases that trap heat in the atmosphere. Some greenhouse gases such as carbon dioxide occur naturally and are emitted into the atmosphere through natural processes and human activities. Other greenhouse gases (e.g., fluorinated gases) are created and emitted solely through human activities.

H-2A: An agricultural work program that provides admission of alien guest workers to the United States on a nonimmigrant basis to perform agricultural work of a seasonal or temporary nature.

Healthy, Hunger-Free Kids Act of 2010: Authorizes funding for federal child nutrition programs and increases access to healthy food for low-income children. The bill that reauthorizes these programs is often referred to by shorthand as the child nutrition reauthorization bill.

High fructose corn syrup (HFCS): A natural sweetener created by converting glucose in corn starch to fructose. HFCS production expanded during the 1980s as a substitute for higher-cost beet and cane sugar used in soft drinks.

Hunger: A condition in which people do not get enough food to provide the nutrients (carbohydrate, fat, protein, vitamins, and minerals) for fully productive, active and healthy lives.

Income support: Programs providing direct, income-supplementing payments to farmers and intended to protect farm income without affecting market prices.

Know Your Farmer, Know Your Food: A USDA-wide effort to strengthen local and regional food systems.

Let's Move: Program developed by First Lady Michelle Obama to solve the epidemic of childhood obesity within a generation.

Local and regional purchase: Sourcing food aid nearer to the location of the recipients, providing the ability to act quickly and effectively in cases where a rapid food aid response is critical to saving lives.

Low birth weight: Children born weighing 2,500 grams (5 pounds, 8 ounces) or less, being especially vulnerable to illness and death during the first months of life.

Malnutrition: The condition that occurs when people's diets do not provide adequate nutrients for growth and maintenance or they are unable to fully utilize the food they eat due to illness. Malnutrition includes being underweight for one's age, too short for one's age (stunting), dangerously thin for one's height (wasting), deficient in vitamins and minerals (micronutrient deficiencies), and severely overweight (obesity).

Micronutrients: The vitamins, major minerals and trace elements needed for a healthy, balanced diet.

Millennium Development Goals (MDGs): A set of objectives to improve the quality of life for all people, first laid out in a series of international conferences in the 1990s, then officially adopted by the United Nations in 2000 with the Millennium Declaration. The goals serve as a road map for development by 2015.

Monetization: The process of selling U.S. food aid in local markets of developing countries to get the cash needed for development programs. These programs may be run by well-meaning organizations, but monetization has the effect of distorting local markets and thereby hurting farmers in these countries.

National School Lunch Program: Provides nutritionally balanced, low-cost lunches that are free to children in households with incomes at or below 130 percent of poverty and reduced price for those in households with incomes between 130 and 185 percent of poverty.

Organic farming: An approach to farming based on biological methods that avoid the use of synthetic crop or livestock production inputs and on a broadly defined philosophy of farming that puts value on ecological harmony, resource efficiency, and non-intensive animal husbandry practices.

Poverty-focused development assistance: Foreign assistance that directly affects the lives of hungry and poor people such as programs that immunize children, train teachers, build water wells, schools, and rural roads, and provide agricultural training to help farmers increase their productivity.

Producer: An owner, operator, landlord, tenant, or sharecropper who shares in the risk of producing a crop and is entitled to share in the crop available for marketing from the farm, or would have shared had the crop been produced.

Program crops: Crops for which Federal support programs are available to producers, including wheat, corn, barley, grain sorghum, oats, extralong staple and upland cotton, rice, oilseeds, peanuts, and sugar.

Recommended Daily Allowance (RDA): The daily dietary intake level of a nutrient that is considered sufficient to meet the requirements of nearly all healthy individuals in each life-stage and gender group.

Renewable fuels: Broadly, renewable fuels are made from replenishing feedstocks (such as biomass, sunlight, wind, water, and waste products) in contrast to exhaustible (nonrenewable) feedstocks such as petroleum and coal. Renewable fuels are a subset of alternative fuels.

Renewable Fuel Standard (RFS): A policy proposal whereby motor fuels in the United States would be required to contain a certain percentage or volume of renewable fuels.

Revenue insurance: Provides farmers protection against losses in revenue. Revenue is determined by the income earned from all farm activities, minus operating costs. Operating costs include capital-intensive investments such as farm equipment and inputs like seeds, fertilizer and fuel to run the equipment. Land prices also must be accounted for when determining revenue. Revenue insurance makes up the difference when revenues fall below the break-even point.

Safety nets: Government policies and charitable programs designed to ensure basic needs are met among low-income, disabled and other vulnerable social groups. Safety nets may also provide protection against risks, such as lost income, limited access to credit or devastation from natural disaster.

School Breakfast Program: Provides nutritional meals to students at participating schools (and to children in a few residential child care institutions). Certified low-income students receive free or reduced-price breakfasts

Section 32: USDA program that distributes surplus agricultural commodities, mostly to child nutrition programs.

Smallholder farmer: A farmer who works a small plot of land, generally less than five acres. The greatest number of people living in extreme poverty consists of smallholder farmers and their families.

Special Supplemental Nutrition Program for Women, Infants and Children (WIC): Safeguards the health of low-income women, infants, and children up to age 5 who are at nutritional risk. The WIC program provides monthly packages of nutritious foods, information on healthy eating, and referral to health care.

Specialty crops: Fruits, vegetables, tree nuts, dried fruits, nursery crops, and horticulture crops.

Stunting: Failure to grow to normal height caused by chronic undernutrition during the formative years of childhood.

Supplemental Nutrition Assistance Program (SNAP): Previously the Food Stamp Program, SNAP supplements the food budgets of low-income households with monthly benefits in the form of an electronic benefits card that they can use like cash at authorized retail stores.

Sustainable agriculture: A systematic approach to farming intended to reduce agricultural pollution, enhance natural resource and financial sustainability, and improve efficiency.

Undernutrition: A condition resulting from inadequate consumption of calories, protein and/or nutrients to meet the basic physical requirements for an active and healthy life.

Value-added: Agricultural products that have increased in value because of processing; such products include wheat flour and soybean oil. Livestock are considered value added products because they have increased the value of pasture and feed grains going into them.

Value chain: The full sequence of activities or functions required to bring a product or service from conception, through intermediary steps of production, transformation, marketing, and delivery to the final consumers.

Wasting: A condition in which a person is seriously below the normal weight for his or her height due to acute malnutrition or a medical condition.

World Food Program (WFP): The specialized agency of the United Nations providing logistical support necessary to get food to the right people at the right time in response to emergency food shortages and in development work.

World Trade Organization (WTO): The international organization established to oversee international trade agreements and settle disputes between member countries. Currently there are 153 member countries.

2012 DATA TABLES: USER GUIDE

Tables 1 and 2 provide the most recent data at the time of this printing on global development indicators. **Table 3 and 4** provide the most recent data at the time of this printing on U.S. poverty, hunger, and national nutrition programs.

Table 1 and **Table 2** include countries with more than 300,000 people. Regional data in Table 1 include all countries in a region, including those with fewer than 300,000 people. In Table 2, only low- and middle-income countries are represented in the regional data. Names of countries, regions, and income groupings adhere to World Bank definitions.

Note that Korea, Dem. Rep. is commonly known as North Korea, and West Bank and Gaza are often called the Occupied Palestinian Territories; data for Sudan usually include South Sudan, and data for China do not include Hong Kong Special Administrative Region of China, Macao Special Administrative Region of China, or Taiwan Province of China.

Low- & middle-income countries had Gross National Income per capita of less than $12,196 in 2009. High income countries had Gross National Income per capita of $12,196 or more in 2009.

On the Web

For updates to the data tables throughout the year, visit:
www.bread.org/go/hunger2012

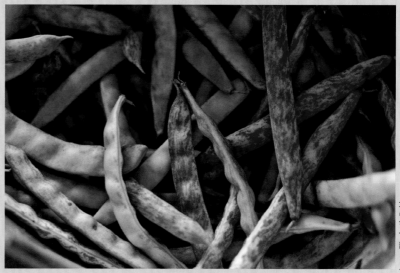

Laura Elizabeth Pohl

TABLE 1 – World Demographics

| | Population | | | | | Life expectancy at birth (years) 2009 | HDI index 2010 | Employment to pop. ratio for people above age 15 (% of total population) 2008-2009 | Workers' remittances & compensation received by employees (current US$) 2009 | Refugee population 2009 | |
	total 2010	ages 0-14 (% of total pop.) 2009	growth (annual %) 2010	density (people per sq. km of land area) 2010	rural (% of total pop.) 2009	urban (% of total pop.) 2009					by country or territory of origin	by country or territory of asylum
World	6,855,208,767	27.2	1.2	53	49.7	50.3	69	..	60.7	416,120,432,082	15,163,210	15,163,210
High-income countries	1,122,975,925	17.5	0.6	33	22.7	77.3	80	..	55.8	108,466,802,770	90,034	1,984,101
Low- & middle-income countries	5,732,232,842	29.0	1.3	60	54.9	45.1	67	..	61.8	307,653,629,312	9,986,904	13,179,109
Sub-Saharan Africa	862,324,301	42.6	2.5	37	63.1	36.9	53	..	65.1	20,748,702,263	2,666,143	2,089,538
Angola	18,992,707	45.0	2.6	15	42.4	57.6	48	0.40	76.4	82,084,000d	141,021	14,734
Benin	9,211,741	43.1	3.1	83	58.4	41.6	62	0.44	71.6	242,532,800	411	7,205
Botswana	1,977,569	33.3	1.4	3	39.7	60.3	55	0.63	46.0	87,863,150	30	3,022
Burkina Faso	16,286,706	46.3	3.3	60	80.0	20.0	53	0.31	81.9	99,300,000	990	543
Burundi	8,518,862	38.4	2.6	332	89.3	10.7	51	0.28	84.2	28,232,150	94,239	24,967
Cameroon	19,958,351	40.9	2.2	42	42.4	57.6	51	0.46	59.1	147,579,500	14,766	99,957
Cape Verde	512,582	36.2	1.4	127	39.6	60.4	71	0.53	55.7	146,162,200	24	..
Central African Rep.	4,505,945	40.6	1.9	7	61.3	38.7	47	0.32	72.6	..	159,554	27,047
Chad	11,506,130	45.7	2.6	9	72.9	27.1	49	0.29	69.7	..	55,014	338,495
Comoros	675,000	38.1	2.4	363	71.9	28.1	66	0.43	69.4	11,345,750	268	1b
Congo, Dem. Rep.	67,827,495	46.7	2.7	30	65.4	34.6	48	0.24	66.7	..	455,852	185,809
Congo, Rep.	3,758,678	40.5	2.0	11	38.3	61.7	54	0.49	64.6	13,671,710	20,544	111,411
Cote d'Ivoire	21,570,746	40.6	2.3	68	50.6	49.4	58	0.40	60.4	185,470,800	23,153	24,604
Equatorial Guinea	693,385	41.0	2.5	25	60.5	39.5	51	0.54	62.6	..	344	..
Eritrea	5,223,994	41.5	2.9	52	78.8	21.2	60	..	65.6	..	209,168	4,751
Ethiopia	84,975,606	43.5	2.6	85	82.7	17.3	56	0.33	80.6	261,602,000	62,889	121,886
Gabon	1,501,266	36.1	1.8	6	14.5	85.5	61	0.65	58.2	10,336,600	144	8,845
Gambia, The	1,750,732	42.3	2.6	175	42.7	57.3	56	0.39	72.1	79,801,170	1,973	10,118
Ghana	24,332,755	38.4	2.1	107	49.2	50.8	57	0.47	65.2	114,455,700	14,893	13,658
Guinea	10,323,755	42.8	2.5	42	65.1	34.9	58	0.34	81.2	63,690,000	10,920	15,325
Guinea-Bissau	1,647,380	42.6	2.2	59	70.1	29.9	48	0.29	66.9	46,685,631	1,109	7,898
Kenya	40,862,900	42.8	2.6	72	78.1	21.9	55	0.47	73.0	1,686,228,000	9,620	358,928
Lesotho	2,084,182	38.8	0.8	69	73.8	26.2	45	0.43	54.1	414,088,400	10	..
Liberia	4,101,767	42.7	3.6	43	39.2	60.8	59	0.30	65.9	54,243,430	71,599	6,952
Madagascar	20,146,442	42.9	2.6	35	70.1	29.9	61	0.43	83.3	10,290,640	274	..
Malawi	14,900,841	46.2	3.1	158	80.7	19.3	54	0.38	72.1	873,950	130	5,443
Mali	15,369,809	44.2	3.0	13	67.3	32.7	49	0.31	47.0	404,674,100	2,926	13,538
Mauritania	3,365,675	39.5	2.3	3	58.8	41.2	57	0.43	47.2	1,881,330	39,143	26,795
Mauritius	1,282,000	22.6g	0.5	632	57.5	42.5	73	0.70	53.8	211,174,400	23	..
Mozambique	23,405,670	44.0	2.2	30	62.4	37.6	48	0.28	77.9	111,125,300	136	3,547
Namibia	2,212,037	36.9	1.9	3	62.6	37.4	62	0.61	42.9	13,605,110	921	7,163
Niger	15,891,482	49.9	3.9	13	83.4	16.6	52	0.26	59.8	89,135,337	822	325
Nigeria	158,258,917	42.5	2.3	174	50.9	49.1	48	0.42	51.8	9,584,753,000	15,609	9,127
Rwanda	10,277,212	42.3	2.8	417	81.4	18.6	51	0.39	80.3	92,617,970	129,109	54,016
São Tomé & Principe	165,397	40.7	1.6	172	38.6	61.4	66	0.49	..	2,000,000	33	..
Senegal	12,860,717	43.6	2.6	67	57.4	42.6	56	0.41	66.0	1,364,716,895	16,305	22,151
Sierra Leone	5,835,664	43.4	2.4	81	61.9	38.1	48	0.32	64.8	46,706,090	15,417	9,051
Somalia	9,358,602	44.9	2.4	15	63.0	37.0	50	..	66.5	..	678,309	1,815
South Africa	49,962,243	30.5	1.3	41	38.8	61.2	52	0.60	41.1	902,262,500	384	47,974
Sudan	43,551,941	39.1	2.5	18	55.7	44.3	58	0.38	47.3	2,992,686,000	368,195	186,292
Swaziland	1,201,904	39.3	1.4	70	74.8	25.2	46	0.50	50.4	93,457,760	32	759
Tanzania	45,039,573	44.7	2.9	51	74.0	26.0	56	0.40	78.0	23,288,820	1,204	118,731
Togo	6,780,030	39.9	2.4	125	57.3	42.7	63	0.43	64.6	306,752,700	18,378	8,531
Uganda	33,796,461	48.9	3.3	171	86.9	13.1	53	0.42	83.0	749,698,000	7,554	127,345
Zambia	12,926,409	46.2	1.6	17	64.4	35.6	46	0.39	61.2	41,260,000	206	56,785
Zimbabwe	12,644,041	39.9	1.0	33	62.2	37.8	45	0.14	64.9	..	22,449	3,995
Middle East & North Africa	383,545,468	30.9	1.8	35	39.2	60.8	71	..	46.4	35,011,470,410	2,017,484	7,834,349
Algeria	35,422,589	27.3	1.5	15	34.1	65.9	73	0.68	49.4	2,058,691,000	8,185	94,137

TABLE 1 – World Demographics

	Gross Domestic Product (GDP) 2009-2010				Public spending (% of GDP)			Exports of goods & services (current million US$) 2007-2010	Imports of goods & services (current million US$) 2007-2010	Food exports	Food imports	Paved roads (% of total roads) 2005-2010	Mobile cellular subscriptions 2009
	total (current million US$)	growth (annual %)	per capita (current US$)	per capita PPP (current int'l$)	education 2007-2010	health 2009	military 2007-2010			as % of merchandise 2005-2010			
World	63,048,775	4.2	9,197	11,128	4.4	6.1	2.7	15,893,554	15,511,170	8.4	7.9	..	4,672,420,222
High-income countries	43,002,153	3.1	38,293	37,283	5.1	7.4	2.9	11,303,217	11,169,728	7.7	7.9	86.9	1,235,569,664
Low- & middle-income countries	19,997,406	7.6	3,489	6,016	3.9	2.9	2.1	4,601,320	4,341,016	11.2	8.1	..	3,436,850,558
Sub-Saharan Africa	1,112,012	4.8	1,290	2,237	3.8	2.9	1.7	297,909	320,039	13.7	11.1	..	313,618,084
Angola	84,391	2.3	4,443	6,064	2.6	4.1	4.2	39,432	34,901	..	..	..	8,109,421
Benin	6,633	3.0	720	1,514	3.5	2.3	1.0	922	1,875	40.6	30.7	..	5,033,349
Botswana	14,857	7.2	7,513	13,991	8.9	8.2	3.1	3,971	5,273	5.1	13.1	32.6	1,874,101
Burkina Faso	8,820	9.2	542	1,260	4.6	3.9	1.3	665	1,547	26.8	15.7	..	3,299,000
Burundi	1,611	3.9	189	399	8.3	6.0	3.8	99	432	67.5	12.5	..	838,414
Cameroon	22,394	2.6	1,122	2,223	3.7	1.6	1.5	5,896	6,856	12.0	18.0	..	7,397,159
Cape Verde	1,648	5.4	3,215	3,826	5.9	2.9	0.6	366	1,013	72.6	29.4	..	392,000
Central African Republic	2,013	3.3	447	765	1.3	1.6	1.8	290	449	0.8	17.1	..	168,000
Chad	7,588	4.3	659	1,327	3.2	3.9	6.4	2,879	4,794	..	..	..	2,686,000
Comoros	541	2.1	802	1,185	7.6	2.1	..	79	258	13.8	19.5	..	100,000
Congo, Dem. Rep.	13,145	7.2	194	335	..	4.9	1.1	1,017	2,298	..	..	..	10,163,391
Congo, Rep.	11,898	8.8	3,165	4,532	1.8[a]	1.6	1.2	6,884	4,876	..	..	7.1	2,171,000
Cote d'Ivoire	22,780	3.0	1,056	1,725	4.6	1.0	1.6	9,722	7,866	48.2	23.2	7.9	13,345,890
Equatorial Guinea	14,007	0.9	20,200	34,824	..	3.4	..	7,713	4,328	..	..	..	445,000
Eritrea	2,117	2.2	405	545	2.0	1.0	..	84	379	..	..	..	141,130
Ethiopia	29,717	10.1	350	1,009	5.5	2.0	1.3	3,011	8,229	77.5	10.9	13.7	4,051,703
Gabon	13,011	5.7	8,667	14,968	..	1.7	1.1	5,773	3,685	0.8	16.6	..	1,373,000
Gambia, The	807	5.0	461	1,382	..	3.0	0.7	223	368	53.0	34.3	..	1,433,000
Ghana	31,306	6.6	1,287	1,629	5.4[a]	3.1	0.4	7,982	10,820	63.5	14.8	14.9	15,108,916
Guinea	4,511	1.9	437	1,047	2.4	0.9	..	1,671	1,865	2.5	13.2	..	5,607,000
Guinea-Bissau	879	3.5	533	1,083	..	1.6	2.1[a]	..	..	98.7	50.7	..	560,345
Kenya	31,409	5.3	769	1,621	7.0	1.5	1.9	7,413	11,253	44.0	15.4	..	19,364,560
Lesotho	2,132	3.3	1,023	1,598	12.4	5.6	2.8	809	1,764	..	..	..	661,000
Liberia	986	5.5	240	405	2.8	5.3	0.8	262	1,454	..	..	..	842,000
Madagascar	8,721	1.6	433	989	3.0	2.8	1.1	2,447	4,484	28.8	10.7	..	5,997,436
Malawi	5,106	7.1	343	876	..	3.6	1.2	1,420	1,783	86.6	13.1	..	2,400,000
Mali	9,251	4.5	602	1,057	4.4	2.7	2.0	1,871	2,542	28.1	12.4	19.0	3,742,000
Mauritania	3,636	5.0	1,080	1,984	2.9	1.6	3.8	1,504	2,043	12.5	28.2	26.8	2,182,249
Mauritius	9,729	4.0	7,589	13,568	3.2	2.1	0.2	4,161	5,074	32.4	21.7	98.0	1,086,748
Mozambique	9,586	7.2	410	934	5.0[b]	4.1	0.9	2,454	4,287	23.3	15.4	20.8	5,970,781
Namibia	12,170	4.8	5,502	6,633	6.4	4.0	3.3	4,319	5,548	22.5	13.9	..	1,217,000
Niger	5,549	8.8	349	705	4.5	3.5	1.0[a]	512[a]	824[a]	18.3	24.9	20.7	2,599,000
Nigeria	193,669	7.9	1,224	2,365	..	2.1	0.9	62,054	46,999	4.5	11.8	..	73,099,312
Rwanda	5,628	7.5	548	1,194	4.1	3.9	1.4	610	1,524	42.3	12.4	..	2,429,252
São Tomé & Príncipe	197	4.5	1,190	1,880	..	2.9	..	..	..	92.4	35.9	..	64,000
Senegal	12,954	4.2	1,007	1,853	5.8	3.1	1.6	3,082	5,637	29.5	24.2	..	6,901,492
Sierra Leone	1,905	4.9	326	825	4.3	0.9	2.3	305	554	..	..	..	1,160,000
Somalia	..	..	..	..	..	..	..	..	..	..	..	..	641,000
South Africa	363,704	2.8	7,280	10,492	5.4	3.4	1.4	77,883	80,328	10.2	6.5	..	46,436,000
Sudan	62,046	4.5	1,425	2,239	..	2.0	4.2	8,230	11,391	5.6	14.9	..	15,339,895
Swaziland	3,645	1.1	3,033	4,966	7.8	4.0	2.1	1,794	2,295	21.1	20.5	..	656,000
Tanzania	23,057	7.0	527	1,423	6.8	3.8	1.0	4,963	7,511	35.5	8.9	7.4	17,469,486
Togo	3,153	3.4	465	881	4.6	1.7	2.0	1,048	1,561	15.7	14.6	21.0	2,187,334
Uganda	17,011	5.2	503	1,249	3.2	1.6	2.2	3,753	5,557	63.0	13.0	..	9,383,734
Zambia	16,193	7.6	1,253	1,550	1.3	2.5	1.7	4,560	4,118	7.5	6.5	..	4,406,682
Zimbabwe	7,474	9.0	591	..	..	..	2.8	2,040	3,678	19.3	22.4	..	2,991,000
Middle East & North Africa	2,176,845	2.6	5,781	9,984	5.1	2.9	6.3	1,366,201	949,268	2.1	11.1	71.0	295,860,955
Algeria	159,426	3.0	4,501	8,333	4.3	5.0	3.8	56,798	50,772	0.3	16.3	73.5	32,729,824

TABLE 1 – World Demographics

| | Population | | | | | | Life expectancy at birth (years) 2009 | HDI index 2010 | Employment to pop. ratio for people above age 15 (% of total population) 2008-2009 | Workers' remittances & compensation received by employees (current US$) 2009 | Refugee population 2009 | |
	total 2010	ages 0-14 (% of total pop.) 2009	growth (annual %) 2010	density (people per sq. km of land area) 2010	rural (% of total pop.) 2009	urban (% of total pop.) 2009					by country or territory of origin	by country or territory of asylum
Bahrain	807,131	26.4	2.0	1,062	11.4	88.6	76	0.80	61.0	..	79	139
Djibouti	879,053	36.1	1.7	38	12.3	87.7	56	0.40	..	32,466,620	622	12,111
Egypt, Arab Rep.	84,474,427	32.3	1.8	85	57.2	42.8	70	0.62	43.2	7,149,600,000	6,990	94,406
Iran, Islamic Rep.	73,864,000	24.1	1.3	45	31.0	69.0	72	0.70	48.9	1,044,671,000	72,774	1,070,488
Iraq	32,297,391	41.1	2.5	74	33.5	66.5	68	..	37.1	70,900,000[d]	1,785,212	35,218
Israel	7,577,000	27.7	1.8	350	8.3	91.7	82	0.87	50.4	1,267,000,000	1,310	17,736
Jordan	6,093,000	34.5	2.4	69	21.5	78.5	73	0.68	37.9	3,597,042,000	2,129	2,434,489
Kuwait	2,863,000	23.4	2.4	161	1.6	98.4	78	0.77	65.3	..	938	221
Lebanon	4,254,583	25.3	0.7	416	12.9	87.1	72	..	45.9	7,558,139,000	16,260	476,053
Libya	6,545,619	30.1	1.9	4	22.3	77.7	75	0.75	48.6	14,380,730	2,202	9,005
Morocco	32,381,283	28.4	1.2	73	43.6	56.4	72	0.57	46.1	6,269,542,000	2,286	773
Oman	2,905,114	31.5	2.1	9	28.3	71.7	76	..	51.4	39,011,700	64	26
Qatar	1,508,322	16.0	6.8	130	4.3	95.7	76	0.80	76.9	..	68	29
Saudi Arabia	25,988,900	32.4	2.3	13	17.7	82.3	73	0.75	47.2	217,440,000	633	575
Syrian Arab Republic	21,615,919	35.0	2.5	118	45.4	54.6	74	0.59	44.8	1,332,498,000	17,914	1,526,575
Tunisia	10,535,100	23.2	1.0	68	33.1	66.9	74	0.68	41.0	1,964,489,000	2,260	92
United Arab Emirates	4,707,307	19.2	2.3	56	22.1	77.9	78	0.82	75.9	..	414	279
West Bank & Gaza	4,152,102	44.9	2.7	690	28.0	72.0	74	..	30.2	1,260,806,000	95,201	1,885,188
Yemen, Rep.	24,255,928	43.8	2.8	46	68.8	31.2	63	0.44	39.0	1,160,000,000	1,934	170,854
South Asia	**1,590,678,804**	**32.2**	**1.5**	**333**	**70.2**	**29.8**	**64**	**..**	**56.3**	**75,060,596,700**	**3,192,116**	**2,263,369**
Afghanistan	30,605,401	46.1	2.7	47	75.6	24.4	44	0.35	55.2	..	2,887,123	37
Bangladesh	164,425,491	31.5	1.3	1,263	72.4	27.6	67	0.47	67.9	10,523,100,000	10,432	228,586
Bhutan	708,484	30.5	1.6	18	64.4	35.6	67	..	61.1	..	89,070	..
India	1,170,938,000	31.3	1.3	394	70.2	29.8	64	0.52	55.6	49,468,370,000	19,514	185,323
Maldives	313,920	28.0	1.4	1,046	60.8	39.2	72	0.60	57.3	3,714,700	16	..
Nepal	29,852,682	36.5	1.8	208	82.3	17.7	67	0.43	61.5	2,985,612,000	5,108	108,461
Pakistan	173,383,000	36.9	2.1	225	63.4	36.6	67	0.49	51.5	8,717,000,000	35,132	1,740,711
Sri Lanka	20,451,826	24.3	0.7	326	84.9	15.1	74	0.66	54.7	3,362,800,000	145,721	251
East Asia & Pacific	**2,196,942,469**	**21.8**	**0.7**	**90**	**52.0**	**48.0**	**73**	**..**	**68.2**	**97,113,930,779**	**997,571**	**514,077**
Australia	22,327,200	19.0[h]	2.0	3	11.1	88.9	82	0.94	59.4	4,089,076,000	28	22,548
Brunei Darussalam	407,045	26.8	1.8	77	24.7	75.3	78	0.80	63.3	..	1	..
Cambodia	14,138,255	33.3	1.1	80	77.8	22.2	62	0.49	74.6	337,824,000	17,025	135
China	1,338,300,000	20.2	0.5	143	56.0	44.0	73	0.66	71.0	48,729,430,000	200,638	300,989
Fiji	854,098	31.3	0.6	47	47.1	52.9	69	0.67	56.3	153,642,700	1,892	2
Hong Kong SAR, China	7,041,270	12.0	0.5	6,757	0.0	100.0	83	0.86	56.6	347,792,400	12	86
Indonesia	232,516,771	27.0	1.1	128	47.4	52.6	71	0.60	61.8	6,792,907,000	18,213	798
Japan	127,380,000	13.3	-0.1	349	33.4	66.6	83	0.88	54.2	1,776,459,000	150	2,332
Kiribati	99,547	..	1.5	123	56.1	43.9	61[a]	..	..	8,183,240	33	..
Korea, Dem. Rep.	23,990,703	21.7	0.4	199	37.0	63.0	67	..	63.9	..	881	..
Korea, Rep.	48,875,000	16.8	0.3	504	18.3	81.7	80	0.88	58.1	2,522,000,000	573	268
Lao PDR	6,436,093	37.5	1.8	28	68.0	32.0	65	0.50	77.7	37,576,340	8,398	..
Macao SAR, China	547,591	12.9	1.8	19,557	0.0	100.0	81	..	63.9	724,792,700	9	6
Malaysia	27,913,990	29.5	1.6	85	28.7	71.3	75	0.74	60.5	1,130,872,000	532	66,137
Mongolia	2,701,117	26.0	1.1	2	42.7	57.3	67	0.62	51.6	199,618,700	1,495	11
Myanmar	50,495,672	26.8	0.9	77	66.8	33.2	62	0.45	74.4	137,314,300	406,669	..
New Zealand	4,370,700	20.4	1.3	17	13.3	86.7	80	0.91	62.7	627,738,700	10	3,289
Papua New Guinea	6,888,387	39.8	2.3	15	87.5	12.5	61	0.43	70.2	12,013,890	70	9,703
Philippines	93,616,853	33.9	1.8	314	34.3	65.7	72	0.64	60.1	19,766,000,000	993	95
Samoa	178,943	39.4	0.1	63	76.8	23.2	72	..	..	124,390,900	4[d]	..
Singapore	5,140,300	16.3	3.0	7,343	0.0	100.0	81	0.85	61.6	..	80	7
Solomon Islands	535,699	39.1	2.4	19	81.7	18.3	67	0.49	64.5	2,380,829	66	..
Thailand	68,139,238	21.7	0.6	133	66.3	33.7	69	0.65	71.5	1,637,093,000	502	105,297
Timor-Leste	1,124,355	45.0	2.2	76	72.3	27.7	62	0.50	66.8	..	7	1
Tuvalu	9,827	..	0.2	328	50.1	49.9	..	..	..	..	..	..

TABLE 1 – World Demographics

	Gross Domestic Product (GDP) 2009-2010				Public spending (% of GDP)			Exports of goods & services (current million US$) 2007-2010	Imports of goods & services (current million US$) 2007-2010	Food exports	Food imports	Paved roads (% of total roads) 2005-2010	Mobile cellular subscriptions 2009
	total (current million US$)	growth (annual %)	per capita (current US$)	per capita PPP (current int'l$)	education 2007-2010	health 2009	military 2007-2010			as % of merchandise 2005-2010			
Bahrain	20,595	6.3d	26,021	35,006d	2.9	3.1	3.6	21,213	16,277	0.4	5.2	81.5	1,578,000
Djibouti	1,049	5.0	1,214	2,309	8.4	5.3	3.7	484	654	0.4	29.3	..	128,776
Egypt, Arab Rep.	218,912	5.2	2,591	6,031	3.8	2.1	2.1	47,185	60,048	10.7	17.2	86.9	55,352,232
Iran, Islamic Rep.	331,015	1.8	4,540	11,504	4.7	2.2	2.7	92,050	61,612	4.3	1.9	73.3	52,555,000
Iraq	82,150	0.8	2,544	3,506	..	2.8	6.3	..	..	0.0	..	..	19,722,000
Israel	217,334	4.7	28,683	28,726	5.9	4.5	6.9	67,707	62,942	3.4	7.6	100.0	9,022,000
Jordan	27,574	3.1	4,525	5,663	..	6.0	5.5	10,915	16,300	16.6	17.0	100.0	6,014,366
Kuwait	148,023d	4.4c	54,260d	48,403c	3.8	2.8	3.2	98,345	37,956	0.3	14.7	..	2,907,000d
Lebanon	39,155	7.0	9,203	13,859	1.8	4.0	4.1	7,688	16,234	16.4	15.3	..	1,526,000
Libya	62,360	2.1	9,714	16,425	..	2.6	1.2	62,780	25,589	..	..	..	5,004,000
Morocco	91,196	3.3	2,771	4,607	5.6	1.9	3.3	26,121	36,088	22.1	11.2	67.8	25,310,760
Oman	46,114	12.8d	16,207	25,341d	3.9	2.4	8.7	35,750	22,887	3.1	10.9	43.5	3,970,563
Qatar	98,313	8.6	69,754	90,950	..	2.0	2.2	45,958	30,692	0.0	6.0	..	2,472,130
Saudi Arabia	375,766	0.6	14,799	23,369	5.6	3.3	11.0	201,963	160,639	0.5	11.3	21.5	44,864,356
Syrian Arab Republic	59,103	3.2	2,734	4,964	4.9	0.9	4.2	17,680	18,636	22.0	14.0	91.0	9,697,061
Tunisia	44,291	3.7	4,204	8,536	7.1	3.4	1.4	20,568	21,894	9.2	8.6	75.2	9,753,926
United Arab Emirates	230,252	-0.7	50,070	57,473	1.2	1.9	5.6	180,885	132,498	0.8	6.6	..	10,671,878
West Bank & Gaza	4,015a	6.3a	1,123a	2465a	..	..	..	564a	2,738a	..	..	100.0	1,224,000
Yemen, Rep.	26,365	3.8	1,118	2,458	5.2	1.6	4.4	..	..	5.7	27.8	8.7	3,842,000
South Asia	**2,088,236**	**8.8**	**1,313**	**3,202**	**2.9**	**1.3**	**2.6**	**319,465**	**404,597**	**11.4**	**6.8**	**51.8**	**712,967,921**
Afghanistan	11,757d	3.4d	405d	1,070d	..	1.6	1.8	1,831	5,603	54.7	18.3	29.3	12,000,000
Bangladesh	100,076	5.8	609	1,486	2.4	1.1	1.1	17,360	23,727	6.5	22.5	..	50,400,000
Bhutan	1,516	7.4	2,140	5,420	4.8	4.5	..	741	617	6.1	14.6	..	327,052
India	1,729,010	9.7	1,477	3,586	3.1	1.4	2.7	269,732	330,849	8.0	4.2	49.3	525,089,984
Maldives	1,480	4.8	4,714	5,719	11.2	5.2	..	988	1,388	98.4	15.9	100.0	457,770
Nepal	15,701	4.6	526	1,194	4.6	2.1	1.6	1,968	4,689	25.1	15.4	55.9	7,617,769
Pakistan	174,799	4.4	1,008	2,677	2.7	0.9	3.0	20,805	33,002	16.7	11.4	65.4	102,980,000
Sri Lanka	49,552	8.0	2,423	5,141	..	1.8	3.5	8,969	11,700	26.4	15.7	..	14,095,346
East Asia & Pacific	**16,219,241**	**7.1**	**7,383**	**9,668**	**3.1**	**4.2**	**1.6**	**4,266,537**	**3,871,270**	**4.8**	**6.6**	**65.0**	**1,435,767,036**
Australia	924,843	1.3	42,279	39,545	4.5	5.6	1.9	205,671	224,588	14.1	5.8	..	24,220,000
Brunei Darussalam	10,732	-1.8	26,852	48,522	..	2.6	2.6	8,238	2,893	0.1	17.0	77.2	426,323
Cambodia	11,343	6.7	802	2,150	2.1	1.6	1.2	6,228	6,546	0.7	7.0	..	5,593,000
China	5,878,629	10.3	4,393	7,536	..	2.3	2.0	1,333,300	1,113,200	2.9	4.9	53.5	747,000,000
Fiji	3,009	0.1	3,524	4,527	..	2.5	1.4	1,330	1,744	70.2	20.6	..	640,000
Hong Kong SAR, China	224,458	7.0	31,877	46,331	4.5	..	..	408,132	393,067	6.9	4.4	100.0	12,206,910
Indonesia	706,558	6.1	3,039	4,429	2.8	1.2	0.9	130,339	115,226	17.3	8.9	59.1	159,247,632
Japan	5,497,813	5.1	43,161	34,013	3.5	6.7	1.0	636,143	620,791	0.7	10.5	79.6	114,917,000
Kiribati	151	1.8	1,519	2,450	..	10.3	..	..	..	82.4	42.3	..	1,000
Korea, Dem. Rep.	..	..	..	..	..	..	..	..	..	..	..	2.8	69,261
Korea, Rep.	1,014,483	6.2	20,757	29,004	4.2	3.5	2.9	415,427	382,813	1.1	5.0	78.5	47,944,224
Lao PDR	7,491	8.4	1,164	2,449	2.3	0.8	0.4	1,791	2,429	..	..	13.5	3,234,642
Macao SAR, China	21,736	1.3	40,404	59,870	2.2	..	..	19,475	9,152	9.3	17.1	100.0	1,037,380
Malaysia	237,804	7.2	8,519	14,845	4.1	2.2	2.0	186,175	144,582	11.3	8.1	82.8	30,379,000
Mongolia	6,083	6.1	2,252	4,079	5.6	4.0	1.4	2,347	2,632	1.7	11.8	..	2,249,023
Myanmar	..	12.7	..	..	..	0.2	..	..	..	..	..	11.9	448,000
New Zealand	126,679	2.5	29,352	29,895	6.1	7.8	1.1	35,729	33,603	55.7	10.7	65.9	4,700,000
Papua New Guinea	9,480	8.0	1,376	2,443	..	2.5	0.5	4,572	4,509	..	..	..	900,000
Philippines	199,589	7.6	2,132	3,925	2.8	1.3	0.8	51,039	49,641	7.7	11.6	..	74,489,000
Samoa	565	1.0	3,159	4,468	5.7	6.1	..	166	291	21.4	30.1	..	151,000
Singapore	222,699	14.5	43,324	56,794	3.0	1.6	4.3	426,358	391,657	2.1	3.3	100.0	6,652,000
Solomon Islands	679	7.0	1,267	2,701	..	5.1	..	220	308	..	..	..	30,000
Thailand	318,847	7.8	4,679	8,612	4.1	3.3	1.8	180,335	152,588	15.1	5.5	..	83,057,000
Timor-Leste	701	7.4	623	921	16.8	8.8	11.8	..	..	96.3	17.6	..	..
Tuvalu	..	..	..	..	..	9.9	..	..	..	..	21.5	..	2,000

TABLE 1 – World Demographics

	Population						Life expectancy at birth (years) 2009	HDI index 2010	Employment to pop. ratio for people above age 15 (% of total population) 2008-2009	Workers' remittances & compensation received by employees (current US$) 2009	Refugee population 2009	
	total 2010	ages 0-14 (% of total pop.) 2009	growth (annual %) 2010	density (people per sq. km of land area) 2010	rural (% of total pop.) 2009	urban (% of total pop.) 2009					by country or territory of origin	by country or territory of asylum
Vanuatu	239,651	38.6	2.5	20	74.8	25.2	71	..	..	6,472,110	..	4
Vietnam	88,361,983	25.7	1.2	285	71.7	28.3	75	0.57	69.4	6,625,908,000	339,289	2,357
Europe & Central Asia	**893,314,336**	**17.4**	**0.4**	**33**	**30.2**	**69.8**	**75**	**..**	**52.8**	**128,417,503,990**	**738,922**	**1,649,545**
Albania	3,169,087	23.5	0.4	116	52.6	47.4	77	0.72	46.2	1,317,469,000	15,711	70
Armenia	3,090,379	20.3	0.2	109	36.2	63.8	74	0.70	38.1	769,453,200	18,000	3,607
Austria	8,381,780	14.9	0.2	102	32.6	67.4	80	0.85	54.5	3,285,937,000	12	38,906
Azerbaijan	8,883,200	24.2	1.2	108	47.9	52.1	70	0.71	60.0	1,273,725,000	16,939	1,642
Belarus	9,645,000	14.7	-0.2	48	26.1	73.9	70	0.73	52.3	357,800,000	5,525	580
Belgium	10,866,560	16.8	0.7	359	2.6	97.4	81	0.87	46.5	10,436,870,000	71	15,545
Bosnia & Herzegovina	3,759,633	15.4	-0.2	73	52.0	48.0	75	0.71	41.5	2,080,799,000	70,018	7,132
Bulgaria	7,561,910	13.4	-0.3	70	28.6	71.4	73	0.74	46.3	1,557,790,000	2,745	5,393
Croatia	4,430,003	15.1	-0.0	79	42.5	57.5	76	0.77	43.3	1,476,479,000	76,478	1,238
Cyprus	879,723	17.8	1.0	95	29.9	70.1	80	0.81	57.5	153,388,600	11	2,888
Czech Republic	10,534,920	14.1	0.4	136	26.5	73.5	77	0.84	54.3	1,200,799,000	1,067	2,323
Denmark	5,565,020	18.2	0.6	131	13.1	86.9	79	0.87	60.3	894,261,300	10	20,355
Estonia	1,340,200	15.1	-0.0	32	30.5	69.5	75	0.81	54.5	324,556,200	248	24
Finland	5,362,610	16.7k	0.5	18	36.4	63.6	80	0.87	54.7	859,404,700	6	7,447
France	64,876,618l	18.4	0.5	118	22.4	77.6	81	0.87	47.9	15,550,500,000	87	196,364
Georgia	4,452,800	16.8	0.9	78	47.2	52.8	72	0.70	54.3	714,335,400	15,020	870
Germany	81,635,580	13.5	-0.3	234	26.3	73.7	80	0.88	51.7	10,878,940,000	170	593,799
Greece	11,329,170	14.2	0.4	88	38.8	61.2	80	0.85	48.4	2,020,324,000	62	1,695
Hungary	10,004,970	14.8	-0.2	112	32.1	67.9	74	0.80	44.8	2,129,965,000	1,537	6,044
Iceland	318,450	20.6	-0.2	3	7.7	92.3	81	0.87	71.2	23,482,590	4	62
Ireland	4,451,310	20.7	0.0	65	38.4	61.6	80	0.89	57.8	575,684,400	7	9,571
Italy	60,574,530	14.2	0.6	206	31.8	68.2	81	0.85	43.6	2,682,861,000	45	54,965
Kazakhstan	16,316,050	23.7	2.4	6	41.8	58.2	68	0.71	63.5	123,657,600	3,744	4,340
Kosovo	1,815,000	..	0.6	167	..	..	70	..	..	..	..	..
Kyrgyz Republic	5,365,167	29.4	0.8	28	63.6	36.4	67	0.60	58.3	991,799,800	2,612	423
Latvia	2,242,830	13.8	-0.5	36	31.8	68.2	73	0.77	55.0	591,100,000	791	43
Lithuania	3,318,970	14.9	-0.6	53	32.9	67.1	73	0.78	50.2	1,169,199,000	501	793
Luxembourg	506,640	17.8	1.7	196	17.7	82.3	80	0.85	51.2	1,584,703,000	2c	3,230
Macedonia, FYR	2,060,563	18.0	0.2	82	32.6	67.4	74	0.70	34.8	381,064,500	7,926	1,542
Malta	417,700	15.6	0.7	1,305	5.5	94.5	80	0.81	45.2	45,693,360	9	5,955
Moldova	3,562,062	16.9	-0.1	124	58.5	41.5	69	0.62	44.7	1,210,760,000	5,925	141
Montenegro	625,516	19.4	0.2	47	40.2	59.8	74	0.77	..	..	2,582	24,019
Netherlands	16,622,560	17.8	0.6	492	17.6	82.4	81	0.89	59.3	3,691,353,000	44	76,008
Norway	4,882,930m	19.0	1.2	16	22.5	77.5	81	0.94	62.3	631,471,300	4	37,826
Poland	38,177,910	15.0	0.1	125	38.7	61.3	76	0.79	48.2	8,126,000,000	2,059	15,320
Portugal	10,641,710	15.3	0.1	116	39.9	60.1	79	0.79	55.7	3,584,702,000	31	389
Romania	21,449,980	15.2	-0.2	93	45.6	54.4	73	0.77	48.1	4,929,000,000	4,358	1,069
Russian Federation	141,750,000	14.8	-0.1	9	27.2	72.8	69	0.72	56.7	5,358,730,000	109,455	4,880
Serbia	7,289,300	17.7	-0.4	82	47.8	52.2	74	0.74	44.4	5,406,200,000	195,626	86,351
Slovak Republic	5,429,970	15.4	0.2	113	43.3	56.7	75	0.82	52.6	1,670,910,000	334	401
Slovenia	2,065,110	13.8	1.1	103	51.7	48.3	79	0.83	54.1	279,075,600	39	289
Spain	46,217,400	14.8	0.6	93	22.7	77.3	82	0.86	48.6	9,904,310,000	34	3,970
Sweden	9,394,130	16.6	1.0	23	15.4	84.6	81	0.88	57.6	651,515,800	19	81,356
Switzerland	7,790,010	15.3	0.8	195	26.5	73.5	82	0.87	61.2	2,524,300,000	18	46,203
Tajikistan	7,074,845	36.9	1.7	51	73.5	26.5	67	0.58	55.4	1,748,152,000	562	2,679
Turkey	75,705,147	26.8	1.2	98	30.9	69.1	72	0.68	42.3	970,000,000	146,387	10,350
Turkmenistan	5,176,502	29.5	1.3	11	50.9	49.1	65	0.67	58.3	..	743	60
Ukraine	45,759,961	13.9	-0.5	79	32.0	68.0	69	0.71	53.5	5,073,000,000	24,522	7,334
United Kingdom	62,246,610	17.4	0.7	257	10.0	90.0	80	0.85	56.3	7,251,676,000	156	269,363
Uzbekistan	28,160,361	29.3	1.4	66	63.1	36.9	68	0.62	57.5	..	6,669	555

TABLE 1 – World Demographics

	Gross Domestic Product (GDP) 2009-2010				Public spending (% of GDP)			Exports of goods & services (current million US$) 2007-2010	Imports of goods & services (current million US$) 2007-2010	Food exports	Food imports	Paved roads (% of total roads) 2005-2010	Mobile cellular subscriptions 2009
	total (current million US$)	growth (annual %)	per capita (current US$)	per capita PPP (current int'l$)	education 2007-2010	health 2009	military 2007-2010			as % of merchandise 2005-2010			
Vanuatu	729	3.0	3,042	4,574	4.8	3.3	..	264	343	61.5	21.3	..	126,452
Vietnam	103,572	6.8	1,172	3,130	5.3	2.8	2.2	66,375	76,434	20.0	7.0	47.6	88,566,000
Europe & Central Asia	**20,075,279**	**2.2**	**22,473**	**24,273**	**4.9**	**7.3**	**2.0**	**7,145,311**	**6,815,441**	**8.9**	**9.6**	**89.1**	**1,075,388,296**
Albania	11,786	3.5	3,719	8,915	..	2.8	2.1	3,443	6,533	5.6	17.1	..	4,161,615
Armenia	9,265	1.0	2,998	5,357	3.0	2.0	4.0	1,045	3,176	19.9	19.3	90.5	2,620,000
Austria	376,162	2.0	44,879	39,712	5.4	8.2	0.9	192,567	175,270	7.4	7.9	100.0	11,773,000
Azerbaijan	51,092	5.0	5,752	10,052	2.8	1.4	3.5	22,583	10,658	3.6	15.7	50.6	7,757,120
Belarus	54,713	7.6	5,673	13,951	4.5	4.1	1.8	24,884	30,461	10.7	7.8	88.6	9,686,200
Belgium	467,472	2.2	43,019	37,491	6.0	8.1	1.1	343,775	330,868	9.7	9.4	78.2	12,419,000
Bosnia & Herzegovina	16,888	0.8	4,492	8,752	..	6.7	1.5	5,699	9,881	7.7	19.0	52.3	3,257,239
Bulgaria	47,714	0.2	6,310	13,746	4.1	4.4	2.3	23,305	27,165	16.6	10.0	98.4	10,617,148
Croatia	60,852	-1.2	13,736	19,490	4.6	6.6	1.8	22,748	24,843	12.8	10.1	86.9	6,035,070
Cyprus	25,039	-1.0	31,280	30,710	4.1	2.5	2.2	11,736	14,570	37.1	15.5	64.6	977,521
Czech Republic	192,152	2.3	18,239	25,276	4.2	6.1	1.5	132,277	121,390	4.5	6.3	..	14,258,404
Denmark	310,405	2.1	55,778	39,409	7.8	9.0	1.4	147,894	136,104	18.9	13.3	100.0	7,406,000
Estonia	18,674	1.8	13,934	20,024	4.8	5.3	2.3	13,473	12,449	10.2	12.5	28.8	2,720,538
Finland	238,801	3.1	44,531	36,667	5.9	7.0	1.5	88,935	83,086	2.3	7.3	65.5	7,700,000
France	2,560,002	1.5	39,460	33,820	5.6	9.0	2.4	610,680	662,142	12.4	9.3	100.0	59,543,000
Georgia	11,667	6.4	2,620	5,035	3.2	2.9	5.6	3,172	5,267	17.7	15.3	94.1	2,837,000
Germany	3,309,669	3.6	40,542	37,622	4.5	8.6	1.4	1,359,727	1,195,136	5.6	7.9	..	105,000,000
Greece	304,865	-4.5	26,910	28,129	4.0ª	6.7	4.0	61,522	96,552	25.4	12.8	..	13,295,093
Hungary	130,419	1.2	13,035	20,315	5.2	5.1	1.3	125,977	124,080	7.9	5.3	37.7	11,792,475
Iceland	12,594	-3.5	39,548	34,834	7.4	6.7	0.1	6,429	5,364	43.5	11.5	36.6	348,984
Ireland	203,892	-1.0	45,805	39,996	4.9	7.8	0.6	201,130	167,231	8.8	12.0	100.0	4,871,098
Italy	2,051,412	1.3	33,866	31,508	4.3	7.3	1.7	506,414	514,810	8.1	10.2	..	90,613,000
Kazakhstan	142,987	7.0	8,764	12,050	2.8	2.7	1.2	48,444	38,956	3.8	8.5	89.9	14,995,325
Kosovo	5,591	4.0	3,080	..	4.3	..	..	758	2,929	..	..	..	..
Kyrgyz Republic	4,616	-1.4	860	2,257	5.9	3.5	3.6	2,283	3,697	23.9	16.9	..	4,487,123
Latvia	24,010	-0.3	10,705	16,312	5.0	3.9	2.6	11,048	11,293	17.3	16.6	100.0	2,243,000
Lithuania	36,306	1.3	10,939	18,193	4.7	4.5	1.7	28,388	33,778	18.9	14.0	28.6	4,961,499
Luxembourg	55,096	3.5	108,747	89,626	..	5.8	0.7	88,594	71,210	8.5	12.0	..	719,000
Macedonia, FYR	9,118	0.7	4,425	11,072	..	4.6	2.1	4,085	6,203	18.2	13.2	56.5	1,943,216
Malta	7,987	-2.1	19,248	24,703	6.4	5.6	0.6	5,925	5,883	4.7	15.6	87.5	422,083
Moldova	5,809	6.9	1,631	3,087	9.6	6.4	0.5	1,991	3,967	74.2	15.2	85.8	2,784,832
Montenegro	4,004	1.1	6,401	12,797	..	6.7	1.4	1,357	2,728	..	..	..	752,000
Netherlands	783,413	1.8	47,130	42,448	5.3	8.3	1.5	550,049	492,587	14.7	10.9	..	21,182,000
Norway	414,462	0.4	84,880	56,921	6.8	7.6	1.5	160,418	104,367	6.3	8.4	80.5	5,336,000
Poland	468,585	3.8	12,274	19,752	4.9	4.9	2.0	167,206	166,778	11.0	7.9	68.2	44,553,136
Portugal	228,538	1.3	21,476	25,575	5.2	7.9	2.0	65,116	82,991	11.3	13.1	..	15,178,000
Romania	161,624	0.9	7,535	14,282	4.3	4.3	1.4	53,687	64,838	7.4	9.1	..	25,377,000
Russian Federation	1,479,819	4.0	10,440	19,840	3.9	3.5	4.3	341,648	250,911	3.2	17.0	80.1	230,500,000
Serbia	39,128	1.8	5,368	11,493	4.7	6.3	2.2	11,800	18,889	18.6	5.8	47.7	9,912,339
Slovak Republic	89,034	0.5	16,397	23,912	3.6	5.7	1.5	87,169	90,921	4.7	6.9	87.0	5,497,719
Slovenia	47,763	1.2	23,129	27,392	5.7	6.4	1.8	28,561	27,823	4.2	8.9	100.0	2,100,435
Spain	1,407,405	-0.1	30,452	31,976	4.3	7.0	1.3	342,247	373,729	16.0	11.2	..	50,991,056
Sweden	458,004	5.5	48,754	38,885	6.6	7.8	1.3	196,955	169,066	4.9	9.9	23.6	11,426,000
Switzerland	523,772	2.6	67,236	46,424	5.2	6.7	0.8	254,229	200,401	3.9	6.3	100.0	9,255,000
Tajikistan	5,640	3.8	797	2,087	3.5	1.8	..	668	2,805	..	..	..	4,900,000
Turkey	735,264	8.9	9,712	14,741	..	5.1	2.8	142,853	150,082	10.8	4.4	..	62,779,552
Turkmenistan	21,074	8.1	4,071	7,628	..	1.2	..	15,079	9,145	..	..	..	1,500,000
Ukraine	137,929	4.2	3,014	6,674	5.3	3.8	2.9	52,578	54,543	23.8	10.5	97.8	55,333,216
United Kingdom	2,246,079	1.3	36,084	35,844	5.5	7.8	2.7	601,632	653,159	6.6	10.8	100.0	80,375,368
Uzbekistan	38,982	8.5	1,384	3,090	..	2.5	..	11,679	11,698	..	..	..	16,417,914

TABLE 1 – World Demographics

| | Population | | | | | Life expectancy at birth (years) 2009 | HDI index 2010 | Employment to pop. ratio for people above age 15 (% of total population) 2008-2009 | Workers' remittances & compensation received by employees (current US$) 2009 | Refugee population 2009 | |
	total 2010	ages 0-14 (% of total pop.) 2009	growth (annual %) 2010	density (people per sq. km of land area) 2010	rural (% of total pop.) 2009	urban (% of total pop.) 2009					by country or territory of origin	by country or territory of asylum
Latin America & Caribbean	**584,452,890**	**28.1**	**1.0**	**29**	**21.1**	**78.9**	**74**	**..**	**60.4**	**56,821,227,940**	**462,235**	**367,437**
Argentina	40,665,732	25.1	1.0	15	7.8	92.2	76	0.78	56.5	658,251,200	608	3,230
Bahamas, The	345,736	25.5	1.2	35	16.1	83.9	74	0.78	65.4	..	15	..
Belize	344,700	35.2	3.4	15	47.8	52.2	77	0.69	56.9	80,489,150	17	230
Bolivia	10,030,832	36.2	1.7	9	34.0	66.0	66	0.64	70.7	1,068,649,000	..	679
Brazil	194,946,470	25.9	0.9	23	14.0	86.0	73	0.70	63.9	4,234,281,000	973	4,232
Chile	17,134,708	22.7	1.0	23	11.3	88.7	79	0.78	49.6	4,400,000	1,312	1,539
Colombia	46,300,196	29.2	1.4	42	25.2	74.8	73	0.69	62.0	4,179,615,000	389,753	196
Costa Rica	4,639,827	25.9	1.3	91	36.2	63.8	79	0.72	57.2	513,091,800	344	19,116
Cuba	11,204,351	17.7	0.0	105	24.3	75.7	79	..	54.4	..	7,549	454
Dominican Republic	10,225,482	31.5	1.3	212	30.2	69.8	73	0.66	53.3	3,466,700,000	230	..
Ecuador	13,774,909	31.1	1.1	55	33.8	66.2	75	0.70	60.5	2,502,339,000	1,027	116,557
El Salvador	6,194,126	32.3	0.5	299	39.0	61.0	71	0.66	54.3	3,482,401,000	5,051	30
Guatemala	14,376,881	41.9	2.5	134	51.0	49.0	71	0.56	62.4	4,019,300,000	5,768	131
Guyana	761,442	29.7	-0.1	4	71.6	28.4	68	0.61	57.8	253,025,500	727	..
Haiti	9,958,175	36.3	-0.7	361	51.8	48.2	61	0.40	55.4	1,375,540,000	24,116	3
Honduras	7,615,584	37.4	2.0	68	51.7	48.3	72	0.60	56.3	2,520,245,000	1,166	19
Jamaica	2,712,091	29.4	0.5	250	46.5	53.5	72	0.69	56.2	1,911,999,000	909	26
Mexico	108,523,000	28.5	1.0	56	22.5	77.5	75	0.75	57.1	21,952,530,000	6,435	1,235
Nicaragua	5,822,265	35.1	1.4	48	43.0	57.0	73	0.57	58.3	768,400,000	1,478	120
Panama	3,508,475	29.3	1.6	47	26.0	74.0	76	0.75	58.7	175,400,000	105	16,923
Paraguay	6,459,727	34.0	1.7	16	39.1	60.9	72	0.64	72.8	609,200,000	77	89
Peru	29,496,120	30.3	1.1	23	28.5	71.5	73	0.72	68.8	2,377,792,000	6,271	1,108
Suriname	524,345	28.9	0.9	3	24.7	75.3	69	0.65	46.5	4,800,000	45	1
Trinidad & Tobago	1,343,725	20.7	0.4	262	86.4	13.6	70	0.74	60.7	99,299,940	240	37
Uruguay	3,356,584	22.8	0.3	19	7.6	92.4	76	0.77	56.4	100,757,000	188	168
Venezuela, RB	28,834,000	29.8	1.6	33	6.3	93.7	74	0.70	61.3	131,000,000	6,221	201,313
North America	**343,950,500**	**19.9**	**0.9**	**19**	**18.1**	**81.9**	**79**	**..**	**59.1**	**2,947,000,000**	**2,467**	**444,895**
Canada	34,173,900	16.5	1.3	4	19.5	80.5	81	0.89	61.2	..	99	169,434
United States	309,712,000	20.3	0.9	34	18.0	82.0	79	0.90	59.2	2,947,000,000	2,368	275,461

..   Data not available.
0   Zero, or rounds to zero at the displayed number of decimal places.
a   Data refers to 2005.
b   Data refers to 2006.
c   Data refers to 2007.
d   Data refers to 2008.
e   Data refers to 2009.
f   Data refers to 2010.
g   Including Agalega, Rodrigues, and Saint Brandon.
h   Including Christmas Island, Cocos (Keeling) Islands, and Norfolk Island.
k   Including Åland Islands.
l   Including overseas departments.
m   Including Svalbard and Jan Mayen Islands.

Notes and Sources for Tables on pages 182-184.

TABLE 1 – World Demographics

	Gross Domestic Product (GDP) 2009-2010				Public spending (% of GDP)			Exports of goods & services (current million US$) 2007-2010	Imports of goods & services (current million US$) 2007-2010	Food exports	Food imports	Paved roads (% of total roads) 2005-2010	Mobile cellular subscriptions 2009
	total (current million US$)	growth (annual %)	per capita (current US$)	per capita PPP (current int'l$)	education 2007-2010	health 2009	military 2007-2010			as % of merchandise 2005-2010			
Latin America & Caribbean	**5,181,851**	**6.2**	**8,866**	**11,429**	**4.0**	**3.9**	**1.5**	**929,646**	**960,234**	**17.9**	**8.2**	**..**	**517,247,930**
Argentina	368,712	9.2	9,067	15,794	4.9	6.3	0.8	65,581	49,152	50.5	3.7	..	51,891,000
Bahamas, The	7,538	0.9	21,803	24,987	..	3.2	..	3,278	4,928	20.1	18.4	..	358,812
Belize	1,432	2.0	4,153	6,566	5.7	3.6	1.1	844	952	57.3	12.7	..	161,783
Bolivia	19,786	4.2	1,973	4,768	6.3	3.1	1.6	6,194	5,706	19.6	9.2	..	7,148,400
Brazil	2,087,890	7.5	10,710	11,127	5.1	4.1	1.6	177,332	178,223	34.2	5.3	..	173,959,360
Chile	203,443	5.2	11,873	15,026	4.0	3.8	3.1	62,417	49,694	20.8	7.2	..	16,450,223
Colombia	288,189	4.3	6,224	9,391	4.8	5.4	4.1	38,045	42,877	15.5	10.3	..	42,159,612
Costa Rica	34,564	3.5	7,450	11,398	6.3	7.1	..	12,659	12,309	25.1	7.2	25.3	1,950,318
Cuba	62,704[d]	4.3[d]	5,596[d]	..	13.6	11.0	3.2	12,555	11,381	10.5	11.9	..	443,000
Dominican Republic	51,577	7.8	5,044	9,010	2.3	2.4	0.6	10,409	14,154	25.1	14.4	..	8,629,815
Ecuador	58,910	3.6	4,277	8,511	..	2.9	3.3	21,261	27,532	35.6	9.5	14.8	13,634,768
El Salvador	21,796	1.0	3,519	6,691	3.6	3.8	0.6	4,696	7,966	23.0	18.9	..	7,566,245
Guatemala	41,190	2.6	2,865	4,744	3.2	2.6	0.4	8,722	12,364	44.3	13.7	..	17,307,460
Guyana	2,222	4.4	2,918	3,064	6.1	7.2	..	698[a]	983[a]	59.9	15.1	..	281,368[a]
Haiti	6,710	-5.1	674	1,106	..	1.4	..	921	2,845	..	..	..	3,648,000
Honduras	15,400	2.6	2,022	3,883	..	3.4	0.8	6,028	8,701	54.2	18.8	..	7,714,000
Jamaica	13,995	-0.5	5,160	7,811	5.8	2.8	0.6	4,190	6,436	27.1	18.1	73.3	2,971,254
Mexico	1,039,662	5.5	9,580	15,224	4.8	3.1	0.5	243,584	256,171	7.0	7.3	35.3	83,527,872
Nicaragua	6,551	4.5	1,125	2,749	..	5.4	0.7	2,157	3,758	87.2	17.6	12.0	3,204,367
Panama	26,777	7.5	7,632	13,910	3.8	5.9	..	19,037	15,102	84.2	11.6	38.1	5,677,107
Paraguay	18,475	15.3	2,860	5,148	4.0	3.0	0.9	6,624	7,346	84.8	8.2	..	5,618,639
Peru	153,845	8.8	5,216	9,335	2.7	2.7	1.2	30,696	25,706	22.8	11.0	13.9	24,700,360
Suriname	3,252	3.1	6,257	7,597	..	3.7	..	545[a]	810[a]	2.2	11.7	..	763,912
Trinidad & Tobago	20,398	0.1	15,180	25,496	..	2.7	..	17,728	10,210	3.2	10.1	..	1,970,000
Uruguay	40,265	8.5	11,996	14,277	2.8	4.7	1.6	8,346	8,047	64.3	10.1	..	3,802,000
Venezuela, RB	387,852	-1.9	13,451	11,956	3.7	2.4	1.3	59,523	66,759	0.2	16.2	..	28,123,570
North America	**16,162,456**	**2.9**	**46,991**	**46,266**	**5.2**	**7.8**	**4.4**	**1,962,101**	**2,372,293**	**10.6**	**5.9**	**67.4**	**321,570,000**
Canada	1,574,052	3.1	46,060	38,841	4.9	7.5	1.4	383,652	406,545	11.5	8.1	..	23,081,000
United States	14,582,400	2.9	47,084	47,084	5.5	7.9	4.7	1,578,400	1,964,700	10.2	5.5	67.4	298,404,000

Millennium Development Goals: Progress Chart to Date

This chart provides an overview of progress on the eight Millennium Development Goals. Progress or lack of progress differs in every state, so regional overviews provide a snapshot at an aggregated level. In some instances, trends are driven by high performance or lack of performance by one or a small group of countries.

| Goals and Targets | Africa | | Asia | | | | Oceania | Latin America & Caribbean | Caucasus & Central Asia |
	Northern	sub-Saharan	Eastern	S. Eastern	Southern	Western			
GOAL 1: Eradicate extreme poverty and hunger									
Reduce extreme poverty by half	On Track	Off Track	On Track	On Track	Off Track	No Progress	No Data	Off Track	Off Track
Reduce hunger by half	On Track	Off Track	On Track	On Track	No Progress	No Progress	No Data	On Track	Off Track
GOAL 2: Achieve universal primary education									
Universal primary schooling	On Track	Off Track	Off Track	Off Track	On Track	Off Track	No Data	On Track	No Progress
GOAL 3: Promote gender equality and empower women									
Equal girls' enrollment in primary school	On Track	On Track	On Track	On Track	On Track	On Track	No Progress	On Track	On Track
Women's share of paid employment	Off Track	Off Track	On Track	Off Track	Off Track	Off Track	Off Track	On Track	On Track
Women's equal representation in national parliaments	Off Track	Off Track	No Progress	Off Track	Off Track	Off Track	Off Track	Off Track	Off Track
GOAL 4: Reduce child mortality									
Reduce mortality of under-five-year-olds by two-thirds	On Track	Off Track	On Track	Off Track	Off Track	Off Track	On Track	Off Track	Off Track
GOAL 5: Improve maternal health									
Reduce maternal mortality by three-quarters	On Track	No Progress	On Track	Off Track	Off Track	Off Track	Off Track	On Track	On Track
GOAL 6: Combat HIV/AIDS, malaria, and other diseases									
Halt and reverse spread of HIV/AIDS	No Progress	On Track	Off Track	Off Track	On Track	Off Track	On Track	Off Track	No Progress
Halt and reverse spread of tuberculosis	On Track	Off Track	On Track	On Track	On Track	On Track	On Track	On Track	Off Track
GOAL 7: Ensure environmental sustainability									
Reverse loss of forests	On Track	Off Track	On Track	No Progress	No Progress	On Track	No Progress	Off Track	No Progress
Halve proportion without improved drinking water	On Track	Off Track	On Track	On Track	On Track	Off Track	No Progress	On Track	Off Track
Halve proportion without sanitation	On Track	Off Track	Off Track	On Track	Off Track	Off Track	No Progress	Off Track	On Track
Improve the lives of slum-dwellers	On Track	Off Track	On Track	On Track	On Track	No Progress	No Progress	On Track	No Data
GOAL 8: Develop a global partnership for development									
Internet users	On Track	Off Track	On Track	Off Track	Off Track	On Track	Off Track	On Track	On Track

On Track • Target already met or expected to be met by 2015.
Off Track • Progress insufficient to reach the target if prevailing trends persist.
No progress or deterioration.
Missing or insufficient data.

* Red color refers to insufficient progress (i.e. MMR has declined less than 2 percent annually).

Source: Adapted from U.N. Statistics Division (2011), *The Millennium Development Goals Report 2011.*

TABLE 2A – MDG 1: Eradicate Extreme Poverty and Hunger

	People living in poverty 2005-2010			Employed people living below $1 PPP per day (%) 2005-2007	Distribution of income by quintiles (% of total income) 2005-2010					Population undernourished 2006	
	below national poverty line (% of total population)	below national rural poverty line (% of rural population)	below national urban poverty line (% of urban population)		lowest 20%	second 20%	third 20%	fourth 20%	highest 20%	million(s)	% of total population
World	..	..	..	..	..	..	..	..	..	..	..
High-income countries	..	..	..	..	..	..	..	..	..	..	..
Low- & middle-income countries	..	..	..	..	..	..	..	..	..	..	..
Sub-Saharan Africa	..	..	..	..	..	..	..	..	..	..	..
Angola	..	..	..	..	..	..	..	..	..	7	41.0
Benin	..	..	..	..	..	..	..	..	..	1	12.0
Botswana	..	..	..	..	..	..	..	..	..	1	25.0
Burkina Faso	..	..	..	..	..	..	..	..	..	1	9.0
Burundi	66.9	68.9	34.0	..	9.0	11.9	15.4	21.0	42.8	5	62.0
Cameroon	39.9	55.0	12.2	..	..	..	..	..	..	4	21.0
Cape Verde	26.6	44.3	13.2	..	..	..	..	..	..	0	10.0
Central African Republic	62.0	69.4	49.6	..	..	..	..	..	..	2	40.0
Chad	..	..	..	..	..	..	..	..	..	4	37.0
Comoros	..	..	..	..	..	..	..	..	..	0	46.0
Congo, Dem. Rep.	71.3	75.7	61.5	..	5.5	9.2	13.8	20.9	50.6	42	69.0
Congo, Rep.	50.1	57.7	..	..	5.0	8.4	13.0	20.5	53.1	1	15.0
Cote d'Ivoire	42.7	54.2	29.4	..	5.6	10.1	14.9	21.8	47.6	3	14.0
Eritrea	..	..	..	..	..	..	..	..	..	3	64.0
Ethiopia	..	..	..	..	9.3	13.2	16.8	21.4	39.4	32	41.0
Gabon	32.7	44.6	29.8	3.6	6.1	10.1	14.6	21.2	47.9	..	..
Gambia, The	..	..	..	..	..	..	..	..	..	0	19.0
Ghana	28.5	39.2	10.8	..	5.2	9.8	14.8	21.9	48.3	1	5.0
Guinea	53.0	63.0	30.5	..	6.4	10.5	15.1	21.9	46.2	2	17.0
Guinea-Bissau	..	..	..	..	..	..	..	..	..	0	22.0
Kenya	45.9	49.1	33.7	15.4	4.7	8.8	13.3	20.3	53.0	11	31.0
Lesotho	..	..	..	..	..	..	..	..	..	0	14.0
Liberia	63.8	67.7	55.1	83.8	6.4	11.4	15.7	21.6	45.0	1	33.0
Madagascar	68.7	73.5	52.0	64.1	6.2	9.6	13.1	17.7	53.5	5	25.0
Malawi	..	..	..	..	..	..	..	..	..	4	28.0
Mali	47.4	57.6	25.5	51.3	6.5	10.7	15.2	21.6	46.0	2	12.0
Mauritania	..	..	..	..	..	..	..	..	..	0	7.0
Mauritius	..	..	..	..	..	..	..	..	..	0	5.0
Mozambique	54.7	56.9	49.6	..	5.2	9.5	13.7	20.1	51.5	8	38.0
Namibia	..	..	..	..	..	..	..	..	..	0	19.0
Niger	59.5	63.9	36.7	61.7	8.3	12.0	15.8	21.1	42.8	3	20.0
Nigeria	..	..	..	..	..	..	..	..	..	9	6.0
Rwanda	58.5	64.2	23.2	..	4.2	7.7	11.7	18.2	58.2	3	34.0
São Tomé & Principe	..	..	..	..	..	..	..	..	..	..	..
Senegal	50.8	61.9	35.1	..	6.2	10.6	15.3	22.0	45.9	2	17.0
Sierra Leone	..	..	..	..	..	..	..	..	..	2	35.0
Somalia	..	..	..	..	..	..	..	..	..	..	..
South Africa	23.0	..	..	..	..	..	..	..	..	..	..
Sudan	..	..	..	..	..	..	..	..	..	9	22.0
Swaziland	..	..	..	..	..	..	..	..	..	0	18.0
Tanzania	33.4	37.4	..	..	6.8	11.1	15.6	21.7	44.8	14	34.0
Togo	61.7	74.3	36.8	35.8	5.4	10.3	15.2	22.0	47.1	2	30.0
Uganda	24.5	27.2	9.1	47.8	5.8	9.6	13.8	20.0	50.7	6	21.0
Zambia	59.3	76.8	26.7	..	..	..	..	..	..	5	43.0
Zimbabwe	..	..	..	..	..	..	..	..	..	4	30.0
Middle East & North Africa	..	..	..	..	..	..	..	..	..	..	..
Algeria	..	..	..	..	..	..	..	..	..	..	..
Djibouti	..	..	..	..	..	..	..	..	..	0	28.0

TABLE 2A – MDG 1: Eradicate Extreme Poverty and Hunger

	People living in poverty 2005-2010			Employed people living below $1 PPP per day (%) 2005-2007	Distribution of income by quintiles (% of total income) 2005-2010					Population undernourished 2006	
	below national poverty line (% of total population)	below national rural poverty line (% of rural population)	below national urban poverty line (% of urban population)		lowest 20%	second 20%	third 20%	fourth 20%	highest 20%	million(s)	% of total population
Egypt, Arab Rep.	22.0	30.0	10.6	..	9.0	12.6	16.1	20.9	41.5	..	..
Iran, Islamic Rep.	..	..	..	..	6.4	10.9	15.6	22.2	45.0	..	..
Iraq	22.9	39.3	16.1	..	..	..	..	..	..	..	..
Jordan	13.3	19.0	12.0	..	7.2	11.1	15.2	21.1	45.4	..	..
Lebanon	..	..	..	..	..	..	..	..	..	..	..
Libya	..	..	..	..	..	..	..	..	..	..	..
Morocco	9.0	14.5	4.8	..	6.5	10.5	14.5	20.6	47.9	..	..
Syrian Arab Republic	..	..	..	..	..	..	..	..	..	..	..
Tunisia	3.8	..	..	..	..	..	..	..	..	..	..
West Bank & Gaza	21.9	..	..	..	..	..	..	..	..	1	18.0
Yemen, Rep.	34.8	40.1	20.7	..	7.2	11.3	15.3	21.0	45.3	7	31.0
South Asia	..	..	..	..	..	..	..	..	..	..	..
Afghanistan	36.0	37.5	29.0	..	9.0	13.1	16.9	22.3	38.7	..	..
Bangladesh	40.0	43.8	28.4	50.1	9.4	12.6	16.1	21.1	40.8	42	27.0
Bhutan	23.2	30.9	1.7	..	..	..	..	..	..	..	..
India	27.5	28.3	25.7	39.2	8.1	11.3	14.9	20.4	45.3	238	21.0
Maldives	..	..	..	..	..	..	..	..	..	0	7.0
Nepal	..	..	..	..	..	..	..	..	..	5	16.0
Pakistan	22.3	27.0	13.1	19.3	9.0	12.4	15.8	20.7	42.1	43	26.0
Sri Lanka	15.2	15.7	6.7	..	6.9	10.4	14.4	20.5	47.8	4	19.0
East Asia & Pacific	..	..	..	..	..	..	..	..	..	..	..
Cambodia	30.1	34.5	11.8	..	6.6	9.4	13.1	19.2	51.7	3	22.0
China	..	2.5	..	..	5.7	9.8	14.7	22.0	47.8	130	10.0
Fiji	31.0	43.3	18.6	..	..	..	..	..	..	..	..
Indonesia	13.3	16.6	9.9	..	7.6	11.3	15.1	21.1	44.9	30	13.0
Kiribati	..	..	..	..	..	..	..	..	..	..	..
Korea, Dem. Rep.	..	..	..	..	..	..	..	..	..	8	33.0
Lao PDR	27.6	31.7	17.4	..	7.6	11.3	15.3	20.9	44.8	1	23.0
Malaysia	3.8	8.2	1.7	..	4.5	8.7	13.7	21.6	51.5	..	..
Mongolia	35.2	46.6	26.9	..	7.1	11.2	15.6	22.1	44.0	1	26.0
Myanmar	..	..	..	..	..	..	..	..	..	8	16.0
Papua New Guinea	..	..	..	..	..	..	..	..	..	..	..
Philippines	26.5	..	..	..	5.6	9.1	13.7	21.2	50.4	13	15.0
Samoa	..	..	..	..	..	..	..	..	..	..	..
Solomon Islands	..	..	..	..	..	..	..	..	..	0	10.0
Thailand	8.1	10.4	3.0	..	3.9	7.0	11.4	19.2	58.6	11	16.0
Timor-Leste	49.9	..	..	..	9.0	12.5	16.1	21.2	41.3	0	31.0
Tuvalu	..	..	..	..	..	..	..	..	..	..	..
Vanuatu	..	..	..	..	..	..	..	..	..	0	7.0
Vietnam	14.5	18.7	3.3	20.4	7.3	10.9	15.1	21.3	45.4	10	11.0
Europe & Central Asia	..	..	..	..	..	..	..	..	..	..	..
Albania	12.4	14.6	10.1	..	8.1	12.1	15.9	20.9	43.0	..	..
Armenia	26.5	25.5	26.9	..	8.8	12.8	16.7	21.9	39.8	1	22.0
Azerbaijan	15.8	18.5	14.8	..	8.0	12.1	16.2	21.7	42.1	..	..
Belarus	5.4	..	..	..	9.2	13.8	17.8	22.9	36.4	..	..
Bosnia & Herzegovina	14.0	17.8	8.2	..	6.7	11.3	16.1	22.7	43.2	..	..
Bulgaria	..	..	..	..	5.0	9.1	13.9	21.0	51.0	..	..
Georgia	23.6	29.7	18.3	..	5.3	10.3	15.2	22.1	47.2	..	..
Kazakhstan	..	..	..	..	8.7	12.8	16.7	22.0	39.9	..	..
Kosovo	45.0	49.2	37.4	..	..	..	..	..	..	..	..
Kyrgyz Republic	43.1	50.8	29.8	..	8.8	11.8	15.5	21.2	42.8	1	10.0
Latvia	..	..	..	..	6.8	11.7	16.3	22.4	42.9	..	..
Lithuania	..	..	..	..	6.6	11.1	15.7	22.1	44.4	..	..

TABLE 2A – MDG 1: Eradicate Extreme Poverty and Hunger

	People living in poverty 2005-2010			Employed people living below $1 PPP per day (%) 2005-2007	Distribution of income by quintiles (% of total income) 2005-2010					Population undernourished 2006	
	below national poverty line (% of total population)	below national rural poverty line (% of rural population)	below national urban poverty line (% of urban population)		lowest 20%	second 20%	third 20%	fourth 20%	highest 20%	million(s)	% of total population
Macedonia, FYR	19.0	21.3	17.7	..	5.4	9.3	14.0	21.0	50.3	..	..
Moldova	29.0	..	..	..	6.8	10.9	15.4	21.7	45.3	..	..
Montenegro	4.9	8.9	2.4	..	8.5	13.1	17.2	22.4	38.8	..	..
Romania	13.8	22.3	6.8	..	8.1	12.8	17.1	22.7	39.3	..	..
Russian Federation	11.1	21.2	7.4	..	6.0	9.8	14.3	20.9	48.9	..	..
Serbia	6.6	9.8	4.3	..	9.1	13.5	17.5	22.5	37.4	..	..
Tajikistan	47.2	49.2	41.8	..	..	..	..	..	..	2	30.0
Turkey	18.1	38.7	8.9	..	5.7	10.8	15.6	22.1	45.8	..	..
Turkmenistan	..	..	..	..	..	..	..	..	..	0	6.0
Ukraine	7.9	11.3	6.3	..	9.4	13.6	17.5	22.5	37.1	..	..
Uzbekistan	..	..	..	..	..	..	..	..	..	3	11.0
Latin America & Caribbean	..	..	..	..	..	..	..	..	..	..	..
Argentina	..	..	13.2	..	4.1	8.9	14.3	22.2	50.5	..	..
Belize	..	..	..	..	..	..	..	..	..	0	5.0
Bolivia	60.1	77.3	50.9	..	2.8	6.4	11.1	18.8	61.0	3	27.0
Brazil	21.4	..	..	2.7	3.3	7.2	11.9	19.5	58.1	12	6.0
Chile	15.1	12.9	15.5	..	4.1	7.9	12.1	18.8	57.0	..	..
Colombia	45.5	64.3	39.6	..	2.5	6.0	10.7	18.7	62.1	4	10.0
Costa Rica	21.7	23.0	20.7	..	4.2	7.8	12.5	20.1	55.4	..	..
Cuba	..	..	..	..	..	..	..	..	..	..	..
Dominican Republic	50.5	57.1	45.3	..	4.4	8.4	13.1	20.5	53.6	2	24.0
Ecuador	36.0	57.5	25.0	..	4.2	8.3	13.2	20.4	53.9	2	15.0
El Salvador	37.8	46.5	33.3	..	4.3	9.0	13.9	20.9	51.9	1	9.0
Guatemala	51.0	70.5	30.0	..	3.4	7.2	12.0	19.5	57.8	3	21.0
Guyana	..	..	..	..	..	..	..	..	..	0	7.0
Haiti	..	..	..	..	..	..	..	..	..	6	57.0
Honduras	60.0	65.4	54.3	..	2.0	6.0	11.3	20.0	60.8	1	12.0
Jamaica	9.9	..	..	..	..	..	..	..	..	0	5.0
Mexico	47.4	60.8	39.8	..	3.9	7.9	12.5	19.4	56.2	..	..
Nicaragua	46.2	67.9	29.1	12.8	3.8	7.7	12.3	19.4	56.9	1	19.0
Panama	32.7	59.8	17.7	..	3.6	7.4	12.2	20.1	56.8	1	15.0
Paraguay	35.1	49.8	24.7	..	3.8	7.7	12.4	19.7	56.5	1	11.0
Peru	34.8	60.3	21.1	..	3.9	8.4	13.6	21.5	52.6	4	15.0
Suriname	..	..	..	..	..	..	..	..	..	0	14.0
Uruguay	20.5	22.2	20.3	..	5.6	9.8	14.5	21.4	48.6	..	..
Venezuela, RB	29.0	..	..	..	4.9	9.6	14.7	21.8	49.0	2	8.0

..   Data not available.
0   Zero, or rounds to zero at the displayed number of decimal places.

Notes and Sources for Tables on pages 182-184.

TABLE 2B – MDG 2: Achieve Universal Primary Education
MDG 3: Promote Gender Equality and Empower Women

| | MDG 2 | | | | | | MDG 3 | | | | | | |
| | School enrollment 2007-2010 | | | Persistence to grade 5 (% of cohort) 2007-2010 | Literacy rate 2005-2009 | | School enrollment ratio (female to male) 2007-2010 | | | Literacy ratio (female to male) 2005-2009 | | Women employed in non-agricultural sector (% of non-ag. employment) 2005-2010 | Seats held by women in national parliaments (%) 2010 |
	primary (% net)	secondary (% net)	tertiary (% gross)		youth ages 5-24 (%)	adults above age 15 (%)	primary	secondary	tertiary	youth ages 15-24	adults above age 15		
World	**87.8**	**59.8**	**26.9**	..	**89.3**	**83.7**	**0.96**	**0.97**	**1.08**	**0.94**	**0.90**	..	**19.3**
High-income countries	**94.9**	**90.3**	**69.7**	..	**99.5**	**98.4**	**1.00**	**0.99**	**1.23**	**1.00**	**0.99**	**46.5**	**22.9**
Low- & middle-income countries	**86.9**	**55.7**	**21.2**	..	**88.0**	**80.3**	**0.96**	**0.96**	**1.02**	**0.94**	**0.87**	..	**18.0**
Sub-Saharan Africa	**75.1**	**27.0**	**6.2**	..	**71.9**	**62.3**	**0.92**	**0.79**	**0.63**	**0.88**	**0.76**	..	**19.6**
Angola	..	..	2.8	..	73.1	70.0	0.81	..	..	0.81	0.70	..	38.6
Benin	94.7	..	5.8	..	54.3	41.7	0.88	0.57[a]	..	0.67	0.54	..	10.8
Botswana	86.9	59.9	7.6	89.1[a]	95.2	84.1	0.97	1.05	1.15	1.03	1.01	43.4	7.9
Burkina Faso	63.3	15.4	3.4	75.1	39.3	28.7	0.89	0.74	0.49	0.71	0.59	..	15.3
Burundi	98.9	9.1	2.7	72.6	76.6	66.6	0.97	0.72	0.43	0.99	0.84	..	32.1
Cameroon	91.6	..	9.0	77.7	83.1	70.7	0.86	0.83	0.79	0.87	0.80	..	13.9
Cape Verde	82.6	63.3	14.9	89.7	98.2	84.8	0.93	1.18	1.27	1.02	0.89	..	18.1
Central African Republic	66.7	10.4	2.5	53.6	64.7	55.2	0.71	0.56	0.43	0.79	0.61	..	9.6
Chad	..	..	2.0	38.0[a]	46.3	33.6	0.70	0.41	0.17	0.73	0.52	..	5.2
Comoros	87.3	..	5.2	..	85.3	74.2	0.92	0.76[a]	..	0.99	0.86	..	3.0
Congo, Dem. Rep.	..	..	6.0	77.6	67.7	67.0	0.85	0.56	0.35	0.85	0.69	..	8.4
Congo, Rep.	58.9	..	6.4	76.9	80.5[a]	..	0.94	..	0.21	0.90[a]	..	..	7.3
Cote d'Ivoire	57.2	..	8.4	66.1	66.6	55.3	0.81	..	0.50	0.85	0.70	..	8.9
Eritrea	35.7	27.4	2.0	73.1	88.7	66.6	0.83	0.71	0.32	0.94	0.72	..	22.0
Ethiopia	82.7	..	3.6	45.9	44.6	29.8	0.91	0.77	0.31	0.60	0.43	47.3	27.8
Gabon	..	..	..	..	97.6	87.7	..	..	..	0.98	0.92	..	14.7
Gambia, The	68.7	41.6	4.6	71.5	65.5	46.5	1.06	0.94	..	0.85	0.62	..	7.5
Ghana	75.9	46.1	8.6	79.0	80.1	66.6	0.99	0.89	0.62	0.97	0.83	..	8.3
Guinea	72.9	29.2	9.2	68.6	61.1	39.5	0.86	0.59	0.34	0.79	0.55	..	19.3[d]
Guinea-Bissau	..	..	2.9	..	70.9	52.2	..	..	..	0.81	0.57	..	10.0
Kenya	82.6	49.6	4.1	..	92.7	87.0	0.98	0.90	0.70	1.02	0.92	..	9.8
Lesotho	73.1	28.8	3.6	62.2	92.0	89.7	1.00	1.38	1.19	1.14	1.15	..	24.2
Liberia	..	..	..	59.8	75.6	59.1	0.90	..	..	1.15	0.86	..	12.5
Madagascar	98.5	23.8	3.6	49.4	64.9	64.5	0.98	0.94	0.90	0.97	0.91	37.7	7.9[d]
Malawi	90.8	25.0	0.5	50.7	86.5	73.7	1.03	0.88	0.51	0.99	0.83	..	20.8
Mali	72.9	30.1	6.0	86.9	38.8	26.2	0.84	0.65	0.41	0.65	0.52	..	10.2
Mauritania	76.3	16.3	3.8	49.4	67.7	57.5	1.08	0.89	0.41	0.91	0.78	..	22.1
Mauritius	94.0	80.1[a]	25.9	97.2	96.5	87.9	1.00	1.02	1.25	1.02	0.94	37.1	18.8
Mozambique	90.6	14.7	1.5[a]	53.7	70.9	55.1	0.90	0.79	0.49[a]	0.82	0.59	..	39.2
Namibia	89.1	54.4	8.9	91.5	93.0	88.5	0.98	1.17	1.32	1.04	0.99	..	24.4
Niger	54.0	8.9	1.4	64.3	36.6[a]	28.7[a]	0.80	0.60	0.34	0.44[a]	0.35	36.1	12.4[e]
Nigeria	61.4	25.8	10.1[a]	..	71.8	60.8	0.88	0.77	0.70[a]	0.84	0.69	21.1	7.0
Rwanda	95.9	..	4.8	48.5	77.2	70.7	1.01	0.95	0.75	1.01	0.89	..	56.3
São Tomé & Príncipe	97.5	32.5	4.1	79.2	95.3	88.8	1.01	1.12	0.93	1.01	0.90	..	18.2
Senegal	73.1	20.8	8.0	69.8	65.0	49.7	1.04	0.79	0.58	0.76	0.63	..	22.7
Sierra Leone	..	24.9	..	..	57.6	40.9	0.88	0.66	..	0.71	0.57	..	13.2
Somalia	..	..	..	..	..	..	0.55	0.46	..	..	..	..	6.8
South Africa	84.7	71.9	..	..	97.6	88.7	0.96	1.05	..	1.01	0.96	44.0	44.5
Sudan	..	..	..	86.0	85.9	70.2	0.90	0.88	..	0.93	0.76	..	25.6
Swaziland	82.8	28.6	4.4	80.3	93.4	86.9	0.93	0.90	0.97	1.03	0.98	..	13.6
Tanzania	96.4	..	1.4[a]	80.9	77.4	72.9	1.00	0.78	0.48[a]	0.97	0.85	30.5	30.7
Togo	93.5	..	5.3	75.7	76.5	56.9	0.94	0.53	..	0.80	0.63	..	11.1
Uganda	92.2	21.6	4.1	57.7	87.4[f]	73.2	1.01	0.84	0.80	0.95[f]	0.78	..	31.5
Zambia	90.7	46.2	..	71.0	74.6	70.9	0.99	0.84	..	0.82	0.76	..	14.0
Zimbabwe	89.9	38.0	3.2	..	98.9	91.9	0.99	0.92	0.64	1.01	0.94	..	15.0

TABLE 2ʙ – MDG 2: Achieve Universal Primary Education
MDG 3: Promote Gender Equality and Empower Women

| | MDG 2 | | | | | | MDG 3 | | | | | | |
| | School enrollment 2007-2010 | | | Persistence to grade 5 (% of cohort) 2007-2010 | Literacy rate 2005-2009 | | School enrollment ratio (female to male) 2007-2010 | | | Literacy ratio (female to male) 2005-2009 | | Women employed in non-agricul-tural sector (% of non-ag. employment) 2005-2010 | Seats held by women in national parliaments (%) 2010 |
	primary (% net)	secondary (% net)	tertiary (% gross)		youth ages 5-24 (%)	adults above age 15 (%)	primary	secondary	tertiary	youth ages 15-24	adults above age 15		
Middle East & North Africa	**90.4**	**63.9**	**27.4**	**..**	**90.1**	**74.4**	**0.93**	**0.92**	**0.97**	**0.94**	**0.80**	**16.7**	**9.3**
Algeria	93.8	..	30.6	94.5	91.8	72.6	0.94	1.08ᵃ	1.44	0.94	0.79	13.1	7.7
Djibouti	44.4	24.4	3.5	64.3	..	..	0.89	0.73	0.69	..	..	..	13.8
Egypt, Arab Rep.	93.6	..	28.5	96.8	84.9	66.4	0.95	..	..	0.93	0.77	19.0	1.8
Iran, Islamic Rep.	99.5	..	36.5	94.3	98.7	85.0	0.99	0.95	1.07	1.00	0.90	16.1	2.8
Iraq	87.5	43.1	..	..	82.7	78.1	0.84	0.75	..	0.95	0.81	12.1	25.2
Jordan	89.5	81.9	40.7	..	98.9	92.2	1.01	1.04	1.11	1.00	0.93	15.7	6.4
Lebanon	90.1	75.1	52.5	95.3	98.7	89.6	0.98	1.11	1.19	1.01	0.92	..	3.1
Libya	..	..	..	..	99.9	88.9	0.95	1.17	..	1.00	0.86	..	7.7
Morocco	89.7	..	12.9	84.2	79.5	56.1	0.92	0.86	0.88	0.83	0.64	20.8	10.5
Syrian Arab Republic	..	69.2	..	..	94.4	84.2	0.96	0.99	..	0.97	0.86	16.3	12.4
Tunisia	97.9	71.3	33.7	96.1	96.8	77.6	0.98	1.08	1.49	0.98	0.82	..	27.6
West Bank & Gaza	75.2	84.6	45.7	..	99.2	94.6	1.00	1.07	1.31	1.00	0.94	17.9	..
Yemen, Rep.	72.7	37.4ᵃ	10.2	..	84.1	62.4	0.80	0.49ᵃ	0.42	0.75	0.56	6.2	0.3
South Asia	**86.4**	**..**	**11.4**	**68.9**	**78.7**	**61.1**	**0.95**	**0.88**	**0.69**	**0.85**	**0.68**	**18.5**	**19.2**
Afghanistan	..	26.8	3.6	..	..	..	0.67	0.49	0.24	..	..	..	27.7ᵉ
Bangladesh	86.3	41.5	7.9	66.6	75.5	55.9	1.04	1.12	0.56	1.04	0.84	20.1	18.6
Bhutan	87.4	47.5	6.6	95.5	74.4ᵃ	52.8ᵃ	1.01	0.99	0.59	0.85ᵃ	0.59	16.6	8.5
India	91.4	..	13.5	68.5	81.1	62.8	0.97	0.88	0.70	0.84	0.68	18.1	10.8
Maldives	96.2	69.4	0.0	99.7	99.3	98.4	0.95	1.05	1.00	1.00	1.00	30.0	6.5
Nepal	..	..	..	61.7	82.0	59.1	..	0.89	..	0.88	0.65	..	33.2
Pakistan	66.4	32.7	6.4	60.2	71.1	55.5	0.84	0.79	0.85	0.77	0.58	13.2	22.2
Sri Lanka	95.0	..	..	88.7	98.0	90.6	1.00	..	..	1.01	0.97	31.0	5.3
East Asia & Pacific	**93.3**	**66.8**	**24.2**	**..**	**98.7**	**93.5**	**1.01**	**1.06**	**1.08**	**1.00**	**0.94**	**..**	**18.5**
Cambodia	94.8	34.0	10.0	62.1	87.5	77.6	0.94	0.82	0.54	0.96	0.83	..	21.1
China	..	..	24.5	..	99.4	94.0	1.04	1.07	1.07	1.00	0.94	..	21.3
Fiji	89.5	79.1	15.4ᵃ	91.9	..	..	0.99	1.07	1.20ᵃ	..	..	29.6	11.3
Indonesia	95.3	69.0	23.5	86.1	99.5	92.2	0.97	0.99	0.92	1.00	0.93	32.4	18.0
Kiribati	..	67.5ᵃ	..	..	..	..	1.04	1.11	..	..	..	38.5	4.3
Korea, Dem. Rep.	..	..	..	..	100.0	100.0	..	..	..	1.00	1.00	..	15.6
Lao PDR	92.7	36.0	13.4	67.0	83.9ᵃ	72.7ᵃ	0.91	0.81	0.78	0.88ᵃ	0.77	50.2	25.2
Malaysia	94.1	68.4	36.5	96.6	98.5	92.5	0.99	1.07	1.30	1.00	0.95	39.2	9.9
Mongolia	90.5	82.4	52.7	94.4	96.0	97.5	0.99	1.07	1.55	1.03	1.01	51.1	3.9
Myanmar	..	49.6	10.7	69.6	95.7	92.0	0.98	1.02	1.37	0.99	0.94	..	..
Papua New Guinea	..	..	..	..	67.5	60.1	0.84	..	..	1.09	0.89	..	0.9
Philippines	91.7	60.7	28.7	78.4	97.8	95.4	0.98	1.09	1.24	1.02	1.01	41.7	21.4
Samoa	89.5	..	..	..	99.5	98.8	0.98	1.13	..	1.00	1.00	..	8.2
Solomon Islands	80.6	30.2	..	..	..	..	0.97	0.84	..	..	..	..	0.0
Thailand	90.1	70.7	44.6	..	98.1ᵃ	93.5ᵃ	0.98	1.09	1.24	1.00ᵃ	0.96	45.4	13.3
Timor-Leste	82.0	..	15.2	75.8	..	50.6	0.95	1.00ᵃ	0.71	..	0.73	..	29.2
Tuvalu	..	..	..	..	..	..	0.98	..	..	..	..	..	0.0
Vanuatu	97.3ᵃ	..	..	76.1	94.0	82.0	0.95	1.09	..	1.00	0.96	38.9	3.8
Vietnam	..	..	..	..	96.9	92.8	..	..	..	0.99	0.95	..	25.8
Europe & Central Asia	**91.7**	**81.3**	**55.0**	**..**	**99.2**	**97.9**	**0.99**	**0.97**	**1.22**	**1.00**	**0.98**	**48.0**	**15.5**
Albania	84.7	..	..	..	98.8	95.9	0.97	1.01	..	1.01	0.97	..	16.4
Armenia	84.1	87.2	50.1	..	99.8	99.5	1.03	1.03	1.29	1.00	1.00	44.8	9.2
Azerbaijan	85.2	92.6	19.1	0.0	100.0	99.5	0.99	1.03	0.99	1.00	0.99	43.6	11.4
Belarus	94.4	86.8	77.0	..	99.8	99.7	1.02	1.02	1.44	1.00	1.00	56.0	35.0
Bosnia & Herzegovina	87.1	..	37.0	..	99.7	97.8	1.02	1.02	1.31	1.00	0.97	35.7	19.0
Bulgaria	95.8	83.4	51.0	..	97.5	98.3	1.00	0.96	1.30	1.00	0.99	51.3	20.8

TABLE 2B – MDG 2: Achieve Universal Primary Education
MDG 3: Promote Gender Equality and Empower Women

	MDG 2						MDG 3						
	School enrollment 2007-2010			Persistence to grade 5 (% of cohort) 2007-2010	Literacy rate 2005-2009		School enrollment ratio (female to male) 2007-2010			Literacy ratio (female to male) 2005-2009		Women employed in non-agricul-tural sector (% of non-ag. employment) 2005-2010	Seats held by women in national parliaments (%) 2010
	primary (% net)	secondary (% net)	tertiary (% gross)		youth ages 5-24 (%)	adults above age 15 (%)	primary	secondary	tertiary	youth ages 15-24	adults above age 15		
Georgia	99.6	80.8	25.5	95.5	99.8	99.7	1.00	0.96	1.22	1.00	1.00	46.1	6.5
Kazakhstan	89.0	88.5	41.1	..	99.8	99.7	1.00	0.98	1.45	1.00	1.00	50.0	17.8
Kosovo	..	..	..	..	..	..	..	..	..	..	..	..	..
Kyrgyz Republic	83.5	79.1	50.8	..	99.8	99.2	1.00	1.01	1.32	1.00	0.99	50.8	25.6
Latvia	..	..	69.2	96.0	99.7	99.8	0.96	1.03	1.89	1.00	1.00	52.7	22.0
Lithuania	92.2	91.6	77.3	..	99.8	99.7	0.98	1.00	1.56	1.00	1.00	53.0	19.1
Macedonia, FYR	85.8	81.6[a]	40.4	..	98.7	97.1	1.01	0.97	1.20	1.00	0.97	41.9	32.5
Moldova	87.5	79.6	38.3	..	99.5	98.5	0.98	1.03	1.39	1.00	0.99	54.1	23.8
Montenegro	..	..	..	..	..	..	..	..	..	..	..	43.4	11.1
Romania	90.3	72.8	65.6	..	97.4	97.7	0.99	0.99	1.34	1.00	0.99	45.8	11.4
Russian Federation	..	..	77.2	..	99.7	99.6	1.00	0.97	1.36	1.00	1.00	50.6	14.0
Serbia	94.2	90.2	49.8	..	..	..	0.99	1.03	1.29	..	..	44.0	21.6
Tajikistan	97.3	82.5	19.8	..	99.9	99.7	0.96	0.87	0.41	1.00	1.00	37.1	19.0
Turkey	94.7	73.9	38.4	94.2	97.8	90.8	0.97	0.89	0.78	0.98	0.89	22.4	9.1
Turkmenistan	..	..	..	..	99.8	99.6	..	..	..	1.00	1.00	..	16.8
Ukraine	88.6	85.0	79.4	..	99.8	99.7	1.00	0.98	1.25	1.00	1.00	54.6	8.0
Uzbekistan	87.3	91.7	9.8	..	99.9	99.3	0.98	0.99	0.70	1.00	0.99	39.4	22.0
Latin America & Caribbean	**94.2**	**73.2**	**37.0**	**..**	**97.0**	**91.1**	**0.97**	**1.08**	**1.28**	**1.00**	**0.98**	**41.1**	**23.6**
Argentina	98.5[a]	79.2	67.7	96.3	99.2	97.7	0.99	1.13	1.52	1.00	1.00	45.0	38.5
Belize	97.3	64.8	11.2	95.6	..	..	0.97	1.08	1.85	..	..	37.7	0.0
Bolivia	91.3	68.9	38.3	85.1	99.1	90.7	0.99	0.98	0.84	0.99	0.91	38.1	25.4
Brazil	95.3	51.6	37.6	..	97.8	90.0	0.93	1.11	1.29	1.01	1.00	41.6	8.8
Chile	94.9	84.7	54.8	96.4	99.2	98.6	0.95	1.03	1.03	1.00	1.00	36.2	14.2
Colombia	89.6	73.6	37.0	84.7	97.9	93.2	1.00	1.10	1.05	1.01	1.00	47.5	8.4[e]
Costa Rica	..	..	25.3[a]	95.7	98.2	96.1	0.99	1.06	1.26[a]	1.01	1.00	41.5	38.6
Cuba	99.3	82.8	117.8	95.9	100.0	99.8	0.98	0.99	1.68	1.00	1.00	43.4	43.2
Dominican Republic	87.0	61.5	..	68.5[a]	95.8	88.2	0.86	1.13	..	1.02	1.00	38.8	20.8
Ecuador	97.0	59.2	42.4	81.7	96.8	84.2	1.02	1.05	1.15	1.00	0.93	38.7	32.3
El Salvador	94.0	55.0	24.6	79.8	95.0	84.1	0.97	1.02	1.09	1.01	0.94	48.0	19.0
Guatemala	95.1	39.9	17.7	70.6	86.5	74.5	0.94	0.93	1.00	0.95	0.87	43.0	12.0
Guyana	95.2	..	11.2	86.7	..	..	0.99	1.01	0.96	..	..	..	30.0
Haiti	..	..	..	..	..	48.7	..	..	..	..	0.84	..	4.1
Honduras	96.6	..	18.7	77.8	93.9	83.6	1.00	1.27	1.51	1.03	1.00	33.7	18.0
Jamaica	80.2	76.7	24.2	..	95.2	86.4	0.97	1.04	2.22	1.07	1.12	48.2	13.3
Mexico	98.1	72.4	27.2	93.9	98.5	93.4	0.98	1.06	0.98	1.00	0.97	39.4	26.2
Nicaragua	91.8	45.2	..	51.4	87.0[a]	78.0[a]	0.98	1.13	..	1.04[a]	1.00	38.1	20.7
Panama	97.0	65.6	45.1	89.3	96.4	93.6	0.97	1.08	1.54	1.00	0.99	42.2	8.5
Paraguay	87.4	59.5	28.6	83.7	98.8	94.6	0.97	1.04	1.35	1.00	0.98	39.5	12.5
Peru	94.4	71.1	34.5	87.2	97.4	89.6	1.00	0.99	1.06	0.99	0.89	37.5	27.5
Suriname	90.1	64.6[a]	..	79.8	99.4	94.6	0.95	1.28	..	1.00	0.98	..	9.8
Uruguay	98.6	69.6	64.9	94.5	99.0	98.3	0.97	1.13	1.75	1.01	1.01	45.5	15.2
Venezuela, RB	91.9	71.2	78.6	94.1	98.4	95.2	0.97	1.09	1.69	1.01	1.00	41.6	18.6[e]

..   Data not available.
0   Zero, or rounds to zero at the displayed number of decimal places.
a   Data refers to 2005.
b   Data refers to 2006.
c   Data refers to 2007.
d   Data refers to 2008.
e   Data refers to 2009.
f   Data refers to 2010.

Notes and Sources for Tables on pages 182-184.

TABLE 2c – MDG 4: Reduce Child Mortality

	Mortality rate 2009		Low birth weight newborns (% of births) 2005-2010	Percent of children under-5 suffering from: 2005-2010				Vitamin A supplement coverage rate (% of children 6-59 months) 2005-2010	Measles immunization (% of children 12-23 months) 2009	Consumption of iodized salt (% of households) 2005-2010	Exclusive breastfeeding (% of children under 6 months) 2005-2010
	children under age 1 (per 1,000 live births)	children under age 5 (per 1,000 live births)		underweight		wasting	stunting				
				moderate & severe	severe	moderate & severe	moderate & severe				
World	**43**	**61**	**15.2**	**21.3**	..	..	**31.7**	..	**81.9**	**70.7**	**36.7**
High-income countries	**6**	**7**	..	..	..	..	..	..	**93.0**	..	..
Low- & middle-income countries	**47**	**66**	**15.2**	**22.4**	..	..	**33.3**	..	**80.7**	**70.7**	**36.7**
Sub-Saharan Africa	**81**	**130**	**13.7**	**24.7**	..	..	**42.0**	**80.8**	**68.4**	**52.3**	**33.3**
Angola	98	161	..	..	..	..	..	28.0	77.0	44.7	..
Benin	75	118	14.9	20.2	6.3	8.4	44.7	56.0	72.0	67.2	43.1
Botswana	43	57	13.1	..	..	..	..	89.0	94.0	..	20.3
Burkina Faso	91	166	16.2	26.0	7.0	11.3	35.1	100.0	75.0	33.7	16.0
Burundi	101	166	11.2	..	..	..	..	90.0	91.0	98.0	44.7
Cameroon	95	154	10.8	16.6	5.7	7.3	36.4	95.0	74.0	49.1	21.2
Cape Verde	23	28	6.0	..	..	..	..	..	96.0	..	59.6
Central African Republic	112	171	13.0	..	..	..	..	87.0	62.0	62.3	23.1
Chad	124	209	..	..	..	..	..	71.0	23.0	..	..
Comoros	75	104	..	..	..	..	..	40.0	79.0	..	..
Congo, Dem. Rep.	126	199	9.6	28.2	13.4	14.0	45.8	89.0	76.0	78.9	36.1
Congo, Rep.	81	128	13.1	11.8	3.4	8.0	31.2	8.0	76.0	82.0	19.1
Cote d'Ivoire	83	119	16.7	16.7	5.4	8.6	40.1	88.0	67.0	..	4.3
Eritrea	39	55	..	..	..	..	..	44.0	95.0	..	..
Ethiopia	67	104	20.3	34.6	13.7	12.3	50.7	84.0	75.0	19.9	49.0
Gabon	52	69	..	..	..	..	..	0.0	55.0	..	..
Gambia, The	78	103	19.9	15.8	3.9	7.4	27.6	28.0	96.0	6.6	40.8
Ghana	47	69	13.4	14.3	3.6	8.7	28.6	90.0	93.0	32.4	62.8
Guinea	88	142	12.2	20.8	7.9	8.3	40.0	94.0	51.0	41.1	48.1
Guinea-Bissau	115	193	23.9	17.4	3.9	8.9	47.7	80.0	76.0	0.9	16.1
Kenya	55	84	7.7	16.4	4.1	7.0	35.2	51.0	74.0	97.6	31.9
Lesotho	61	84	..	16.6	..	5.6	45.2	85.0	85.0	..	53.8
Liberia	80	112	13.7	20.4	7.2	7.8	39.4	92.0	64.0	..	29.0
Madagascar	41	58	15.6	..	..	..	49.2	95.0	64.0	52.6	50.7
Malawi	69	110	12.5	15.5	3.9	4.2	53.2	95.0	92.0	49.7	56.7
Mali	101	191	18.7	27.9	11.3	15.3	38.5	100.0	71.0	78.9	37.8
Mauritania	74	117	33.7	16.7	2.6	8.4	24.2	89.0	59.0	23.4	34.7
Mauritius	15	17	..	..	..	..	..	..	99.0	..	..
Mozambique	96	142	15.2	..	..	..	..	97.0	77.0	25.1	36.8
Namibia	34	48	15.7	17.5	4.6	7.5	29.6	68.0	76.0	..	23.9
Niger	76	160	26.7	39.9	16.5	12.4	54.8	95.0	73.0	46.0	9.9
Nigeria	86	138	11.7	26.7	12.7	14.4	41.0	78.0	41.0	..	13.1
Rwanda	70	111	6.3	18.0	4.9	4.8	51.7	94.0	92.0	87.8	88.4
São Tomé & Príncipe	52	78	7.8	13.1	3.1	10.5	29.3	37.0	90.0	36.6	51.4
Senegal	51	93	18.8	14.5	3.9	8.7	20.1	97.0	79.0	41.3	34.1
Sierra Leone	123	192	13.6	21.3	8.0	10.5	37.4	99.0	71.0	58.2	11.2
Somalia	109	180	11.2	32.8	13.1	13.2	42.1	62.0	24.0	1.2	9.1
South Africa	43	62	..	..	..	..	..	39.0	62.0	..	..
Sudan	69	108	..	31.7	16.4	21.0	37.9	84.0	82.0	11.0	34.0
Swaziland	52	73	9.2	6.1	1.5	2.9	29.5	27.0	95.0	79.9	32.7
Tanzania	68	108	9.5	16.7	..	3.5	44.4	94.0	91.0	43.4	50.0
Togo	64	98	11.5	22.3	3.2	16.3	27.8	100.0	84.0	25.4	48.2
Uganda	79	128	14.0	16.4	4.7	6.3	38.7	64.0	68.0	95.8	60.1
Zambia	86	141	11.0	14.9	3.5	5.6	45.8	91.0	85.0	..	60.9
Zimbabwe	56	90	11.4	14.0	4.1	7.3	35.8	..	76.0	90.9	25.9
Middle East & North Africa	**27**	**33**	**10.4**	**6.8**	..	..	**25.0**	..	**86.7**	**68.9**	**31.4**
Algeria	29	32	5.8	3.7	1.3	4.0	15.9	..	88.0	60.7	6.9
Djibouti	75	94	10.2	29.6	14.6	26.0	32.6	94.0	73.0	0.4	1.3
Egypt, Arab Rep.	18	21	12.9	6.8	1.9	7.9	30.7	68.0	95.0	78.7	53.2

TABLE 2c – MDG 4: Reduce Child Mortality

	Mortality rate 2009		Low birth weight newborns (% of births) 2005-2010	Percent of children under-5 suffering from: 2005-2010				Vitamin A supplement coverage rate (% of children 6-59 months) 2005-2010	Measles immunization (% of children 12-23 months) 2009	Consumption of iodized salt (% of households) 2005-2010	Exclusive breastfeeding (% of children under 6 months) 2005-2010
	children under age 1 (per 1,000 live births)	children under age 5 (per 1,000 live births)		underweight		wasting	stunting				
				moderate & severe	severe	moderate & severe	moderate & severe				
Iran, Islamic Rep.	26	31	7.2	..	..	..	..	..	99.0	98.7	23.1
Iraq	35	44	14.8	7.1	2.5	5.8	27.5	0.8	69.0	28.4	25.1
Jordan	22	25	12.6	1.9	0.2	1.6	8.3	..	95.0	..	21.8
Lebanon	11	12	..	..	..	..	..	..	53.0	..	..
Libya	17	19	..	5.6	2.0	6.5	21.0	..	98.0	..	..
Morocco	33	38	..	..	..	..	..	..	98.0	21.2	..
Syrian Arab Republic	14	16	9.4	10.0	3.4	10.3	28.6	..	81.0	..	28.7
Tunisia	18	21	5.3	3.3	0.9	3.4	9.0	..	98.0	..	6.2
West Bank & Gaza	25	30	7.3	2.2	..	1.8	11.8	..	..	85.7	26.5
Yemen, Rep.	51	66	..	..	..	..	..	47.0	58.0	..	..
South Asia	**55**	**71**	**27.3**	**42.5**	**..**	**18.9**	**47.5**	**73.1**	**74.5**	**55.1**	**46.4**
Afghanistan	134	199	..	..	..	..	..	95.0	76.0	..	83.0
Bangladesh	41	52	21.6	41.3	12.1	17.5	43.2	91.0	89.0	84.3	42.9
Bhutan	52	79	9.3	12.0	2.4	4.6	37.5	48.0	98.0	..	..
India	50	66	27.6	43.5	17.4	20.0	47.9	66.0	71.0	51.1	46.4
Maldives	11	13	..	..	..	..	..	52.0	98.0	..	47.8
Nepal	39	48	21.2	38.8	11.0	12.7	49.3	95.0	79.0	..	53.0
Pakistan	71	87	31.6	..	..	..	..	91.0	80.0	..	37.1
Sri Lanka	13	15	16.6	21.6	3.9	11.8	19.2	64.0	96.0	92.4	75.8
East Asia & Pacific	**21**	**26**	**6.0**	**8.8**	**..**	**3.5**	**19.0**	**..**	**91.4**	**86.8**	**28.7**
Cambodia	68	88	8.9	28.8	9.1	8.9	39.5	98.0	92.0	82.7	73.5
China	17	19	2.7	4.5	..	2.9	11.7	..	94.0	96.4	27.6
Fiji	15	18	..	..	..	..	..	..	94.0	..	..
Indonesia	30	39	11.1	17.5	5.1	14.8	35.6	84.0	82.0	62.3	15.3
Kiribati	37	46	..	..	..	..	..	62.0	82.0	..	..
Korea, Dem. Rep.	26	33	..	..	..	..	..	99.0	98.0	..	..
Lao PDR	46	59	10.8	31.6	9.8	7.3	47.6	88.0	59.0	83.8	26.0
Malaysia	6	6	10.5	..	..	..	..	..	95.0	..	..
Mongolia	24	29	5.2	5.3	1.6	2.7	27.5	95.0	94.0	83.1	57.2
Myanmar	54	71	..	..	..	..	..	95.0	87.0	92.9	..
Papua New Guinea	52	68	10.1	18.1	5.2	4.4	43.9	12.0	58.0	91.9	56.1
Philippines	26	33	21.2	..	..	..	..	91.0	88.0	44.5	34.0
Samoa	21	25	..	..	..	..	..	..	49.0	..	..
Solomon Islands	30	36	12.5	11.5	2.4	4.3	32.8	..	60.0	..	73.7
Thailand	12	14	9.2	7.0	0.7	4.7	15.7	..	98.0	47.2	5.4
Timor-Leste	48	56	..	..	..	..	..	45.0	70.0	59.9	51.6
Tuvalu	29	35	..	1.6	0.3	3.3	10.0	..	90.0	..	34.7
Vanuatu	14	16	10.2	11.7	2.4	5.9	25.9	..	52.0	22.9	40.1
Vietnam	20	24	5.3	20.2	5.0	9.7	30.5	99.0	97.0	93.2	16.9
Europe & Central Asia	**19**	**21**	**7.1**	**..**	**..**	**..**	**..**	**..**	**95.6**	**..**	**..**
Albania	14	15	6.9	6.6	1.7	7.3	27.0	..	97.0	75.6	38.6
Armenia	20	22	7.4	4.2	1.1	5.5	18.2	..	96.0	97.0	32.5
Azerbaijan	30	34	9.7	8.4	2.3	6.8	26.8	79.0	67.0	53.8	11.8
Belarus	11	12	3.8	1.3	0.5	2.2	4.5	..	99.0	..	9.0
Bosnia & Herzegovina	13	14	4.5	1.6	0.6	4.0	11.8	..	93.0	62.0	17.6
Bulgaria	8	10	8.9	..	..	..	..	..	96.0	100.0	..
Georgia	26	29	4.9	2.3	1.0	3.0	14.7	..	83.0	99.9	10.9
Kazakhstan	26	29	5.8	4.9	1.7	3.7	17.5	..	99.0	92.0	16.8
Kosovo	..	..	..	..	..	..	..	..	..	..	..
Kyrgyz Republic	32	37	5.3	2.7	0.5	3.4	18.1	99.0	99.0	76.1	31.5
Latvia	7	8	..	..	..	..	..	..	96.0	..	..
Lithuania	5	6	..	..	..	..	..	..	96.0	..	..
Macedonia, FYR	10	11	6.0	1.8	0.6	3.4	11.5	..	96.0	94.0	16.0
Moldova	15	17	6.0	3.2	0.5	5.8	11.3	..	90.0	59.8	45.5
Montenegro	8	9	3.9	2.2	1.1	4.2	7.9	..	86.0	..	19.3

TABLE 2c – MDG 4: Reduce Child Mortality

| | Mortality rate 2009 | | Low birth weight newborns (% of births) 2005-2010 | Percent of children under-5 suffering from: 2005-2010 | | | | Vitamin A supplement coverage rate (% of children 6-59 months) 2005-2010 | Measles immunization (% of children 12-23 months) 2009 | Consumption of iodized salt (% of households) 2005-2010 | Exclusive breastfeeding (% of children under 6 months) 2005-2010 |
| | children under age 1 (per 1,000 live births) | children under age 5 (per 1,000 live births) | | underweight | | wasting | stunting | | | | |
				moderate & severe	severe	moderate & severe	moderate & severe				
Romania	10	12	..	..	..	..	..	..	97.0	..	..
Russian Federation	11	12	6.0	..	..	..	..	..	98.0	..	..
Serbia	6	7	5.8	1.8	0.6	4.5	8.1	..	95.0	32.2	15.1
Tajikistan	52	61	9.7	14.9	4.3	8.7	33.1	87.0	89.0	61.9	25.4
Turkey	19	20	11.0	..	..	..	..	..	97.0	68.9	41.6
Turkmenistan	42	45	4.2	..	..	..	..	..	99.0	86.5	10.9
Ukraine	13	15	4.2	..	..	..	..	..	94.0	18.3	18.0
Uzbekistan	32	36	4.8	4.4	1.4	4.5	19.6	65.0	95.0	53.1	26.4
Latin America & Caribbean	**19**	**23**	**8.4**	**3.8**	**..**	**..**	**14.1**	**..**	**93.1**	**88.7**	**43.7**
Argentina	13	14	7.3	2.3	..	1.2	8.2	..	99.0	..	..
Belize	16	18	13.5	4.9	1.5	1.9	22.2	..	97.0	..	10.2
Bolivia	40	51	6.3	4.5	1.0	1.4	27.2	45.0	86.0	88.8	60.4
Brazil	17	21	8.2	2.2	..	1.6	7.1	..	99.0	95.7	39.8
Chile	7	9	5.8	0.5	..	0.3	2.0	..	96.0	..	84.5
Colombia	16	19	6.0	5.1	..	1.5	16.2	..	95.0	..	46.8
Costa Rica	10	11	6.5	..	..	..	..	..	81.0	..	15.3
Cuba	4	6	5.1	..	..	..	..	..	96.0	88.0	26.4
Dominican Republic	27	32	11.0	3.4	0.6	2.3	10.1	..	79.0	18.5	9.4
Ecuador	20	24	10.0	..	..	..	..	..	66.0	..	..
El Salvador	15	17	..	..	..	..	..	20.0	95.0	..	31.4
Guatemala	33	40	..	..	..	..	..	43.0	92.0	76.0	49.6
Guyana	29	35	18.9	10.8	3.6	8.3	18.2	..	97.0	..	33.2
Haiti	64	87	24.6	18.9	7.3	10.3	29.7	42.0	59.0	3.1	40.7
Honduras	25	30	10.2	8.6	1.6	1.4	29.9	40.0	99.0	..	29.7
Jamaica	26	31	13.7	2.2	..	2.0	3.7	..	88.0	..	15.2
Mexico	15	17	8.0	3.4	0.6	2.0	15.5	68.0	95.0	..	..
Nicaragua	22	26	8.4	4.3	..	0.3	18.8	6.0	99.0	..	30.6
Panama	16	23	..	..	..	..	..	4.0	85.0	..	..
Paraguay	19	23	..	..	..	..	..	..	91.0	94.4	..
Peru	19	21	8.4	5.4	0.5	1.0	29.8	..	91.0	..	69.9
Suriname	24	26	10.9	7.5	1.2	4.9	10.7	..	88.0	..	2.0
Uruguay	11	13	8.4	..	..	..	..	..	94.0	..	57.1
Venezuela, RB	15	18	8.2	3.7	..	5.0	15.6	..	83.0	..	..

.. Data not available.
0 Zero, or rounds to zero at the displayed number of decimal places.

Notes and Sources for Tables on pages 182-184.

TABLE 2D – MDG 5: Improve Maternal Health

	Maternal mortality ratio (per 100,000 live births) 2008	Lifetime risk of maternal death (probability 1 woman in:) 2008	Pregnant women receiving any prenatal care (%) 2005-2010	Pregnant women with anemia (%) 2005-2010	Women with a birth in past 5 years with adequately iodized salt (%) 2005-2010	Births attended by skilled health staff (%) 2005-2010	Nurses, midwives, & physicians (per 1,000 people) 2005-2010	Total fertility rate (births per woman) 2009	Adolescent fertility rate (births per 1,000 women ages 15-19) 2009	Contraceptive prevalence of married women ages 15-49 (%) 2005-2010
World	**260**	**143**	**82.4**	..	..	**65.3**	..	**2.5**	**54**	**61.1**
High-income countries	**15**	**3,891**	..	..	..	..	..	**1.7**	**19**	..
Low- & middle-income countries	**290**	**123**	**82.3**	..	..	**64.1**	..	**2.7**	**58**	**61.0**
Sub-Saharan Africa	**650**	**31**	**71.1**	..	..	**44.4**	..	**5.0**	**110**	**20.9**
Angola	610	29	79.8	..	..	47.3	..	5.6	121	..
Benin	410	43	84.1	..	58.7	74.0	0.8	5.4	108	17.0
Botswana	190	182	94.1	..	..	94.6	3.2	2.8	50	52.8
Burkina Faso	560	28	85.0	..	..	53.5	0.8	5.8	125	17.4
Burundi	970	25	92.4	..	..	33.6	..	4.5	18	9.1
Cameroon	600	35	82.0	..	..	63.0	..	4.5	122	29.2
Cape Verde	94	347	97.6	..	..	77.5	1.9	2.7	89	61.3
Central African Republic	850	27	69.3	..	..	43.7	..	4.7	96	19.0
Chad	1,200	14	..	..	..	..	..	6.1	155	..
Comoros	340	71	75.0	..	..	..	..	3.9	43	..
Congo, Dem. Rep.	670	24	85.3	60.0	..	74.0	..	5.9	191	20.6
Congo, Rep.	580	39	85.8	69.8	81.9	83.4	0.9	4.3	106	44.3
Cote d'Ivoire	470	44	84.8	..	..	56.8	0.6	4.5	122	12.9
Eritrea	280	72	..	..	..	..	..	4.5	62	..
Ethiopia	470	40	27.6	30.6	18.6	5.7	0.3	5.2	94	14.7
Gabon	260	112	..	..	..	..	..	3.2	85	..
Gambia, The	400	49	97.8	..	..	56.8	0.6	5.0	87	..
Ghana	350	66	90.1	70.0	..	57.1	1.1	3.9	61	23.5
Guinea	680	26	88.4	69.4	..	46.1	0.1	5.3	147	9.1
Guinea-Bissau	1,000	18	77.9	..	..	38.8	0.6	5.7	125	10.3
Kenya	530	38	91.5	..	97.7	43.8	..	4.9	101	45.5
Lesotho	530	62	91.8	..	..	61.5	..	3.3	69	47.0
Liberia	990	20	79.3	..	..	46.3	0.3	5.8	136	11.4
Madagascar	440	45	86.3	38.3	49.1	43.9	..	4.6	127	39.9
Malawi	510	36	91.9	..	..	53.6	0.3	5.5	127	41.0
Mali	830	22	70.4	76.9	79.1	49.0	0.3	6.5	155	8.2
Mauritania	550	41	75.4	..	..	60.9	0.8	4.4	82	9.3
Mauritius	36	1,553	..	..	..	99.2	..	1.5	41	..
Mozambique	550	37	89.1	..	..	55.3	0.3	5.0	139	16.2
Namibia	180	163	94.6	..	..	81.4	3.2	3.3	67	55.1
Niger	820	16	46.4	61.5	49.1	32.9	0.2	7.1	152	11.2
Nigeria	840	23	57.7	..	52.5	38.9	2.0	5.6	118	14.6
Rwanda	540	35	95.8	19.8	88.3	52.1	0.5	5.3	35	36.4
São Tomé & Principe	..	..	97.9	..	..	81.7	..	3.7	62	38.4
Senegal	410	46	94.3	69.4	35.8	51.9	0.5	4.7	97	11.8
Sierra Leone	970	21	86.9	62.3	56.9	42.4	0.2	5.2	124	8.2
Somalia	1,200	14	26.1	..	..	33.0	0.1	6.4	69	14.6
South Africa	410	101	..	..	..	..	..	2.5	56	..
Sudan	750	32	63.7	..	..	49.2	1.1	4.1	53	7.6
Swaziland	420	75	84.8	40.2	78.4	69.0	..	3.5	78	50.6
Tanzania	790	23	75.8	..	..	43.4	0.2	5.5	128	26.4
Togo	350	67	84.1	..	..	62.0	0.3	4.2	62	16.8
Uganda	430	35	93.5	64.4	95.8	41.9	1.4	6.3	142	23.7
Zambia	470	38	93.7	..	..	46.5	0.8	5.7	133	40.8
Zimbabwe	790	42	93.4	47.0	..	60.2	..	3.4	61	64.9
Middle East & North Africa	**88**	**382**	**82.6**	..	..	**80.0**	..	**2.7**	**38**	**62.0**
Algeria	120	342	89.4	..	..	95.2	3.2	2.3	7	61.4
Djibouti	300	93	92.3	..	..	92.9	1.0	3.8	21	22.5

TABLE 2ᴅ – MDG 5: Improve Maternal Health

	Maternal mortality ratio (per 100,000 live births) 2008	Lifetime risk of maternal death (probability 1 woman in:) 2008	Pregnant women receiving any prenatal care (%) 2005-2010	Pregnant women with anemia (%) 2005-2010	Women with a birth in past 5 years with adequately iodized salt (%) 2005-2010	Births attended by skilled health staff (%) 2005-2010	Nurses, midwives, & physicians (per 1,000 people) 2005-2010	Total fertility rate (births per woman) 2009	Adolescent fertility rate (births per 1,000 women ages 15-19) 2009	Contraceptive prevalence of married women ages 15-49 (%) 2005-2010
Egypt, Arab Rep.	82	382	73.6	34.2	77.2	78.9	6.4	2.8	37	60.3
Iran, Islamic Rep.	30	1,519	98.3	..	..	97.3	2.5	1.8	17	78.9
Iraq	75	299	83.8	..	..	79.7	2.1	3.9	80	49.8
Jordan	59	507	98.8	25.5	..	99.1	6.5	3.4	24	59.3
Lebanon	26	2,009	..	..	..	..	5.8	1.8	16	..
Libya	64	537	..	..	..	..	8.7	2.6	3	..
Morocco	110	360	..	..	..	..	1.5	2.3	19	..
Syrian Arab Republic	46	611	84.0	..	..	93.0	3.4	3.1	55	58.3
Tunisia	60	860	96.0	..	..	94.6	4.5	2.1	7	60.2
West Bank & Gaza	..	..	98.8	..	..	98.9	..	4.9	73	50.2
Yemen, Rep.	210	91	47.0	..	..	35.7	..	5.1	64	27.7
South Asia	**290**	**111**	**70.1**	**..**	**..**	**46.9**	**1.7**	**2.8**	**75**	**50.7**
Afghanistan	1,400	11	36.0	..	..	24.0	0.7	6.5	117	15.0
Bangladesh	340	113	51.2	..	..	24.4	0.6	2.3	68	52.6
Bhutan	200	173	88.0	..	..	71.4	0.3	2.6	35	35.4
India	230	142	75.2	58.7	..	52.7	1.9	2.7	64	54.0
Maldives	37	1,229	99.6	..	..	97.1	6.0	2.0	13	34.7
Nepal	380	80	43.7	42.4	..	18.7	..	2.8	91	48.0
Pakistan	260	93	60.9	..	..	38.8	1.4	3.9	42	29.6
Sri Lanka	39	1,104	99.4	..	..	98.6	2.4	2.3	29	68.4
East Asia & Pacific	**89**	**583**	**90.7**	**..**	**..**	**88.7**	**2.8**	**1.9**	**19**	**77.1**
Cambodia	290	113	69.3	57.1	..	43.8	1.0	2.9	37	40.0
China	38	1,529	91.0	..	..	99.1	2.8	1.8	10	84.6
Fiji	26	1,335	..	..	..	..	..	2.7	28	43.1
Indonesia	240	187	93.3	..	..	74.9	2.3	2.1	37	56.6
Kiribati	..	..	..	..	..	63.0	..	3.4	..	..
Korea, Dem. Rep.	250	233	..	..	..	..	..	1.9	0	..
Lao PDR	580	49	35.1	..	..	20.3	1.2	3.4	34	38.4
Malaysia	31	1,215	78.8	..	..	98.6	3.7	2.5	12	..
Mongolia	65	734	99.5	..	..	99.4	6.3	2.0	15	55.2
Myanmar	240	176	79.8	..	..	63.9	1.3	2.3	18	41.0
Papua New Guinea	250	94	78.8	..	..	53.0	0.6	4.0	50	32.4
Philippines	94	325	91.0	..	..	62.2	..	3.0	43	50.7
Samoa	..	..	..	..	..	..	1.2	3.9	25	..
Solomon Islands	100	233	73.9	..	..	70.1	1.6	3.8	39	27.0
Thailand	48	1,188	97.8	..	..	97.3	..	1.8	36	76.7
Timor-Leste	370	44	..	27.8	..	..	..	6.4	52	19.8
Tuvalu	..	..	97.4	..	..	97.9	6.5	..	..	30.5
Vanuatu	..	..	84.3	..	..	74.0	1.8	3.9	44	38.4
Vietnam	56	851	90.8	..	..	87.7	2.2	2.0	16	79.5
Europe & Central Asia	**34**	**1,694**	**..**	**..**	**..**	**96.9**	**10.0**	**1.8**	**28**	**69.3**
Albania	31	1,689	97.3	..	..	99.3	5.2	1.9	14	69.3
Armenia	29	1,868	93.0	38.6	98.3	99.9	8.6	1.7	35	53.1
Azerbaijan	38	1,199	76.6	44.7	94.3	88.0	12.2	2.3	33	51.1
Belarus	15	5,098	99.4	..	..	100.0	17.7	1.5	20	72.6
Bosnia & Herzegovina	9	9,323	98.9	..	..	99.6	6.1	1.2	15	35.7
Bulgaria	13	5,754	..	..	..	99.6	8.4	1.6	40	..
Georgia	48	1,327	94.3	..	..	98.3	8.4	1.6	44	47.3
Kazakhstan	45	949	99.9	..	..	99.8	11.6	2.6	29	50.7
Kosovo	..	..	..	..	..	..	..	2.3	..	..
Kyrgyz Republic	81	452	96.9	..	..	97.6	8.0	2.8	32	47.8
Latvia	20	3,565	..	..	..	100.0	7.8	1.3	14	..
Lithuania	13	5,815	..	..	..	100.0	11.0	1.5	20	..

TABLE 2D – MDG 5: Improve Maternal Health

	Maternal mortality ratio (per 100,000 live births) 2008	Lifetime risk of maternal death (probability 1 woman in:) 2008	Pregnant women receiving any prenatal care (%) 2005-2010	Pregnant women with anemia (%) 2005-2010	Women with a birth in past 5 years with adequately iodized salt (%) 2005-2010	Births attended by skilled health staff (%) 2005-2010	Nurses, midwives, & physicians (per 1,000 people) 2005-2010	Total fertility rate (births per woman) 2009	Adolescent fertility rate (births per 1,000 women ages 15-19) 2009	Contraceptive prevalence of married women ages 15-49 (%) 2005-2010
Macedonia, FYR	9	7,322	94.0	..	..	99.7	6.9	1.4	21	13.5
Moldova	32	2,032	98.0	40.4	65.5	99.5[n]	9.3	1.5	33	67.8
Montenegro	15	3,969	97.4	..	..	98.8	7.5	1.6	14	39.4
Romania	27	2,727	..	..	..	98.7	6.1	1.4	29	..
Russian Federation	39	1,857	..	..	..	99.6	12.8	1.6	24	79.5
Serbia	8	7,532	98.2	..	..	99.0	6.5	1.4	21	41.2
Tajikistan	64	426	79.8	..	..	88.4	7.0	3.4	27	37.1
Turkey	23	1,878	95.0	..	..	95.0	3.5	2.1	36	73.0
Turkmenistan	77	500	99.1	..	..	99.5	7.0	2.4	18	48.0
Ukraine	26	2,952	98.5	..	..	98.7	11.6	1.5	27	66.7
Uzbekistan	30	1,358	99.0	..	..	99.9	13.4	2.7	13	64.9
Latin America & Caribbean	**86**	**484**	**95.0**	..	..	**89.4**	..	**2.2**	**73**	**74.8**
Argentina	70	602	99.2	..	..	94.8	..	2.2	56	78.3
Belize	94	327	99.2	..	..	94.9	2.8	2.8	76	34.3
Bolivia	180	150	85.8	49.4	..	71.1	..	3.4	76	60.6
Brazil	58	861	96.7	..	..	97.0	8.2	1.8	74	80.6
Chile	26	2,011	..	..	..	99.7	..	1.9	59	58.4
Colombia	85	455	93.5	..	..	96.4	..	2.4	72	78.2
Costa Rica	44	1,062	89.9	..	..	99.1	..	1.9	67	80.0
Cuba	53	1,381	100.0	..	..	99.9	15.0	1.5	46	77.8
Dominican Republic	100	323	98.9	..	..	97.8	..	2.6	107	72.9
Ecuador	140	266	..	..	..	..	..	2.5	82	..
El Salvador	110	349	94.0	..	..	95.5	2.0	2.3	81	72.5
Guatemala	110	206	..	..	..	51.3	..	4.0	104	54.1
Guyana	270	154	92.1	..	..	91.9	..	2.3	60	42.5
Haiti	300	93	84.5	50.4	3.1	26.1	..	3.4	45	32.0
Honduras	110	239	91.7	21.4	..	66.9	..	3.2	90	65.0
Jamaica	89	451	90.5	..	..	94.5	..	2.4	75	..
Mexico	85	495	94.2	..	..	93.4	..	2.1	63	72.9
Nicaragua	100	301	90.2	..	..	73.7	..	2.7	111	72.4
Panama	71	519	..	..	..	91.5	..	2.5	80	..
Paraguay	95	314	96.3	..	..	81.9	..	3.0	69	79.4
Peru	98	371	94.3	..	..	82.5	2.2	2.5	52	73.2
Suriname	100	403	89.9	..	..	89.8	..	2.4	38	45.6
Uruguay	27	1,710	96.2	..	..	..	9.3	2.0	60	78.0
Venezuela, RB	68	536	..	..	..	..	..	2.5	89	..

.. Data not available.
0   Zero, or rounds to zero at the displayed number of decimal places.
a   Data refers to 2005.
b   Data refers to 2006.
c   Data refers to 2007.
d   Data refers to 2008.
e   Data refers to 2009.
f   Data refers to 2010.
n   Excludes Transnistria region.

Notes and Sources for Tables on pages 182-184.

TABLE 2ᴇ – MDG 6: Combat HIV/AIDS, Malaria, and Other Diseases

	People ages 15-49 living with HIV (%) 2009	Adults ages 15-49 with new HIV cases in 2009 (per 100,000 people)	AIDS deaths in 2009	People with advanced HIV on ARV treatment (%) 2009	People with correct & comprehensive HIV/AIDS knowledge 2005-2010		Notified cases of malaria in 2008 (per 100,000 people)	Malaria deaths in 2008 (per 100,000 people)	Children under age 5 sleeping under insecticide-treated bed nets (%) 2005-2010	Children under age 5 with fever treated with anti-malarial drugs (%) 2005-2010	People with new TB cases in 2009 (per 100,000 people)	TB treatment success (% of new registered cases) 2008
					women ages 15-24 (%)	men ages 15-24 (%)						
World	..	..	..	..	..	..	..	..	..	..	137	85.6
High-income countries	..	..	..	..	..	..	..	..	..	..	14	70.1
Low- & middle-income countries	..	..	..	..	..	..	..	..	..	..	161	85.9
Sub-Saharan Africa	..	..	..	..	..	..	..	..	..	..	344	80.1
Angola	2.0	210	11,000	24.0	..	..	21,593	97	17.7	29.3	298	70.0
Benin	1.2	100	2,700	53.0	15.9	34.8	35,555	113	20.1	54.0	93	89.0
Botswana	24.8	1,560	5,800	83.0	..	..	587	3	..	..	694	65.0
Burkina Faso	1.2	70	7,100	46.0	19.0	..	45,322	163	9.6	48.0	215	76.0
Burundi	3.3	..	15,000	19.0	30.4	..	48,475	73	45.2	17.2	348	90.0
Cameroon	5.3	530	37,000	28.0	32.0	..	27,818	103	13.1	57.8	182	76.0ᶜ
Cape Verde	..	..	..	..	36.0	36.2	23	0	..	..	148	74.0
Central African Republic	4.7	170	11,000	19.0	17.3	26.1	35,786	98	15.1	57.0	327	71.0
Chad	3.4	..	11,000	36.0	..	..	39,508	181	9.8	35.7	283	54.0ᶠ
Comoros	0.1	..	99	18.0	..	..	24,619	98	..	..	39	90.0
Congo, Dem. Rep.	..	..	..	..	15.1	20.7	37,400	156	38.1	39.1	372	87.0
Congo, Rep.	3.4	280	5,100	23.0	8.3	21.9	34,298	120	6.1	48.0	382	76.0
Cote d'Ivoire	3.4	110	36,000	28.0	18.0	27.6	36,482	88	3.0	36.0	399	76.0
Eritrea	0.8	30	1,700	37.0	..	..	762	1	..	..	99	76.0
Ethiopia	..	..	..	..	20.5	33.3	11,509	44	33.1	9.5	359	84.0
Gabon	5.2	430	2,400	47.0	..	..	29,451	83	..	..	501	53.0
Gambia, The	2.0	..	999	18.0	39.3	..	31,925	97	49.0	62.6	269	84.0
Ghana	1.8	150	18,000	24.0	28.3	34.2	31,179	74	28.2	43.0	201	86.0
Guinea	1.3	100	4,700	40.0	16.9	22.8	40,585	140	4.5	73.9	318	78.0
Guinea-Bissau	2.5	210	1,200	30.0	17.7	..	34,043	142	35.5	51.2	229	70.0
Kenya	6.3	530	80,000	48.0	47.5	54.9	30,307	81	46.7	23.2	305	85.0
Lesotho	23.6	2,580	14,000	48.0	38.6	28.7	..	..	..	..	634	73.0
Liberia	1.5	..	3,600	14.0	20.5	27.2	29,994	87	26.4	67.2	288	79.0
Madagascar	0.2	..	1,700	2.0	22.5	26.0	3,735	17	45.8	19.7	261	81.0
Malawi	11.0	950	51,000	46.0	42.1	41.9	33,773	75	56.5	30.9	304	87.0
Mali	1.0	60	4,400	50.0	17.9	22.2	25,366	176	70.2	31.7	324	82.0
Mauritania	0.7	..	999	25.0	4.8	14.0	17,325	80	..	20.7	330	68.0
Mauritius	1.0	..	499	22.0	..	..	..	..	..	..	22	87.0
Mozambique	11.5	1,190	74,000	30.0	35.7	33.7	32,555	80	22.8	36.7	409	84.0
Namibia	13.1	430	6,700	76.0	64.9	61.9	4,589	19	34.0	20.3	727	82.0
Niger	0.8	80	4,300	22.0	13.4	15.9	37,958	154	43.0	33.0	181	81.0
Nigeria	3.6	380	220,000	21.0	22.2	32.6	38,259	151	5.5	33.2	295	78.0
Rwanda	2.9	180	4,100	88.0	50.9	53.6	11,429	40	55.7	5.6	376	87.0
São Tomé & Principe	..	..	..	..	42.6	43.4	1,961	8	56.2	8.4	98	94.0
Senegal	0.9	80	2,600	51.0	19.3	23.7	7,077	83	29.2	9.1	282	84.0
Sierra Leone	1.6	140	2,800	18.0	17.2	27.6	36,141	103	25.8	30.1	644	86.0
Somalia	0.7	..	1,600	6.0	3.7	..	8,711	65	11.4	7.9	285	81.0
South Africa	17.8	1,490	310,000	37.0	..	..	80	0	..	..	971	76.0
Sudan	1.1	..	12,000	5.0	..	..	12,805	106	27.6	54.2	119	81.0
Swaziland	25.9	2,660	7,000	59.0	52.1	52.3	57	0	0.6	0.6	1,257	68.0
Tanzania	5.6	450	86,000	30.0	39.2	41.5	24,088	84	63.8	59.1	183	88.0
Togo	3.2	270	7,700	29.0	15.3	..	30,388	88	38.4	47.7	446	79.0
Uganda	6.5	740	64,000	39.0	31.9	38.2	36,233	149	32.8	59.6	293	70.0
Zambia	13.5	1,170	45,000	64.0	37.8	40.7	13,456	107	49.9	34.0	433	88.0
Zimbabwe	14.3	840	83,000	34.0	53.3	45.6	7,480	33	17.3	23.6	742	74.0
Middle East & North Africa	..	..	..	..	..	..	..	..	..	..	39	86.2
Algeria	0.1	..	999	25.0	13.1	..	..	..	..	..	59	90.0
Djibouti	2.5	250	1,000	14.0	18.4	22.0	467	1	19.9	9.5	620	84.0

TABLE 2ᴇ – MDG 6: Combat HIV/AIDS, Malaria, and Other Diseases

	People ages 15-49 living with HIV (%) 2009	Adults ages 15-49 with new HIV cases in 2009 (per 100,000 people)	AIDS deaths in 2009	People with advanced HIV on ARV treatment (%) 2009	People with correct & comprehensive HIV/AIDS knowledge 2005-2010		Notified cases of malaria in 2008 (per 100,000 people)	Malaria deaths in 2008 (per 100,000 people)	Children under age 5 sleeping under insecticide-treated bed nets (%) 2005-2010	Children under age 5 with fever treated with anti-malarial drugs (%) 2005-2010	People with new TB cases in 2009 (per 100,000 people)	TB treatment success (% of new registered cases) 2008
					women ages 15-24 (%)	men ages 15-24 (%)						
Egypt, Arab Rep.	0.0	..	499	11.0	4.8	18.3	0	0	..	..	19	89.0
Iran, Islamic Rep.	0.2	..	6,400	4.0	..	..	18	0	..	..	19	83.0
Iraq	..	..	..	..	2.9	..	0	0	..	..	64	88.0
Jordan	..	..	..	..	12.9	..	..	..	..	..	6	84.0
Lebanon	0.1	..	499	18.0	..	..	..	..	..	..	15	77.0
Libya	..	..	..	..	..	..	..	..	..	..	40	69.0
Morocco	0.1	..	1,200	27.0	..	..	..	..	..	..	92	85.0
Syrian Arab Republic	..	..	..	..	7.2	..	..	..	..	..	21	86.0
Tunisia	0.0	..	99	53.0	..	..	..	..	..	..	24	86.0
West Bank & Gaza	..	..	..	..	..	..	..	..	..	..	19	94.0
Yemen, Rep.	..	..	..	..	1.5	..	1,106	3	..	..	54	85.0
South Asia	..	..	..	..	..	..	..	..	..	..	**180**	**88.0**
Afghanistan	..	..	..	..	..	..	2,428	0	..	..	189	88.0
Bangladesh	0.0	..	199	23.0	14.6	17.9	1,510	3	..	..	225	91.0
Bhutan	0.2	..	99	14.0	..	..	100	0	..	..	158	91.0
India	0.3	20	170,000	..	19.9	36.1	1,124	2	..	8.2	168	87.0
Maldives	0.0	..	99	17.0	35.0	..	..	..	..	..	39	45.0
Nepal	0.4	30	4,700	11.0	27.6	43.6	103	0	..	0.1	163	89.0
Pakistan	0.1	..	5,800	4.0	3.4	..	881	1	..	3.3	231	90.0
Sri Lanka	0.0	..	199	20.0	..	..	21	0	2.9	0.3	66	85.0
East Asia & Pacific	..	..	..	..	..	..	..	..	..	..	**136**	**91.6**
Cambodia	0.5	10	3,100	94.0	50.1	45.2	1,798	4	4.2	0.2	442	95.0
China	0.1	..	26,000	..	..	..	3	0	..	..	96	94.0
Fiji	0.1	..	99	30.0	..	..	..	..	..	..	19	90.0
Indonesia	0.2	..	8,300	21.0	9.5	14.7	1,645	2	3.3	0.8	189	91.0
Kiribati	..	..	..	..	..	..	..	..	..	..	351	96.0
Korea, Dem. Rep.	..	..	..	0.0	..	..	284	0	..	..	345	89.0
Lao PDR	0.2	..	199	67.0	..	..	327	1	40.5	8.2	89	93.0
Malaysia	0.5	60	5,800	23.0	..	..	75	0	..	..	83	78.0
Mongolia	0.0	..	99	8.0	31.4	..	..	..	..	..	224	87.0
Myanmar	0.6	50	18,000	18.0	..	..	7,943	17	..	..	404	85.0
Papua New Guinea	0.9	70	1,300	52.0	..	..	18,012	36	..	..	250	64.0
Philippines	0.0	..	199	37.0	20.7	..	96	0	..	0.0	280	88.0
Samoa	..	..	..	..	3.0	5.8	..	..	..	..	18	71.0
Solomon Islands	..	..	..	..	29.3	35.1	13,718	19	40.4	19.0	115	94.0
Thailand	1.3	30	28,000	61.0	46.1	..	322	0	..	..	137	82.0
Timor-Leste	..	..	..	..	12.2	19.7	46,380	108	42.0	6.0	498	85.0
Tuvalu	..	..	..	..	39.4	60.7	..	..	..	..	155	78.0
Vanuatu	..	..	..	..	15.4	..	6,036	7	..	..	72	91.0
Vietnam	0.4	..	14,000	34.0	43.6	50.3	55	0	13.0	2.6	200	92.0
Europe & Central Asia	..	..	..	..	..	..	..	..	..	..	**92**	**60.4**
Albania	..	..	..	..	35.9	22.0	..	..	..	..	15	91.0
Armenia	0.1	10	99	24.0	22.6	15.1	0	0	..	..	73	73.0
Azerbaijan	0.1	..	199	21.0	4.8	5.3	1	0	..	..	110	56.0
Belarus	0.3	30	999	29.0	33.5	..	..	..	..	..	39	71.0
Bosnia & Herzegovina	..	..	..	..	43.5	..	..	..	..	..	50	92.0
Bulgaria	0.1	..	199	23.0	17.2	15.3	..	..	..	..	41	85.0
Georgia	0.1	20	99	65.0	15.0	..	0	0	..	..	107	73.0
Kazakhstan	0.1	20	499	27.0	22.4	..	..	..	..	..	163	64.0
Kosovo	..	..	..	..	..	..	..	..	..	..	..	..
Kyrgyz Republic	0.3	80	499	12.0	20.3	..	0	0	..	..	159	84.0
Latvia	0.7	60	999	12.0	..	..	..	..	..	..	45	33.0
Lithuania	0.1	..	99	27.0	..	..	..	..	..	..	71	82.0
Macedonia, FYR	..	..	..	..	26.6	..	..	..	..	..	23	89.0

TABLE 2ᴇ – MDG 6: Combat HIV/AIDS, Malaria, and Other Diseases

	People ages 15-49 living with HIV (%) 2009	Adults ages 15-49 with new HIV cases in 2009 (per 100,000 people)	AIDS deaths in 2009	People with advanced HIV on ARV treatment (%) 2009	People with correct & comprehensive HIV/AIDS knowledge 2005-2010		Notified cases of malaria in 2008 (per 100,000 people)	Malaria deaths in 2008 (per 100,000 people)	Children under age 5 sleeping under insecticide-treated bed nets (%) 2005-2010	Children under age 5 with fever treated with anti-malarial drugs (%) 2005-2010	People with new TB cases in 2009 (per 100,000 people)	TB treatment success (% of new registered cases) 2008
					women ages 15-24 (%)	men ages 15-24 (%)						
Moldova	0.4	40	999	17.0	42.2	39.1	..	..	..	..	178	62.0
Montenegro	..	..	..	..	29.8	..	..	..	..	..	21	85.0
Romania	0.1	..	999	81.0	..	..	..	..	..	..	125	37.0
Russian Federation	1.0	..	999	..	..	..	..	..	..	..	106	57.0
Serbia	0.1	..	199	38.0	42.3	..	..	..	..	..	21	86.0
Tajikistan	0.2	30	499	11.0	2.3	..	9	0	1.3	1.9	202	82.0
Turkey	0.0	..	199	62.0	..	..	0	0	..	..	29	92.0
Turkmenistan	..	..	..	..	4.8	..	0	0	..	..	67	83.0
Ukraine	1.1	..	24,000	10.0	44.8	42.8	..	..	..	..	101	62.0
Uzbekistan	0.1	..	499	..	31.0	..	0	0	..	..	128	81.0
Latin America & Caribbean	..	..	..	..	..	..	..	..	..	..	**45**	**76.6**
Argentina	0.5	40	2,900	70.0	..	..	0	0	..	..	28	44.0
Belize	2.3	200	499	40.0	39.7	..	210	0	..	..	40	83.0
Bolivia	0.2	..	999	19.0	24.3	27.7	365	0	..	..	140	84.0
Brazil	..	..	..	60.0	..	..	210	0	..	..	45	71.0
Chile	0.4	..	..	63.0	..	..	..	..	..	..	11	72.0
Colombia	0.5	..	14,000	17.0	24.1	..	394	0	..	..	35	76.0
Costa Rica	0.3	..	499	68.0	..	..	51	0	..	..	10	89.0
Cuba	0.1	..	99	95.0	51.9	..	..	..	..	..	6	88.0
Dominican Republic	0.9	60	2,300	47.0	40.8	33.7	46	0	..	..	70	75.0
Ecuador	0.4	..	2,200	30.0	..	..	63	0	..	..	68	78.0
El Salvador	0.8	..	1,400	53.0	27.3	..	1	0	..	..	30	91.0
Guatemala	0.8	..	2,600	44.0	..	..	184	0	..	..	62	83.0
Guyana	1.2	..	499	95.0	50.3	47.3	2,194	3	..	..	112	69.0
Haiti	1.9	150	7,100	43.0	33.9	40.4	1,891	5	..	5.1	238	82.0ᶜ
Honduras	0.8	..	2,500	33.0	29.9	..	335	0	..	0.5	58	85.0
Jamaica	1.7	130	1,200	46.0	59.8	..	..	..	..	..	7	64.0
Mexico	0.3	..	..	54.0	..	..	3	0	..	..	17	85.0
Nicaragua	0.2	..	499	40.0	..	..	26	0	..	..	44	89.0
Panama	0.9	60	1,500	37.0	..	..	35	0	..	..	48	79.0
Paraguay	0.3	..	..	37.0	..	..	16	0	..	..	47	81.0
Peru	0.4	..	5,000	37.0	18.7	..	478	0	..	..	113	82.0
Suriname	1.0	60	199	53.0	41.0	..	681	1	..	..	135	59.0
Uruguay	0.5	..	..	49.0	..	..	..	..	..	..	22	83.0
Venezuela, RB	..	..	..	..	..	..	263	0	..	..	33	83.0

..   Data not available.
0   Zero, or rounds to zero at the displayed number of decimal places.
a   Data refers to 2005.
b   Data refers to 2006.
c   Data refers to 2007.
d   Data refers to 2008.
e   Data refers to 2009.
f   Data refers to 2010.

Notes and Sources for Tables on pages 182-184.

TABLE 2F – MDG 7: Ensure Environmental Sustainability

	Nationally protected land (% of land area) 2009	Forest area (% of land area) 2010	Agricultural land (% of land area) 2008	Cereal yield (kg per hectare of harvested land) 2009	Fertilizer consumption (kg per hectare of arable land) 2008	Tractors in use 2007-2010	CO2 emissions (metric ton(s) per capita) 2007	Energy use (kg oil equivalent) per $1,000 GDP (constant 2005 PPP $) 2008	Improved sanitation facilities (% of population with access) 2008	Improved water source 2008 rural (% of rural population with access)	Improved water source 2008 urban (% of urban population with access)	Slum population (% of urban population) 2005-2007
World	12.5	31.1	37.7	3,514	119	..	4.6	..	60.6	77.9	95.8	..
High-income	13.4	28.8	37.3	5,448	109	..	12.5	..	99.5	98.0	99.9	..
Low- & middle-income	12.2	31.9	37.8	3,005	123	..	2.9	..	53.6	76.3	94.4	..
Sub-Saharan Africa	11.7	28.0	44.6	1,302	12	..	0.8	..	31.3	46.8	82.5	..
Angola	12.4	46.9	46.3	588	8	..	1.4	113	57.0	38.0	60.0	86.5
Benin	23.8	41.2	30.7	1,330	0	..	0.5	255	12.0	69.0	84.0	70.8
Botswana	30.9	20.0	45.6	465	..	3,371	2.6	86	60.0	90.0	99.0	..
Burkina Faso	13.9	20.6	45.2	1,035	4	..	0.1	..	11.0	72.0	95.0	59.5
Burundi	4.8	6.7	85.3	1,313	2	..	0.0	..	46.0	71.0	83.0	64.3
Cameroon	9.2	42.1	19.4	1,574	9	..	0.3	185	47.0	51.0	92.0	46.6
Cape Verde	2.5	21.1	23.1	337	..	..	0.6	..	54.0	82.0	85.0	..
Central African Republic	14.7	36.3	8.4	948	..	..	0.1	..	34.0	51.0	92.0	95.0
Chad	9.4	9.2	39.2	812	..	..	0.0	..	9.0	44.0	67.0	90.3
Comoros	0.0	1.6	80.6	1,263	..	..	0.2	..	36.0	97.0	91.0	68.9
Congo, Dem. Rep.	10.0	68.0	9.9	772	1	..	0.0	1,194	23.0	28.0	80.0	76.4
Congo, Rep.	9.4	65.6	30.9	776	1	..	0.4	104	30.0	34.0	95.0	53.4
Cote d'Ivoire	22.6	32.7	63.7	1,724	19	..	0.3	327	23.0	68.0	93.0	56.6
Eritrea	5.0	15.2	75.0	938	0	..	0.1	264	14.0	57.0	74.0	..
Ethiopia	18.4	12.3	34.5	1,652	8	..	0.1	490	12.0	26.0	98.0	79.1
Gabon	14.9	85.4	19.9	1,663	14	..	1.4	106	33.0	41.0	95.0	38.7
Gambia, The	1.5	48.0	65.5	1,053	3	..	0.2	..	67.0	86.0	96.0	45.4
Ghana	14.0	21.7	68.6	1,660	6	1,807[a]	0.4	295	13.0	74.0	90.0	42.8
Guinea	6.8	26.6	56.1	1,711	2	..	0.1	..	19.0	61.0	89.0	45.7
Guinea-Bissau	16.1	71.9	58.0	1,422	..	..	0.2	..	21.0	51.0	83.0	83.1
Kenya	11.6	6.1	47.6	1,204	33	..	0.3	325	31.0	52.0	83.0	54.8
Lesotho	0.5	1.4	77.7	421	..	..	..	..	29.0	81.0	97.0	35.1
Liberia	18.1	44.9	27.2	1,553	..	..	0.2	..	17.0	51.0	79.0	..
Madagascar	2.9	21.6	70.2	2,291	4	..	0.1	..	11.0	29.0	71.0	78.0
Malawi	15.0	34.4	58.2	1,599	2	..	0.1	..	56.0	77.0	95.0	67.7
Mali	2.4	10.2	32.5	1,588	9	1,300	0.0	..	36.0	44.0	81.0	65.9
Mauritania	0.5	0.2	38.5	873	..	390	0.6	..	26.0	47.0	52.0	..
Mauritius	4.5	17.2	48.3	7,895	210	..	3.1	..	91.0	99.0	100.0	..
Mozambique	15.8	49.6	62.0	846	0	..	0.1	538	17.0	29.0	77.0	80.0
Namibia	14.5	8.9	47.1	465	0	..	1.5	138	33.0	88.0	99.0	33.6
Niger	6.8	1.0	34.2	489	0	..	0.1	..	9.0	39.0	96.0	81.9
Nigeria	12.8	9.9	86.2	1,598	13	24,800	0.6	379	32.0	42.0	75.0	64.2
Rwanda	10.0	17.6	81.9	1,097	8	..	0.1	..	54.0	62.0	77.0	68.3
São Tomé & Principe	..	28.1	57.3	2,308	..	..	0.8	..	26.0	88.0	89.0	..
Senegal	24.1	44.0	47.5	1,135	2	..	0.5	141	51.0	52.0	92.0	38.1
Sierra Leone	5.0	38.1	57.7	989	..	..	0.2	..	13.0	26.0	86.0	97.0
Somalia	0.6	10.8	70.2	417	..	1,371[b]	0.1	..	23.0	9.0	67.0	73.5
South Africa	6.9	4.7	81.8	4,395	50	..	9.0	287	77.0	78.0	99.0	28.7
Sudan	4.9	29.4	58.1	587	4	25,564	0.3	189	34.0	52.0	64.0	94.2
Swaziland	3.0	32.7	71.2	560	..	1,550	0.9	..	55.0	61.0	92.0	..
Tanzania	27.7	37.7	39.5	1,224	6	..	0.1	382	24.0	45.0	80.0	65.0
Togo	11.3	5.3	66.7	1,136	5	129	0.2	514	12.0	41.0	87.0	62.1
Uganda	9.7	15.2	66.0	1,539	3	..	0.1	..	48.0	64.0	91.0	63.4
Zambia	36.0	66.5	30.1	2,068	50	..	0.2	466	49.0	46.0	87.0	57.3
Zimbabwe	28.0	40.4	41.2	313	28	..	0.8	..	44.0	72.0	99.0	17.9
Middle East & North Africa	4.0	2.4	23.1	2,352	95	676,471	3.7	..	84.3	80.1	94.7	..
Algeria	6.3	0.6	17.3	1,654	7	104,529	4.1	146	95.0	79.0	85.0	..
Djibouti	0.0	0.3	73.4	1,667	..	6[b]	0.6	..	56.0	52.0	98.0	..
Egypt, Arab Rep.	5.9	0.1	3.6	7,635	724	103,188	2.3	173	94.0	98.0	100.0	17.1

TABLE 2ᶠ – MDG 7: Ensure Environmental Sustainability

	Nationally protected land (% of land area) 2009	Forest area (% of land area) 2010	Agricultural land (% of land area) 2008	Cereal yield (kg per hectare of harvested land) 2009	Fertilizer consumption (kg per hectare of arable land) 2008	Tractors in use 2007-2010	CO_2 emissions (metric ton(s) per capita) 2007	Energy use (kg oil equivalent) per $1,000 GDP (constant 2005 PPP $) 2008	Improved sanitation facilities (% of population with access) 2008	Improved water source 2008 rural (% of rural population with access)	Improved water source 2008 urban (% of urban population with access)	Slum population (% of urban population) 2005-2007
Iran, Islamic Rep.	7.1	6.8	29.7	2,291	91	308,422	7.0	269	..	..	98.0	30.3
Iraq	0.1	1.9	21.6	1,222	44	..	3.3	349	73.0	55.0	91.0	52.8
Jordan	9.4	1.1	11.0	1,044	..	5,483	3.8	239	98.0	91.0	98.0	15.8
Lebanon	0.5	13.4	67.1	2,828	56	..	3.2	114	98.0ᵃ	100.0	100.0	53.1
Libya	0.1	0.1	8.8	623	27	..	9.3	193	97.0	..	..	..
Morocco	1.5	11.5	67.2	1,003	54	..	1.5	118	69.0	60.0	98.0	13.1
Syrian Arab Republic	0.6	2.7	75.7	1,707	88	109,890	3.5	226	96.0	84.0	94.0	10.5
Tunisia	1.3	6.5	63.6	1,401	32	40,438	2.3	121	85.0	84.0	99.0	..
West Bank & Gaza	..	1.5	61.2	1,684ᵈ	..	7,756	0.6	..	89.0	91.0	91.0	..
Yemen, Rep.	0.5	1.0	44.7	1,003	14	..	1.0	147	52.0	57.0	72.0	67.2
South Asia	**6.1**	**17.1**	**54.6**	**2,628**	**148**	**472,552**	**1.2**	**..**	**35.7**	**82.9**	**94.5**	**..**
Afghanistan	0.4	2.1	58.1	1,983	3	925	0.0	..	37.0	39.0	78.0	..
Bangladesh	1.6	11.1	71.4	3,890	165	3,000	0.3	142	53.0	78.0	85.0	70.8
Bhutan	28.3	84.6	14.7	1,899	9	136	0.9	..	65.0	88.0	99.0	..
India	5.3	23.0	60.4	2,471	153	..	1.4	196	31.0	84.0	96.0	32.1
Maldives	..	3.3	30.0	3,917	5	..	3.0	..	98.0	86.0	99.0	..
Nepal	17.0	25.4	29.4	2,374	8	28,971	0.1	333	31.0	87.0	93.0	60.7
Pakistan	10.3	2.2	34.0	2,803	163	439,741	1.0	214	45.0	87.0	95.0	47.5
Sri Lanka	20.8	29.7	42.1	3,722	284	..	0.6	105	91.0	88.0	98.0	..
East Asia & Pacific	**14.9**	**29.6**	**48.0**	**4,843**	**..**	**..**	**4.0**	**..**	**59.0**	**81.4**	**96.0**	**..**
Cambodia	24.0	57.2	31.5	2,947	23	4,611	0.3	199	29.0	56.0	81.0	78.9
China	16.6	22.2	56.0	5,460	468	3,010,658	5.0	280	55.0	82.0	98.0	31.0
Fiji	1.3	55.5	23.4	2,456	47	5,983	1.7	..	..	..	..	..
Indonesia	14.1	52.1	26.6	4,813	189	..	1.8	237	52.0	71.0	89.0	23.0
Kiribati	22.0	14.8	42.0	..	..	..	0.3	..	31.0ᵃ	53.0ᵃ	77.0ᵃ	..
Korea, Dem. Rep.	4.0	47.1	24.5	3,698	..	..	3.0	..	..	100.0	100.0	..
Lao PDR	16.3	68.2	9.6	3,808	..	..	0.3	..	53.0	51.0	72.0	79.3
Malaysia	17.9	62.3	24.0	3,750	930	..	7.3	205	96.0	99.0	100.0	..
Mongolia	13.4	7.0	74.6	1,552	8	3,232	4.0	363	50.0	49.0	97.0	57.9
Myanmar	6.3	48.6	18.4	3,585	3	11,551	0.3	..	81.0	69.0	75.0	45.6
Papua New Guinea	3.1	63.4	2.5	3,727	79	..	0.5	..	45.0	33.0	87.0	..
Philippines	10.9	25.7	39.6	3,229	131	..	0.8	140	76.0	87.0	93.0	43.7
Samoa	3.4	60.4	23.3	..	2	..	0.9	..	100.0	87.0ᵃ	90.0ᵃ	..
Solomon Islands	0.1	79.1	3.0	2,800	..	..	0.4	..	29.0ᵃ	65.0ᵃ	94.0ᵃ	..
Thailand	19.6	37.1	38.5	2,954	131	..	4.1	213	96.0	98.0	99.0	26.0
Timor-Leste	6.0	49.9	25.2	1,276	..	..	0.2	..	50.0	63.0	86.0	..
Tuvalu	0.4	33.3	60.0	..	..	1	..	..	84.0	97.0	98.0	..
Vanuatu	4.3	36.1	15.3	552	..	..	0.4	..	52.0	79.0	96.0	..
Vietnam	6.2	44.5	32.4	5,075	287	..	1.3	267	75.0	92.0	99.0	41.3
Europe & Central Asia	**7.5**	**38.6**	**27.8**	**2,474**	**34**	**2,273,777**	**7.2**	**..**	**89.0**	**89.4**	**98.4**	**..**
Albania	9.8	28.3	43.1	4,315	38	7,438	1.4	91	98.0	98.0	96.0	..
Armenia	8.0	9.2	61.4	2,230	18	14,732	1.6	174	90.0	93.0	98.0	..
Azerbaijan	7.1	11.3	57.6	2,607	21	21,592	3.7	190	45.0	71.0	88.0	..
Belarus	7.3	42.5	43.9	3,372	237	49,517	6.9	250	93.0	99.0	100.0	..
Bosnia & Herzegovina	0.6	42.7	41.6	4,539	12	..	7.7	213	95.0	98.0	100.0	..
Bulgaria	9.1	36.2	47.6	3,413	82	53,100	6.8	216	100.0	100.0	100.0	..
Georgia	3.7	39.5	36.3	1,917	37	27,500	1.4	151	95.0	96.0	100.0	..
Kazakhstan	2.5	1.2	77.0	1,254	3	40,228	14.7	432	97.0	90.0	99.0	..
Kosovo	..	..	52.4ᶜ	..	..	..	..	..	..	..	..	..
Kyrgyz Republic	6.9	5.0	55.9	3,034	19	24,445	1.2	265	93.0	85.0	99.0	..
Latvia	17.8	53.9	29.3	3,075	124	59,562	3.4	127	78.0	96.0	100.0	..
Lithuania	4.5	34.5	42.6	3,450	79	117,580	4.5	156	..	..	..	..
Macedonia, FYR	4.8	39.6	42.4	3,387	56	53,606	5.5	173	89.0	99.0	100.0	..

TABLE 2F – MDG 7: Ensure Environmental Sustainability

	Nationally protected land (% of land area) 2009	Forest area (% of land area) 2010	Agricultural land (% of land area) 2008	Cereal yield (kg per hectare of harvested land) 2009	Fertilizer consumption (kg per hectare of arable land) 2008	Tractors in use 2007-2010	CO_2 emissions (metric ton(s) per capita) 2007	Energy use (kg oil equivalent) per $1,000 GDP (constant 2005 PPP $) 2008	Improved sanitation facilities (% of population with access) 2008	Improved water source 2008 rural (% of rural population with access)	Improved water source 2008 urban (% of urban population with access)	Slum population (% of urban population) 2005-2007
Moldova	1.4	11.7	75.6	2,417	12	35,984	1.3	319	79.0	85.0	96.0	..
Montenegro	13.3	40.4	38.1	2,298	..	..	..	..	92.0	96.0	100.0	..
Romania	7.1	28.6	58.9	2,825	46	174,790	4.4	155	72.0	..	..	..
Russian Federation	9.0	49.4	13.2	2,279	16	364,356	10.8	328	87.0	89.0	98.0	..
Serbia	6.0	30.7	57.2	4,626	115	5,844	..	213	92.0	98.0	99.0	..
Tajikistan	4.1	2.9	33.8	2,250	0	15,951	1.1	207	94.0	61.0	94.0	..
Turkey	1.9	14.7	50.8	2,808	89	1,052,975	4.0	112	90.0	96.0	100.0	14.1
Turkmenistan	3.0	8.8	69.4	2,974	..	..	9.2	605	98.0	72.0a	97.0	..
Ukraine	3.5	16.8	71.3	3,004	33	335,473	6.8	438	95.0	97.0	98.0	..
Uzbekistan	2.3	7.7	62.6	4,578	..	..	4.3	753	100.0	81.0	98.0	..
Latin America & Caribbean	**20.8**	**47.0**	**35.4**	**3,282**	**112**	..	**2.7**	..	**79.3**	**79.7**	**97.1**	..
Argentina	5.4	10.7	48.5	3,167	39	..	4.6	145	90.0	80.0	98.0	23.5
Belize	27.9	61.1	6.7	2,972	50	..	1.4	..	90.0	100.0	99.0	47.3
Bolivia	18.2	52.8	34.0	2,089	5	..	1.4	149	25.0	67.0	96.0	48.8
Brazil	28.0	61.4	31.3	3,526	166	788,053	1.9	135	80.0	84.0	99.0	28.0
Chile	16.5	21.8	21.2	5,472	589	53,915	4.3	140	96.0	75.0	99.0	9.0
Colombia	20.4	54.5	38.4	4,017	492	..	1.4	84	74.0	73.0	99.0	16.1
Costa Rica	20.9	51.0	35.3	3,770	707	..	1.8	104	95.0	91.0	100.0	..
Cuba	6.2	27.0	62.0	2,069	40	72,602	2.4	..	91.0	89.0	96.0	..
Dominican Republic	22.1	40.8	51.7	4,246	..	..	2.1	109	83.0	84.0	87.0	16.2
Ecuador	25.1	39.7	30.0	2,974	214	..	2.2	102	92.0	88.0	97.0	21.5
El Salvador	0.8	13.9	74.9	2,727	118	..	1.1	127	87.0	76.0	94.0	28.9
Guatemala	30.6	34.1	39.4	1,624	92	..	1.0	135	81.0	90.0	98.0	40.8
Guyana	4.9	77.2	8.5	4,139	57	..	2.0	..	81.0	93.0	98.0	33.7
Haiti	0.3	3.7	64.9	961	..	..	0.2	272	17.0	55.0	71.0	70.1
Honduras	18.2	46.4	28.5	1,752	108	..	1.2	174	71.0	77.0	95.0	34.9
Jamaica	18.9	31.1	42.8	1,253	51	..	5.2	227	83.0	89.0	98.0	60.5
Mexico	11.1	33.3	52.7	3,111	45	238,830	4.5	126	85.0	87.0	96.0	14.4
Nicaragua	36.7	25.9	42.8	1,872	32	..	0.8	241	52.0	68.0	98.0	45.5
Panama	18.7	43.7	30.0	2,735	35	..	2.2	72	69.0	83.0	97.0	23.0
Paraguay	5.4	44.3	51.3	2,358	67	25,823	0.7	161	70.0	66.0	99.0	17.6
Peru	13.6	53.1	16.8	3,910	82	..	1.5	65	68.0	61.0	90.0	36.1
Suriname	11.4	94.6	0.5	4,189	526	1,013	4.8	..	84.0	81.0	97.0	3.9
Uruguay	0.3	10.0	84.9	4,047	118	36,465	1.9	107	100.0	100.0	100.0	..
Venezuela, RB	53.7	52.5	24.2	3,826	233	..	6.0	195	91.0a	75.0a	94.0a	32.0

..   Data not available.
0   Zero, or rounds to zero at the displayed number of decimal places.
a   Data refers to 2005.
b   Data refers to 2006.
c   Data refers to 2007.
d   Data refers to 2008.
e   Data refers to 2009.
f   Data refers to 2010.

Notes and Sources for Tables on pages 182-184.

TABLE 2G – MDG 8: Develop a Global Partnership for Development

	Net Official Development Assistance received			Central gov't debt (% of GDP) 2008-2009	Total debt service (% of exports of goods, services, & income) 2008-2009	Present value of external debt (current million US$) 2009	Cumulative debt relief committed under HIPC (million US$ in end-2009 NPV terms) 2009	Net Official Development Assistance provided					Agriculture support for OECD countries (% of their GDP) 2009
	total in 2009 (current million US$)	per capita in 2009 (current US$)	as % of central gov't expense 2008-2009					in 2010 (current million US$)	as % of OECD/ DAC donor's GNI 2010	that is untied (%) 2009	to help build trade capacity (%) 2009	to basic social services in 2009 (current million US$)	
World	127,527	19	..	..	..	..	..	..	..	..	..	..	..
High-income countries	433	0	..	58.1	..	..	..	..	..	..	..	..	..
Low- & middle-income countries	127,093	22	..	..	11.4	3,184,777	..	..	..	..	..	..	..
Sub-Saharan Africa	44,510	53	..	..	5.9	167,925	..	..	..	..	..	..	..
Angola	239	13	..	..	8.4	14,228	..	..	..	..	..	..	..
Benin	683	76	68.2	..	2.1[c]	738	385	..	..	..	..	..	..
Botswana	280	143	..	..	1.2	1,001	..	..	..	..	..	..	..
Burkina Faso	1,084	69	102.5	..	..	1,272	812	..	..	..	..	..	..
Burundi	549	66	..	..	13.3	156	1,009	..	..	..	..	..	..
Cameroon	649	33	..	..	7.4	771	1,861	..	..	..	..	..	..
Cape Verde	196	388	44.9	..	4.2	381	..	..	..	..	..	..	..
Central African Rep.	237	54	..	..	..	222	675	..	..	..	..	..	..
Chad	561	50	..	..	2.8	1,354	241	..	..	..	..	..	..
Comoros	51	77	..	..	..	205	151	..	..	..	..	..	..
Congo, Dem. Rep.	2,354	36	..	..	..	2,384	9,493	..	..	..	..	..	..
Congo, Rep.	283	77	158.0[a]	..	1.7[c]	1,265	1,906	..	..	..	..	..	..
Cote d'Ivoire	2,366	112	57.6	..	9.5	9,738	3,245	..	..	..	..	..	..
Eritrea	145	29	..	..	..	597	..	..	..	..	..	..	..
Ethiopia	3,820	46	104.8[a]	..	3.1	2,931	2,735	..	..	..	..	..	..
Gabon	78	53	..	..	8.1	1,990	..	..	..	..	..	..	..
Gambia, The	128	75	..	..	7.6	203	98	..	..	..	..	..	..
Ghana	1,583	66	33.8	..	2.9	4,235	3,091	..	..	..	..	..	..
Guinea	215	21	..	..	9.6	1,980	801	..	..	..	..	..	..
Guinea-Bissau	146	90	..	..	5.5	848	746	..	..	..	..	..	..
Kenya	1,778	45	27.9	..	5.0	5,689	..	..	..	..	..	..	..
Lesotho	123	60	17.3	..	3.0	388	..	..	..	..	..	..	..
Liberia	505	128	43,884.0	..	142.2	1,977	2,958	..	..	..	..	..	..
Madagascar	445	23	76.2	..	2.3	1,464	1,228	..	..	..	..	..	..
Malawi	772	51	..	..	..	649	1,379	..	..	..	..	..	..
Mali	985	76	74.9	..	2.6	1,200	792	..	..	..	..	..	..
Mauritania	287	87	..	..	..	2,602	913	..	..	..	..	..	..
Mauritius	156	122	8.4	38.9	2.7	589	..	..	..	..	..	..	..
Mozambique	2,013	88	..	..	1.6	1,589	3,147	..	..	..	..	..	..
Namibia	326	150	7.8[b]	..	..	..	..	..	..	..	..	..	..
Niger	470	31	155.5[b]	..	4.5	633	947	..	..	..	..	..	..
Nigeria	1,659	11	8.6	3.0	0.8	5,936	..	..	..	..	..	..	..
Rwanda	934	93	..	..	4.7	353	956	..	..	..	..	..	..
São Tomé & Principe	31	189	..	..	15.7	18	172	..	..	..	..	..	..
Senegal	1,018	81	..	..	6.2[c]	2,492	717	..	..	..	..	..	..
Sierra Leone	437	77	101.9	..	2.2	368	919	..	..	..	..	..	..
Somalia	662	72	..	..	..	3,710	..	..	..	..	..	..	..
South Africa	1,075	22	1.1	..	9.3	42,043	..	..	..	..	..	..	..
Sudan	2,289	54	..	..	5.8	35,082	..	..	..	..	..	..	..
Swaziland	58	49	..	..	2.1	379	..	..	..	..	..	..	..
Tanzania	2,934	67	..	..	3.5	2,648	2,977	..	..	..	..	..	..
Togo	499	75	100.6	..	16.1	1,360	305	..	..	..	..	..	..
Uganda	1,786	55	86.9	32.7	2.0	1,132	1,509	..	..	..	..	..	..
Zambia	1,269	98	79.8[b]	..	3.8	1,172	3,672	..	..	..	..	..	..
Zimbabwe	737	59	..	..	..	6,247	..	..	..	..	..	..	..
Middle East & North Africa	..	..	..	..	..	..	..	..	..	..	..	..	..
Algeria	319	9	0.9	..	1.4	4,719	..	..	..	..	..	..	..
Djibouti	162	188	..	..	6.2	511	..	..	..	..	..	..	..

TABLE 2G – MDG 8: Develop a Global Partnership for Development

| | Net Official Development Assistance received | | | Central gov't debt (% of GDP) 2008-2009 | Total debt service (% of exports of goods, services, & income) 2008-2009 | Present value of external debt (current million US$) 2009 | Cumulative debt relief committed under HIPC (million US$ in end-2009 NPV terms) 2009 | Net Official Development Assistance provided | | | | | Agriculture support for OECD countries (% of their GDP) 2009 |
	total in 2009 (current million US$)	per capita in 2009 (current US$)	as % of central gov't expense 2008-2009					in 2010 (current million US$)	as % of OECD/ DAC donor's GNI 2010	that is untied (%) 2009	to help build trade capacity (%) 2009	to basic social services in 2009 (current million US$)	
Egypt, Arab Rep.	925	11	1.6	79.5	6.5	26,629	..	..	..	..	..	..	..
Iran, Islamic Rep.	93	1	0.1	..	..	11,667	..	..	..	..	..	..	..
Iraq	2,791	89	..	..	..	..	..	..	..	..	..	..	..
Jordan	761	128	10.6	57.9	4.8	5,603	..	..	..	..	..	..	..
Lebanon	641	152	6.3	..	18.0	24,132	..	..	..	..	..	..	..
Libya	39	6	..	..	..	..	..	..	..	..	..	..	..
Morocco	912	28	3.6	46.9	12.5	19,578	..	..	..	..	..	..	..
Syrian Arab Republic	245	12	..	..	3.5	4,413	..	..	..	..	..	..	..
Tunisia	474	45	4.0	47.1	10.1	19,650	..	..	..	..	..	..	..
West Bank & Gaza	3,026	748	..	..	..	..	..	..	..	..	..	..	..
Yemen, Rep.	500	21	..	..	2.7	4,052	..	..	..	..	..	..	..
South Asia	**14,332**	**9**	**..**	**56.5c**	**6.8**	**283,528**	**..**	**..**	**..**	**..**	**..**	**..**	**..**
Afghanistan	6,070	204	112.5	..	0.4	596	654	..	..	..	..	..	..
Bangladesh	1,227	8	12.2	..	5.6	14,697	..	..	..	..	..	..	..
Bhutan	125	180	42.6	56.2	11.4	625	..	..	..	..	..	..	..
India	2,393	2	1.1	53.0	5.9	212,262	..	..	..	..	..	..	..
Maldives	33	107	5.4	52.3	8.3	630	..	..	..	..	..	..	..
Nepal	855	29	34.1a	43.7	10.4	2,728	..	..	..	..	..	..	..
Pakistan	2,781	16	10.6	..	15.0	38,732	..	..	..	..	..	..	..
Sri Lanka	704	35	9.3	85.0c	15.6	13,257	..	..	..	..	..	..	..
East Asia & Pacific	**10,278**	**5**	**..**	**..**	**4.8**	**752,871**	**..**	**..**	**..**	**..**	**..**	**..**	**..**
Cambodia	722	49	62.9	..	0.8	3,544	..	..	..	..	..	..	..
China	1,132	1	..	..	2.9	404,026	..	..	..	..	..	..	..
Fiji	71	84	6.8b	..	1.2	390	..	..	..	..	..	..	..
Indonesia	1,049	5	1.2	28.3	18.4	140,615	..	..	..	..	..	..	..
Kiribati	27	277	..	..	..	..	..	..	..	..	..	..	..
Korea, Dem. Rep.	67	3	..	..	..	..	..	..	..	..	..	..	..
Lao PDR	420	66	62.5	..	15.2c	3,963	..	..	..	..	..	..	..
Malaysia	144	5	0.3	53.3	5.2	60,881	..	..	..	..	..	..	..
Mongolia	372	139	30.7	64.8	4.8	1,497	..	..	..	..	..	..	..
Myanmar	357	7	0.2a	..	1.3b	5,187	..	..	..	..	..	..	..
Papua New Guinea	414	61	..	..	11.7	1,287	..	..	..	..	..	..	..
Philippines	310	3	1.0	..	18.5	54,814	..	..	..	..	..	..	..
Samoa	77	433	..	..	4.3c	136	..	..	..	..	..	..	..
Solomon Islands	206	394	..	..	4.0	110	..	..	..	..	..	..	..
Thailand	..	..	..	28.6	6.8	54,554	..	..	..	..	..	..	..
Timor-Leste	217	191	..	..	..	..	..	..	..	..	..	..	..
Tuvalu	18	881a	..	..	..	..	..	..	..	..	..	..	..
Vanuatu	103	431	..	..	1.5c	96	..	..	..	..	..	..	..
Vietnam	3,744	43	..	..	1.8	21,704	..	..	..	..	..	..	..
Europe & Central Asia	**8,101**	**20**	**..**	**..**	**26.9**	**1,012,513**	**..**	**..**	**..**	**..**	**..**	**..**	**..**
Albania	358	113	..	..	6.9	3,683	..	..	..	..	..	..	..
Armenia	528	171	25.6	..	20.9	3,656	..	..	..	..	..	..	..
Azerbaijan	232	26	3.3	..	1.7	3,701	..	..	..	..	..	..	..
Belarus	98	10	0.6	18.1	5.0	15,228	..	..	..	..	..	..	..
Bosnia & Herzegovina	415	110	5.9	..	10.5	7,925	..	..	..	..	..	..	..
Bulgaria	..	..	..	..	21.3	36,959	..	..	..	..	..	..	..
Georgia	908	213	27.3	34.7	7.3	3,064	..	..	..	..	..	..	..
Kazakhstan	298	19	1.5	9.5	80.2	97,124	..	..	..	..	..	..	..
Kosovo	788	437	..	..	20.8	223	..	..	..	..	..	..	..
Kyrgyz Republic	315	59	35.7	..	14.0	1,576	..	..	..	..	..	..	..
Latvia	..	..	..	41.8	..	..	..	..	..	..	..	..	..
Lithuania	..	..	..	33.3	31.0	28,939	..	..	..	..	..	..	..
Macedonia, FYR	193	95	6.9	..	14.8	5,188	..	..	..	..	..	..	..

TABLE 2G – MDG 8: Develop a Global Partnership for Development

| | Net Official Development Assistance received | | | Central gov't debt (% of GDP) 2008-2009 | Total debt service (% of exports of goods, services, & income) 2008-2009 | Present value of external debt (current million US$) 2009 | Cumulative debt relief committed under HIPC (million US$ in end-2009 NPV terms) 2009 | Net Official Development Assistance provided | | | | | Agriculture support for OECD countries (% of their GDP) 2009 |
	total in 2009 (current million US$)	per capita in 2009 (current US$)	as % of central gov't expense 2008-2009					in 2010 (current million US$)	as % of OECD/ DAC donor's GNI 2010	that is untied (%) 2009	to help build trade capacity (%) 2009	to basic social services in 2009 (current million US$)	
Moldova	245	68	11.8	24.4	14.9	3,157	..	..	..	..	..	..	..
Montenegro	75	121	..	..	4.4	2,025	..	..	..	..	..	..	..
Romania	..	..	..	..	31.4	94,557	..	..	..	..	..	..	..
Russian Federation	..	..	..	8.6	17.7	348,913	..	..	..	..	..	..	..
Serbia	608	83	3.8	..	37.1	30,484	..	..	..	..	..	..	..
Tajikistan	409	59	..	..	38.4	1,792	..	..	..	..	..	..	..
Turkey	1,362	18	0.8	51.4	41.6	231,439	..	..	..	..	..	..	4.0
Turkmenistan	40	8	..	..	..	525	..	..	..	..	..	..	..
Ukraine	668	15	1.4	..	36.2	89,029	..	..	..	..	..	..	..
Uzbekistan	190	7	..	..	..	3,329	..	..	..	..	..	..	..
Latin America & Caribbean	**9,104**	**16**	**..**	**..**	**17.9**	**846,986**	**..**	**..**	**..**	**..**	**..**	**..**	**..**
Argentina	128	3	..	..	17.3	119,952	..	..	..	..	..	..	..
Belize	28	84	..	..	13.6	811	..	..	..	..	..	..	..
Bolivia	726	74	31.0[b]	..	14.4	2,446	1,949	..	..	..	..	..	..
Brazil	338	2	0.1	61.0	23.4	260,697	..	..	..	..	..	..	..
Chile	80	5	0.2	..	22.6	65,749	..	..	..	..	..	..	..
Colombia	1,060	23	2.3	59.3	22.4	44,370	..	..	..	..	..	..	..
Costa Rica	109	24	1.4	..	9.6	7,573	..	..	..	..	..	..	..
Cuba	116	10	..	..	..	..	..	..	..	..	..	..	..
Dominican Republic	120	12	2.1	..	12.1	9,248	..	..	..	..	..	..	..
Ecuador	209	15	..	..	40.8	11,816	..	..	..	..	..	..	..
El Salvador	277	45	53.2	48.5	25.2	10,198	..	..	..	..	..	..	..
Guatemala	376	27	8.0	23.3	18.4	12,013	..	..	..	..	..	..	..
Guyana	173	228	..	..	2.6	668	897	..	..	..	..	..	..
Haiti	1,120	112	..	..	4.6	989	164	..	..	..	..	..	..
Honduras	457	61	13.3	..	6.8	1,775	816	..	..	..	..	..	..
Jamaica	150	55	3.0	115.8	33.9	10,991	..	..	..	..	..	..	..
Mexico	185	2	..	..	16.0	176,766	..	..	..	..	..	..	0.8
Nicaragua	774	135	60.2	..	17.2	2,090	4,861	..	..	..	..	..	..
Panama	66	19	..	..	5.5	11,464	..	..	..	..	..	..	..
Paraguay	148	23	6.1	..	6.1	3,760	..	..	..	..	..	..	..
Peru	442	15	2.0	23.6	11.8	26,341	..	..	..	..	..	..	..
Suriname	157	302	..	..	..	..	..	..	..	..	..	..	..
Uruguay	51	15	0.5	49.5	21.0	10,868	..	..	..	..	..	..	..
Venezuela, RB	67	2	0.1[a]	..	6.4	54,906	..	..	..	..	..	..	..
High-income countries													
Australia	..	..	..	24.1	..	..	..	3,849	0.3	90.8	14.3	281	0.2
Austria	..	..	..	70.7	..	..	..	1,199	0.3	55.2	22.4	23	..
Bahamas, The	..	..	..	34.1[c]	..	..	..	..	..	..	..	..	..
Bahrain	..	..	..	14.7	..	..	..	..	..	..	..	..	..
Belgium	..	..	..	92.4	..	..	..	3,000	0.6	95.5	38.3	187	..
Brunei Darussalam	..	..	..	..	..	..	..	..	..	..	..	..	..
Canada	..	..	..	53.2	..	..	..	5,132	0.3	98.3	16.7	834	0.8
Croatia	169	38	0.7	..	..	..	..	..	..	..	..	..	..
Cyprus	..	..	..	97.3	..	..	..	..	..	..	..	..	..
Czech Republic	..	..	..	31.9	..	..	..	..	..	..	..	..	..
Denmark	..	..	..	41.0	..	..	..	2,867	0.9	96.6	26.2	285	..
Equatorial Guinea	32	47	..	..	..	..	..	..	..	..	..	..	..
Estonia	..	..	..	9.1	..	..	..	..	..	..	..	..	..
Finland	..	..	..	36.2	..	..	..	1,335	0.6	90.3	38.5	54	..
France	..	..	..	82.8	..	..	..	12,916	0.5	89.2	24.7	546	..
Germany	..	..	..	47.2	..	..	..	12,723	0.4	97.1	31.8	723	..
Greece	..	..	..	138.5	..	..	..	500	0.2	49.8	8.2	25	..
Hong Kong SAR, China	..	..	..	30.5	..	0	..	..	..	..	..	..	..

TABLE 2G – MDG 8: Develop a Global Partnership for Development

| | Net Official Development Assistance received | | | Central gov't debt (% of GDP) 2008-2009 | Total debt service (% of exports of goods, services, & income) 2008-2009 | Present value of external debt (current million US$) 2009 | Cumulative debt relief committed under HIPC (million US$ in end-2009 NPV terms) 2009 | Net Official Development Assistance provided | | | | | Agriculture support for OECD countries (% of their GDP) 2009 |
	total in 2009 (current million US$)	per capita in 2009 (current US$)	as % of central gov't expense 2008-2009					in 2010 (current million US$)	as % of OECD/ DAC donor's GNI 2010	that is untied (%) 2009	to help build trade capacity (%) 2009	to basic social services in 2009 (current million US$)	
Hungary	..	..	..	81.7	..	..	..	..	..	..	..	..	..
Iceland	..	..	..	104.7	..	..	..	..	..	..	..	..	1.1
Ireland	..	..	..	69.2	..	..	..	895	0.5	100.0	12.6	161	..
Israel	..	..	..	..	..	..	..	..	..	..	..	..	..
Italy	..	..	..	118.9	..	..	..	3,111	0.2	56.2	37.1	99	..
Japan	..	..	..	157.7	..	..	..	11,045	0.2	94.8	55.4	2,060	1.1
Korea, Rep.	..	..	..	..	..	..	..	1,168	0.1	48.4	66.7	94	2.4
Kuwait	..	..	..	..	..	..	..	..	..	..	..	..	..
Luxembourg	..	..	..	12.7	..	..	..	399	1.1	100.0	16.6	66	..
Macao SAR, China	..	..	..	..	..	..	..	..	..	..	..	..	..
Malta	..	..	..	81.1	..	..	..	..	..	..	..	..	..
Netherlands	..	..	..	58.3	..	..	..	6,351	0.8	80.8	17.9	446	..
New Zealand	..	..	..	37.9c	..	..	..	353	0.3	90.1	14.8	51	0.2
Norway	..	..	..	36.3	..	..	..	4,582	1.1	100.0	28.4	598	1.1
Oman	212	75	..	..	..	..	..	..	..	..	..	..	..
Poland	..	..	..	48.1	..	..	..	..	..	..	..	..	..
Portugal	..	..	..	84.4	..	..	..	648	0.3	27.9	32.8	10	..
Qatar	..	..	..	..	..	..	..	..	..	..	..	..	..
Saudi Arabia	24	1b	..	..	..	..	..	..	..	..	..	..	..
Singapore	..	..	..	113.3	..	..	..	..	..	..	..	..	..
Slovak Republic	..	..	..	38.1	..	..	..	..	..	..	..	..	..
Slovenia	..	..	..	..	..	..	..	..	..	..	..	..	..
Spain	..	..	..	46.5	..	..	..	5,917	0.4	76.6	30.4	737	..
Sweden	..	..	..	44.0	..	..	..	4,527	1.0	99.9	21	176	..
Switzerland	..	..	..	28.9	..	..	..	2,295	0.4	99.2	21.2	84	1.4
Trinidad & Tobago	7	5	0.1	14.1	..	..	..	..	..	..	..	..	..
United Arab Emirates	..	..	..	..	..	..	..	..	..	..	..	..	..
United Kingdom	..	..	..	73.2	..	..	..	13,763	0.6	100.0	23.9	1,738	..
United States	..	..	..	67.1	..	..	..	30,154	0.2	69.8	20.7	7,413	0.9

.. Data not available.
0 Zero, or rounds to zero at the displayed number of decimal places.
a Data refers to 2005.
b Data refers to 2006.
c Data refers to 2007.
d Data refers to 2008.
e Data refers to 2009.
f Data refers to 2010.

Notes and Sources for Tables on pages 182-184.

TABLE 3 – United States: State Hunger and Poverty in 2010

	Food insecure (%) average 2008-2010		Poverty rate (below 100% of the poverty level)		Deep poverty rate (below 50% of the poverty level)		SNAP (average monthly participation)	WIC program (total participation)	School breakfast program (total participation)	National school lunch program (total participation)	Summer food service program (average daily attendance)
	total	with hunger	all	children under age 18	all	children under age 18					
United States	**14.6**	**5.6**	**15.3**	**21.6**	**6.8**	**9.6**	**40,301,878**	**9,176,736**	**11,669,577**	**31,746,724**	**2,304,413**
Alabama	17.3	7.0	19.0	27.7	8.1	12.9	805,095	145,001	217,549	579,210	26,657
Alaska	13.6	4.9	9.9	12.9	4.1	4.5	76,445	27,020	18,668	54,723	4,498
Arizona	15.3	5.9	17.4	24.4	8.3	11.7	1,018,171	206,765	253,182	669,254	17,508
Arkansas	18.6	7.5	18.8	27.6	7.8	11.8	466,598	98,963	157,164	353,466	18,884
California	15.9	5.8	15.8	22.0	6.8	9.3	3,238,548	1,459,460	1,245,046	3,240,289	117,957
Colorado	13.4	5.4	13.4	17.4	6.0	7.5	404,679	109,643	113,574	400,254	10,229
Connecticut	12.7	4.8	10.1	12.8	4.7	6.2	336,064	58,108	71,661	303,655	9,068
Delaware	9.7	4.0	11.8	18.1	5.4	7.6	112,513	23,625	34,527	91,998	14,260
District of Columbia	13.0	4.5	19.2	30.4	10.7	16.2	118,493	16,946	22,438	46,367	35,034
Florida	16.1	6.6	16.5	23.5	7.4	10.4	2,603,185	509,731	644,891	1,609,077	129,804
Georgia	16.9	6.4	17.9	24.8	8.2	11.3	1,591,078	311,993	581,528	1,303,254	70,218
Hawaii	13.1	5.0	10.7	13.9	5.6	7.2	138,166	37,029	36,058	117,353	6,244
Idaho	12.4	4.6	15.7	19.0	6.3	7.5	194,033	47,046	70,972	170,081	21,365
Illinois	12.9	4.5	13.8	19.4	6.1	8.6	1,645,722	307,278	336,675	1,167,636	56,194
Indiana	13.0	5.4	15.3	21.7	7.0	9.8	813,403	174,119	228,866	807,786	54,765
Iowa	12.1	4.9	12.6	16.3	5.3	6.7	340,304	74,685	84,856	397,681	10,463
Kansas	14.5	5.0	13.6	18.4	5.9	7.9	269,710	77,363	99,594	360,637	18,147
Kentucky	15.6	5.7	19.0	26.3	8.2	12.6	778,114	139,100	245,999	556,263	50,137
Louisiana	12.6	4.0	18.7	27.3	8.1	12.3	825,918	155,619	254,106	595,935	25,907
Maine	15.4	6.8	12.9	17.8	4.7	6.3	229,731	27,153	40,242	110,693	7,630
Maryland	12.5	5.1	9.9	13.0	4.9	6.9	560,848	147,848	157,977	433,614	49,585
Massachusetts	10.8	4.5	11.4	14.3	5.3	6.6	749,121	125,637	139,114	544,130	51,810
Michigan	14.7	5.7	16.8	23.5	7.6	10.8	1,776,368	257,388	326,187	920,101	64,732
Minnesota	10.3	4.4	11.6	15.2	5.0	6.4	430,346	138,562	156,634	630,764	65,380
Mississippi	19.4	6.9	22.4	32.5	9.7	15.5	575,674	102,224	204,472	405,577	25,438
Missouri	15.8	6.6	15.3	20.9	6.6	9.6	901,349	151,224	241,681	649,539	24,877
Montana	14.1	5.6	14.6	20.1	6.3	9.6	113,570	20,742	26,494	87,476	7,304
Nebraska	12.7	5.2	12.9	18.2	5.2	7.2	162,817	45,267	59,637	246,266	9,260
Nevada	14.7	5.4	14.9	22.0	7.0	10.0	278,105	74,344	55,293	188,017	5,964
New Hampshire	9.6	4.1	8.3	10.0	3.8	4.8	104,375	17,897	23,567	109,991	4,604
New Jersey	12.1	4.2	10.3	14.5	4.6	6.4	622,022	171,060	181,185	721,587	46,265
New Mexico	15.4	5.6	20.4	30.0	8.7	13.0	356,822	65,472	130,147	227,526	37,964
New York	12.9	5.1	14.9	21.2	6.8	10.1	2,757,836	512,547	601,915	1,826,027	382,071
North Carolina	15.7	5.2	17.5	24.9	7.8	11.5	1,346,495	272,759	370,705	955,810	66,533
North Dakota	7.1	2.7	13.0	16.2	5.9	7.9	59,888	14,621	20,991	82,443	2,747
Ohio	16.4	6.6	15.8	23.3	7.3	11.6	1,607,422	297,672	380,652	1,136,344	69,095
Oklahoma	16.4	7.5	16.9	24.7	7.2	10.7	582,492	133,002	218,255	449,220	11,665
Oregon	13.7	6.1	15.8	21.6	7.2	9.5	705,035	114,140	141,179	315,224	38,595
Pennsylvania	12.5	5.0	13.4	19.1	5.9	8.4	1,574,783	262,269	319,242	1,159,852	99,943
Rhode Island	14.7	5.9	14.0	19.0	6.0	8.3	138,966	25,525	24,587	78,531	7,543
South Carolina	14.8	5.0	18.2	26.1	8.4	13.3	797,110	134,001	256,104	501,965	58,733
South Dakota	12.3	5.4	14.4	18.2	6.3	7.8	95,336	22,778	26,193	108,050	4,986
Tennessee	15.0	6.0	17.7	25.7	7.9	12.2	1,224,023	170,588	293,349	699,875	29,892
Texas	18.8	6.9	17.9	25.7	7.4	10.6	3,551,581	1,036,220	1,635,587	3,352,829	162,502
Utah	13.0	4.8	13.2	15.7	5.6	6.5	247,405	75,389	69,794	339,326	16,777
Vermont	13.8	6.1	12.7	16.7	5.7	7.2	85,538	16,804	22,231	55,144	2,913
Virginia	9.6	3.3	11.1	14.5	4.8	6.2	786,157	160,400	245,058	757,862	50,767
Washington	14.7	6.1	13.4	18.2	6.1	7.8	956,004	194,352	176,918	543,940	36,737
West Virginia	14.1	5.3	18.1	25.5	7.2	10.9	341,156	51,798	95,984	212,390	16,959
Wisconsin	11.8	4.3	13.2	19.1	5.6	7.7	715,213	126,535	151,534	602,502	90,626
Wyoming	11.6	4.3	11.2	14.3	4.7	4.7	34,799	13,687	15,226	56,540	3,779
Puerto Rico	..	..	45.0	56.3	25.3	36.6	..	192,084	131,817	352,447	44,103

.. Data not available.

Notes and Sources for Tables on pages 182-184.

TABLE 4 – United States: National Hunger and Poverty Trends

	2000	2001	2002	2003	2004	2005	2006	2007	2008	2009	2010
Total population (millions)	**281.4**	**284.8**[a]	**288.0**[a]	**290.8**[a]	**293.6**[a]	**296.4**[a]	**299.4**[a]	**301.6**[a]	**301.0**[a]	**303.8**[a]	**305.7**
Food insecurity prevalence (%)											
All U.S. households	10.5	10.7	11.1	11.2	11.9	11.0	10.9	11.1	14.6	14.7	14.5
with hunger[b]	3.1	3.3	3.5	3.5	3.9	3.9	4.0	4.1	5.7	5.7	5.4
Adults	10.1	10.2	10.5	10.8	11.3	10.4	10.4	10.6	14.4	14.5	14.2
with hunger[b]	2.8	3.0	3.0	3.1	3.4	3.5	3.5	3.7	5.4	5.4	4.9
Children	18.0	17.6	18.1	18.2	19.0	16.9	17.2	16.9	22.5	23.2	21.6
with hunger[b]	0.8	0.6	0.8	0.6	0.7	0.8	0.6	0.9	1.5	1.3	1.3
Percent of federal budget spent on food assistance[c]	**1.8**	**1.8**	**1.9**	**2.0**	**2.0**	**2.1**	**2.0**	**2.0**	**2.0**	**2.2**	**2.7**
Total infant mortality rate (per 1,000 live births)	**6.9**	**6.9**	**7.0**	**6.9**	**6.8**	**6.9**	**6.7**	**6.8**	**..**	**..**	**..**
White	5.7	5.7	5.8	5.7	5.7	5.7	5.6	5.6	..	..	..
White, non-Hispanic	5.7	5.7	5.8	5.7	5.7	5.8	5.6	5.6	..	..	..
Hispanic	5.6	5.4	5.6	5.7	5.6	5.6	5.4	5.5	..	..	..
African American	14.1	13.3	14.4	14.0	13.8	13.7	12.9	13.3	..	..	..
Asian/Pacific Islander	4.9	4.7	4.8	4.8	4.7	4.9	4.6	4.8	..	..	..
American Indian/Alaska Native	8.3	9.7	8.6	8.7	8.5	8.1	8.3	9.2	..	..	..
Total poverty rate (%)	**11.3**	**11.7**	**12.1**	**12.5**	**12.7**	**12.6**	**12.3**	**12.5**	**13.2**	**14.3**	**15.1**
Northeast	10.3	10.7	10.9	11.3	11.6	11.3	11.5	11.4	11.6	12.2	12.8
Midwest	9.5	9.4	10.3	10.7	11.6	11.4	11.2	11.1	12.4	13.3	13.9
South	12.5	13.5	13.8	14.1	14.1	14.0	13.8	14.2	14.3	15.7	16.9
West	11.9	12.1	12.4	12.6	12.6	12.6	11.6	12.0	13.5	14.8	15.3
White	9.4	9.9	10.2	10.6	10.8	10.6	10.3	10.5	11.2	12.3	13.0
White, non-Hispanic	7.5	7.8	8.0	8.2	8.6	8.3	8.2	8.2	8.6	9.4	9.9
Hispanic	21.2	21.4	21.8	22.5	21.9	21.8	20.6	21.5	23.2	25.3	26.6
African American	22.1	22.7	24.1	24.3	24.7	24.9	24.3	24.5	24.7	25.8	27.4
Asian[d]	10.8	10.2	10.2	11.8	9.8	11.1	10.1	10.2	11.6	12.5	12.1
American Indian/Alaska Native	25.9[e]	..	..	20.0[f]	..	..	..	..	..	..	..
Elderly (65 years and older)	10.2	10.1	10.4	10.2	9.8	10.1	9.4	9.7	9.7	8.9	9.0
Female-headed households	24.7	26.4	26.5	28.0	28.4	28.7	28.3	28.3	28.7	29.9	31.6
Children under age 6 in households	17.8	18.2	18.5	19.8	20.0	20.0	20.0	20.8	21.3	23.8	25.3
Total child poverty rate (18 years and under) (%)	**16.2**	**16.3**	**16.7**	**17.6**	**17.8**	**17.6**	**17.4**	**18.0**	**19.0**	**20.7**	**22.0**
White	13.0	13.4	13.6	14.3	14.8	14.4	14.1	14.9	15.8	17.7	18.7
White, non-Hispanic	9.4	9.5	9.4	9.8	10.5	10.0	10.0	10.1	10.6	11.9	12.4
Hispanic	28.0	28.0	28.6	29.7	28.9	28.3	26.9	28.6	30.6	33.1	35.0
African American	30.9	30.2	32.3	34.1	33.6	34.5	33.4	34.5	33.9	35.4	38.2
Asian[d]	14.5	11.5	11.7	12.5	10.0	11.1	11.4	11.9	13.3	13.3	13.6
Total unemployment rate (%)	**4.0**	**4.7**	**5.8**	**6.0**	**5.5**	**5.1**	**4.6**	**4.6**	**5.8**	**9.3**	**9.6**
White	3.5	4.2	5.1	5.2	4.8	4.4	4.0	4.1	5.2	8.5	8.7
Hispanic	5.7	6.6	7.5	7.7	7.0	6.0	5.2	5.6	7.6	12.1	12.5
African American	7.6	8.6	10.2	10.8	10.4	10.0	8.9	8.3	10.1	14.8	16.0
Asian[d]	3.6	4.5	5.9	6.0	4.4	4.0	3.0	3.2	4.0	7.3	7.5

TABLE 4: United States – National Hunger and Poverty Trends

	2000	2001	2002	2003	2004	2005	2006	2007	2008	2009	2010
Household income distribution (%)											
Total population											
Lowest 20 percent	3.6	3.5	3.5	3.4	3.4	3.4	3.4	3.4	3.4	3.4	3.3
Second quintile	8.9	8.7	8.8	8.7	8.7	8.6	8.6	8.7	8.6	8.6	8.5
Third quintile	14.8	14.6	14.8	14.8	14.7	14.6	14.5	14.8	14.7	14.6	14.6
Fourth quintile	23.0	23.0	23.3	23.4	23.2	23.0	22.9	23.4	23.3	23.2	23.4
Highest 20 percent	49.6	50.1	49.7	49.8	50.1	50.4	50.5	49.7	50.0	50.3	50.2
Ratio of highest 20 percent to lowest 20 percent	13.8	14.3	14.2	14.6	14.7	14.8	14.8	14.6	14.7	14.8	15.2
White											
Lowest 20 percent	3.7	3.7	3.7	3.6	3.6	3.6	3.7	3.7	3.6	3.7	3.5
Second quintile	9.0	8.9	9.0	8.9	8.8	8.9	8.9	8.9	8.8	8.9	8.7
Third quintile	14.9	14.7	15.0	14.8	14.8	14.7	14.6	14.9	14.8	14.8	14.8
Fourth quintile	22.9	22.9	23.2	23.2	23.1	22.9	22.9	23.3	23.3	23.2	23.3
Highest 20 percent	49.4	49.8	49.2	49.4	49.6	49.9	49.9	49.2	49.4	49.5	49.7
Ratio of highest 20 percent to lowest 20 percent	13.4	13.5	13.2	21.4	13.8	13.9	13.4	13.3	13.7	13.4	14.2
Hispanic											
Lowest 20 percent	4.3	4.0	3.9	3.9	3.8	3.9	3.8	3.9	3.7	3.7	3.5
Second quintile	9.8	9.4	9.4	9.4	9.3	9.5	9.3	9.5	9.2	9.0	9.0
Third quintile	15.7	15.2	14.8	15.0	14.9	15.2	15.0	15.2	14.7	14.7	14.7
Fourth quintile	23.8	23.2	22.9	23.1	22.9	23.3	22.9	23.5	23.2	23.1	23.4
Highest 20 percent	46.4	48.3	49.0	48.6	49.1	48.1	48.9	47.9	49.2	49.5	49.4
Ratio of highest 20 percent to lowest 20 percent	10.8	12.1	12.6	12.5	12.9	12.3	12.8	12.3	13.3	13.4	14.1
African American											
Lowest 20 percent	3.2	3.0	2.9	2.9	2.8	2.8	2.8	2.8	3.0	2.9	2.7
Second quintile	8.6	8.6	8.2	8.2	8.3	8.0	8.1	8.1	8.4	8.2	7.9
Third quintile	15.2	15.0	14.5	14.7	14.6	14.5	14.3	14.5	14.6	14.3	14.2
Fourth quintile	23.8	24.2	23.3	24.0	23.8	23.7	23.2	23.7	23.5	23.5	23.6
Highest 20 percent	49.3	49.2	51.1	50.2	50.5	50.9	51.6	50.8	50.6	51.1	51.6
Ratio of highest 20 percent to lowest 20 percent	15.4	16.4	17.6	17.3	18.0	18.2	18.4	18.1	16.9	17.6	19.1

..	Data not available.
a	U.S. Census estimate.
b	Data from 2005 onward is referred to by the USDA as "very low food security" instead of "food insecure with hunger."
c	Data refer to fiscal year.
d	Reclassified from "Asian and Pacific Islander" in 2002.
e	3-year average: 1998, 1999, and 2000.
f	3-year average: 2001, 2002, and 2003.

Notes and Sources for Tables on pages 182-184.

Notes and Sources for Tables

TABLE 1

HDI Index: Human Development Index (HDI) is a summary composite index that measures a country's average achievements in three basic aspects of human development: health, knowledge, and income. It was developed by the late Pakistani economist Mahbub ul Haq with the collaboration of the Nobel laureate Amartya Sen and other leading development thinkers for the first Human Development Report in 1990. It was introduced as an alternative to conventional measures of national development, such as level of income and the rate of economic growth.

Workers' remittances & compensation received by employees (current US$): comprise current transfers by migrant workers and wages/salaries earned by nonresident workers. Data are the sum of three items defined in the fifth edition of the IMF's Balance of Payments Manual: workers' remittances, compensation of employees, and migrants' transfers.

Gross Domestic Product (GDP): the sum of gross value added by all resident producers in the economy plus any product taxes and minus any subsidies not included in the value of the products. It is calculated without making deductions for depreciation of fabricated assets or for depletion and degradation of natural resources.

Gross Domestic Product per capita (current US$): Gross Domestic Product divided by midyear population.

Gross Domestic Product per capita PPP (current int'l$): PPP GDP is Gross Domestic Product converted to international dollars using purchasing power parity rates. An international dollar has the same purchasing power over GDP as the U.S. dollar has in the United States.

Exports/Imports of goods & services (current million US$): the value of all goods and other market services provided to/received from the rest of the world. They include the value of merchandise, freight, insurance, transport, travel, royalties, license fees, and other services, such as communication, construction, financial, information, business, personal, and government services. They exclude compensation of employees, investment income, and transfer payments.

SOURCES

Columns 1-7 and 9-25: World Bank (2011), World Development Indicators 2011. Column 8: United Nations Development Program (2011), International Human Development Indicators.

TABLE 2A

Employed people living below $1 PPP per day (%): the proportion of employed persons living below $1 (PPP) per day, or working poor, is the share of individuals who are employed, but nonetheless live in a household whose members are estimated to be living below the international poverty line of $1.25 a day, measured at 2005 international prices, adjusted for Purchasing Power Parity (PPP).

Population undernourished: people whose dietary energy consumption is continuously below a minimum dietary energy requirement for maintaining a healthy life and carrying out light physical activity, with an acceptable weight for their height.

SOURCES

Columns 1-3 and 5-9: World Bank (2011), World Development Indicators 2011. Columns 4, 10 and 11: United Nations (2011), Millennium Development Goals Indicators.

TABLE 2B

School enrollment (% net): net enrollment ratio is the ratio of children of school age based on the International Standard Classification of Education 1997 who are enrolled in school to the entire population of the corresponding age group.

School enrollment (% gross): gross enrollment ratio is the ratio of total enrollment, regardless of age, to the population of the age group that corresponds to the level of education shown.

Persistence to grade 5 (% of cohort): is the share of children enrolled in the first grade of primary school who eventually reach grade 5.

Literacy rate: the percentage of people who can read with understanding and write a short, simple statement on their everyday life.

SOURCE

Columns 1-13: World Bank (2011), World Development Indicators 2011.

TABLE 2C

Low birth weight newborns (% of births): newborns weighing less than 2,500 grams (5.5 pounds), with the measurement taken within the first hours of life, before significant postnatal weight loss has occurred.

Percent of children under-5 suffering from underweight, moderate & severe: children whose weight for age is more than two standard deviations below the median for the international reference population ages 0-59 months.

Percent of children under-5 suffering from underweight, severe: children whose weight for age is more than three standard deviations below the median for the international reference population ages 0-59 months.

Percent of children under-5 suffering from wasting, moderate & severe: children whose weight for height is more than two standard deviations below the median for the international reference population ages 0-59 months.

Percent of children under-5 suffering from stunting, moderate & severe: children whose height for age (stunting) is more than two standard deviations below the median for the international reference population ages 0-59 months. For children up to two years old, height is measured by recumbent length. For older children, height is measured standing.

Vitamin A supplement coverage rate (% of children 6-59 months): the percentage of children 6-59 months old who received at least one high-dose vitamin A capsule in the previous six months.

SOURCES

Columns 1-4 and 6-11: World Bank (2011), World Development Indicators 2011. Column 5: United Nations (2011), Millennium Development Goals Indicators.

TABLE 2D

Pregnant women receiving any prenatal care (%): the percentage of women attended by skilled health personnel at least once during pregnancy for reasons related to pregnancy.

Births attended by skilled health staff (%): the percentage of deliveries attended by personnel trained to give the necessary supervision, care, and advice to women during pregnancy, labor, and the postpartum period; to attend to deliveries on their own; and to care for newborns.

Contraceptive prevalence of married women ages 15-49 (%): the percentage of women who are practicing, or whose sexual partners are practicing, any form of contraception. It is usually measured for married women ages 15-49 only.

SOURCES

Columns 1-3, 6, and 8-10: World Bank (2011), World Development Indicators 2011. Columns 4, 5, and 7: United Nations (2011), Millennium Development Goals Indicators.

TABLE 2E

People with advanced HIV on ARV treatment (%): the percentage of adults and children with advanced HIV infection currently receiving antiretroviral (ARV) therapy according to nationally approved treatment protocols (or

WHO/Joint U.N. Program on HIV and AIDS standards), out of the estimated number of people with advanced HIV infection. The human immunodeficiency virus (HIV) is a virus that weakens the immune system, ultimately leading to Acquired Immunodeficiency Syndrome (AIDS). The number of adults with advanced HIV infection who should start treatment is estimated based on the assumption that the average time from HIV seroconversion (becoming HIV-positive) to eligibility for antiretroviral therapy is eight years and that, without antiretroviral therapy, the average time from eligibility to death is three years.

People with new TB cases in 2009 (per 100,000 people): the incidence of Tuberculosis is the estimated number of new pulmonary, smear positive, and extra-pulmonary tuberculosis cases.

SOURCES

Columns 1-3 and 6-10: United Nations (2011), Millennium Development Goals Indicators. Columns 4 and 5: Demographic and Health Surveys (2011), STATcompiler. Columns 11 and 12: World Bank (2011), World Development Indicators.

TABLE 2F

Agricultural land (% of land area): the share of land area that is arable, under permanent crops, and under permanent pastures. Arable land includes land defined by the FAO as land under temporary crops (double-cropped areas are counted once), temporary meadows for mowing or for pasture, land under market or kitchen gardens, and land temporarily fallow. Land abandoned as a result of shifting cultivation is excluded. Land under permanent crops is land cultivated with crops that occupy the land for long periods and need not be replanted after each harvest, such as cocoa, coffee, and rubber. This category includes land under flowering shrubs, fruit trees, nut trees, and vines, but excludes land under trees grown for wood or timber. Permanent pasture is land used for five or more years for forage, including natural and cultivated crops.

Cereal yield (kg per hectare of harvested land): includes wheat, rice, maize, barley, oats, rye, millet, sorghum, buckwheat, and mixed grains. Production data on cereals relate to crops harvested for dry grain only. Cereal crops harvested for hay; harvested green for food, feed, or silage; or used for grazing are excluded. One hectare is 2.5 acres.

Fertilizer consumption (kg per hectare of arable land): the quantity of plant nutrients used per unit of arable land. Fertilizer products include nitrogenous, potash, and phosphate fertilizers (including ground rock phosphate). Traditional nutrients (animal and plant manures) are not included. Arable land includes land defined by the FAO as land under temporary crops (double-cropped areas are counted once), temporary meadows for mowing or for pasture, land under market or kitchen gardens, and land temporarily fallow. Land abandoned as a result of shifting cultivation is excluded.

CO_2 emissions (metric ton(s) per capita): emissions stemming from the burning of fossil fuels and the manufacture of cement. They include carbon dioxide produced during consumption of solid, liquid, and gas fuels and gas flaring.

Energy use (kg of oil equivalent) per $1,000 GDP (constant 2005 PPP $): is the kilogram of oil equivalent of energy use per $1,000 of Gross Domestic Product converted to 2005 constant international dollars using Purchasing Power Parity rates. Energy use refers to use of primary energy before transformation to other end-use fuels. It is calculated as indigenous production, plus imports and stock changes, minus exports and fuels supplied to ships and aircraft engaged in international transport.

Improved sanitation facilities (% of population with access): the percentage of the population with at least adequate access to excreta disposal facilities that can effectively prevent human, animal, and insect contact with excreta. Improved facilities range from simple but protected pit latrines to flush toilets with a sewerage connection. To be effective, facilities must be correctly constructed and properly maintained.

Improved water source: the percentage of the population with reasonable

access to an adequate amount of water from an improved source, such as a household connection, public standpipe, borehole, protected well or spring, or rainwater collection. Unimproved sources include vendors, tanker trucks, and unprotected wells and springs. Reasonable access is defined as the availability of at least 20 liters a person a day from a source within one kilometer of the dwelling.

Slum population (% of urban population): the proportion of urban population living in slum households, usually defined as a group of individuals living under the same roof and lacking one or more of the following: access to improved water, access to improved sanitation, sufficient-living area, housing of sufficient durability.

SOURCES

Columns 1-7 and 9-11: World Bank (2011), World Development Indicators 2011. Columns 8 and 12: United Nations (2011), Millennium Development Goals Indicators.

TABLE 2G

MDG 8 includes targets to address the special needs of least developed countries, landlocked developing countries, and small island developing states. Below you will find the countries in each of these special-needs categories, according to the United Nations' listings within the World Bank's classifications of low- & middle-income (United Nations Statistics Division (2011), "Composition of macro geographical (continental) regions, geographical sub-regions, and selected economic groupings").

Least developed countries: Sub-Saharan Africa: Angola, Benin, Burkina Faso, Burundi, Central African Republic, Chad, Comoros, Dem. Rep. Congo, Eritrea, Ethiopia, the Gambia, Guinea, Guinea-Bissau, Lesotho, Liberia, Madagascar, Malawi, Mali, Mauritania, Mozambique, Niger, Rwanda, Saõ Tomé & Principe, Senegal, Sierra Leone, Somalia, Sudan, Tanzania, Togo, Uganda, and Zambia; Middle East & North Africa: Djibouti and Rep. Yemen; South Asia: Afghanistan, Bangladesh, Bhutan, and Nepal; East Asia & Pacific: Cambodia, Kiribati, Lao PDR, Myanmar, Samoa, Solomon Islands, Timor-Leste, Tuvalu, and Vanuatu; Latin America & the Caribbean: Haiti.

Landlocked developing countries: Sub-Saharan Africa: Botswana, Burkina Faso, Burundi, Central African Republic, Chad, Ethiopia, Lesotho, Malawi, Mali, Niger, Rwanda, Swaziland, Uganda, Zambia, and Zimbabwe; South Asia: Afghanistan, Bhutan, and Nepal; East Asia & Pacific: Lao PDR and Mongolia; Europe & Central Asia: Armenia, Azerbaijan, Kazakhstan, Kyrgyz Republic, FYR Macedonia, Moldova, Tajikistan, Turkmenistan, and Uzbekistan; Latin America & Caribbean: Bolivia and Paraguay.

Small island developing states: Sub-Saharan Africa: Cape Verde, Comoros, Guinea-Bissau, Mauritius, and Saõ Tomé & Principe; South Asia: Maldives; East Asia & Pacific: Fiji, Kiribati, Papua New Guinea, Samoa, Solomon Islands, Timor-Leste, Tuvalu, and Vanuatu; Latin America & Caribbean: Belize, Cuba, Dominican Republic, Guyana, Haiti, Jamaica, and Suriname.

Official Development Assistance (ODA): grants or loans to developing countries and territories—defined as those on the list of aid recipients of the Organization for Economic Cooperation and Development/Development Assistance Committee (OECD/DAC)—that are made by the official sector with the promotion of economic development and welfare as the main objective and at concessional financial terms. It includes loans with a grant element of at least 25 percent (calculated at a discount rate of 10 percent). Technical cooperation is included. Grants, loans, and credits for military purposes are excluded. Also excluded is aid to more advanced developing and transition countries, as categorized by the DAC.

Net Official Development Assistance per capita (current US$): calculated by dividing net ODA received by the midyear population estimate.

Central gov't debt (% of GDP): the entire stock of direct government fixed-term contractual obligations to others that is outstanding on a given date. It includes domestic and foreign liabilities such as currency and money deposits, securities other than shares, and loans. It is the gross amount of government liabilities minus the amount of equity and financial derivatives held by the government. Because debt is a stock rather than a flow, it is measured as of a given date, usually the last day of the fiscal year.

Total debt service (% of exports of goods, services, & income): the sum of principal repayments and interest actually paid in foreign currency, goods, or services on long-term debt, interest paid on short-term debt, and repayments (repurchases and charges) to the IMF.

Present value of external debt (current million US$): the sum of short-term external debt, plus the discounted sum, over the life of existing loans, of total debt service payments due on public, publicly guaranteed, and private nonguaranteed long-term external debt.

Cumulative debt relief committed under HIPC (million US$ in end-2009 NPV terms): the net present value of debt relief committed when a country reaches its decision point under the enhanced HIPC (Heavily Indebted Poor Countries) initiative. It is calculated as the amount needed to bring the net present value (NPV) of the country's debt level down to the thresholds established by the HIPC Initiative (no more than 150 percent of exports or, in certain cases, 250 percent of fiscal revenues). To reach decision point, a country must have a track record of macroeconomic stability, must have prepared an Interim Poverty Reduction Strategy Paper through a participatory process, and must have cleared, or reached an agreement on a process to clear, the outstanding arrears to multilateral creditors. When a country reaches decision point, the amount of debt relief necessary to bring its debt indicators to HIPC thresholds is calculated and the country begins to receive debt relief. The Heavily Indebted Poor Countries (HIPC) initiative is an international effort to improve developing countries' debt sustainability. Launched in 1996 and enhanced in 1999 to broaden and accelerate debt relief, the HIPC initiative is the first joint effort by a united group of multilateral, official bilateral, and commercial creditors to reduce the external debt of the world's most debt-burdened poor countries to sustainable levels.

Net Official Development Assistance provided as % of OECD/DAC donor's GNI: donors' Gross National Income (GNI) at market prices is the total of gross primary incomes that are receivable by resident institutional units and sectors. In contrast to Gross Domestic Product (GDP), GNI is a concept of income rather than value added. GNI is calculated as GDP (the final market price value of the production activity of resident producer units) minus taxes (less subsidies) on production and imports, compensation of employees, and property income payable to the rest of the world, plus the corresponding payments receivable from the rest of the world.

Net Official Development Assistance provided that is untied (%): assistance from one country to another for which the associated goods and services may be fully and freely procured in substantially all countries.

Net Official Development Assistance provided to help build trade capacity (%): assistance that enhances the ability of the recipient country to formulate and implement a trade development strategy; to create an enabling environment for increasing the volume and value-added of exports, diversifying export products and markets, and increasing foreign investment to generate jobs and trade; to stimulate trade by domestic firms and encourage investment in trade-oriented industries; and to benefit from the institutions, negotiations, and processes that shape national trade policy and the rules and practices of international commerce.

Net Official Development Assistance provided to basic social services in 2009 (current million US$): basic social services include basic education, composed of primary education, basic life skills for youth and adults, and early childhood education; and primary health care, composed of basic health care, basic health infrastructure, basic nutrition, infectious disease control, health education, and health personnel development. Basic social services also include basic drinking water supply, basic sanitation, and multi-sector aid for basic social services.

Agriculture support for OECD countries (% of GDP): is the annual monetary value of all gross transfers from taxpayers and consumers, both domestic and foreign, in the form of subsidies arising from policy measures that support agriculture, minus the associated budgetary receipts. Transfers are counted regardless of their objectives and impacts on farm production and income or on consumption of farm products. Agriculture comprises plant and animal products, including tree crops but excluding timber and fish products.

SOURCES

Columns 1-6: World Bank (2011), World Development Indicators 2011. Columns 7-13: United Nations (2011), Millennium Development Goals Indicators.

TABLES 3 AND 4

Food insecure: if a household's access to adequate food is limited by a lack of money and other resources at some time during the year.

Very low food security: the food intake of some household members was reduced and normal eating patterns were disrupted due to limited resources at times during the year.

Poverty: if a family of four, with two adults and two children, has a total money income less than $22,113, then that family and every individual in it are considered in poverty.

SNAP: is the common abbreviation for the Supplemental Nutrition Assistance Program. The number of persons participating is reported monthly. The annual average is the sum of the months divided by twelve.

WIC: is the common abbreviation for Special Supplemental Nutrition Program for Women, Infants, and Children. Participation data are 12-month averages.

School Breakfast Program and National School Lunch Program: participation data are nine-month averages; summer months (June-August) are excluded. Participation is based on average daily meals divided by an attendance factor of 0.927.

Summer food service program: average daily attendance is reported for July only, the peak month of national program activity. Unlike participation data in the National School Lunch and Breakfast programs, average daily attendance is not adjusted for absenteeism.

SOURCES

TABLE 3: *Total population:* U.S. Census Bureau (2011), 2010 Census Data. Data for 2000-2009 come from earlier Census data. *Food insecurity:* Alisha Coleman-Jensen and others (September 2011), Household Food Security in the United States in 2010, Economic Research Report, No. 125, Economic Research Service, U.S. Department of Agriculture. *Federal budget spent on food assistance:* Bread for the World Institute estimate. Data are from spending for U.S. Department of Agriculture's Food and Nutrition Service programs. *Infant mortality rates:* T.J. Mathews and Marian F. MacDorman (June 29, 2011), Infant Mortality Statistics from the 2007 Period: Linked Birth/Infant Death Data Set, National Vital Statistics Reports, Vol. 59, No. 6, Centers for Disease Control and Prevention, U.S. Department of Health and Human Services. *Poverty rates:* Carmen DeNavas-Walt, Bernadette D. Proctor, and Jessica C. Smith (September 2011), Income, Poverty, and Health Insurance Coverage in the United States: 2010, Current Population Reports, U.S. Census Bureau, U.S. Department of Commerce. *Unemployment:* Bureau of Labor Statistics, U.S. Department of Labor (April 2011), "Labor Force Statistics from the Current Population Survey." *Household income distribution:* U.S. Census Bureau, U.S. Department of Commerce (September 2011), Income Inequality: Share of Aggregate Income Received by Each Fifth and Top 5 Percent of....

TABLE 4: Columns 1 and 2: Alisha Coleman-Jensen and others (September 2011), Household Food Security in the United States in 2010, Economic Research Report, No. 125, Economic Research Service, U.S. Department of Agriculture. Columns 3-6: 2010 American Community Survey 1-Year Estimates, American FactFinder, U.S. Department of Commerce (September 2011), "Table S1703: Selected Characteristics of People at Specified Levels of Poverty in the Past 12 Months." Columns 7-11: Food and Nutrition Service, U.S. Department of Agriculture (2011), Data & Statistics: FNS Program Data.

Sponsors

The Hunger Report would not be possible without the generous support of our sponsors.

Co-Publisher
(Donations of $25,000 or more)

Margaret Wallhagen and Bill Strawbridge

Benefactors
(These donors have historically donated $5,000 or more)

American Baptist Churches World Relief supports, enables, and encourages emergency relief, refugee work, disaster rehabilitation, and development assistance. It is funded by the One Great Hour of Sharing offering. It is the responsibility of the World Relief Committee to designate where donations will go in the coming year. Today, One Great Hour of Sharing serves people in over 80 countries around the world. Sponsored by nine Christian U.S. denominations and Church World Service, One Great Hour of Sharing makes sure that it can respond to needs as soon as they happen and that tens of thousands of people receive support for ongoing relief, rehabilitation, and development.

P.O. Box 851
Valley Forge, PA 19482
Phone: (800) 222-3872 ext. 2245
www.abc-oghs.org

Canadian Foodgrains Bank is a partnership of all major Canadian church-based agencies working to end hunger in developing countries. In addition to cash donations, substantial amounts of food grain are donated directly from Canadian farmers and from more than 200 community groups that collectively grow crops for donation to the Canadian Foodgrains Bank. Hunger-related programming is supported by the Foodgrains Bank through its 15 member agencies and includes food aid, food security, nutrition programming, and food justice.

Box 767, 400-393 Portage Avenue
Winnipeg, Manitoba
Canada R3C 2L4
Phone: (204) 944-1993
Toll Free: (800) 665.0377
cfgb@foodgrainsbank.ca
www.foodgrainsbank.ca

Catholic Charities USA includes more than 1,700 local agencies and institutions nationwide, providing help and creating hope for more than 8.5 million people of all faiths. More than half of Catholic Charities services are in food services: food banks and pantries, soup kitchens, congregate dining, and home delivered meals. For more than 280 years, Catholic Charities agencies have been providing vital services in their communities, ranging from day care and counseling to emergency assistance and housing.

Sixty-Six Canal Center Plaza
Suite 600
Alexandria, VA 22314
Phone: (703) 549-1390
www.catholiccharitiesusa.org

Church of the Brethren, Global Food Crisis Fund is the Church of the Brethren's approach to education, advocacy, and action on matters of food security. It crosses cultural and national barriers to serve humanitarian need and to build mutual understanding. It affirms the parallels between the Millennium Development Goals and the Sermon on the Mount. The Global Food Crisis Fund partners with the poor in promoting environmentally sustainable agriculture, raising awareness as to the causes of hunger, and entering into works of compassion that convey the love and fullness of Christ.

1451 Dundee Ave
Elgin, IL 60120
Phone: 1-800-323-8039, ext. 264
www.brethren.org

Church World Service works with local organizations worldwide to support sustainable development, meet emergency needs, help the displaced, and address the root causes of poverty, hunger, and powerlessness. Founded in 1946, Church World Service works in partnership with local organizations worldwide to support sustainable development, meet emergency needs, and address the root causes of poverty and hunger.

475 Riverside Drive, Suite 700
New York, NY 10115-0050
Phone: (800) 297-1516
www.churchworldservice.org

Community of Christ engages the church and others in a response to the needs of hungry people throughout the world. Its primary purpose is to support programs of food production, storage and distribution; fund projects to provide potable water; supply farm animals; instruct in food preparation and nutrition; and educate in marketing strategies for produce. It also seeks to advocate for the hungry and educate about the causes and alleviation of hunger in the world.

1001 W. Walnut
Independence, MO 64050-3562
Phone: (816) 833-1000, ext. 2216
www.cofchrist.org

Cooperative Baptist Fellowship is a fellowship of Baptist Christians and churches who share a passion for the Great Commission of Jesus Christ and a commitment to Baptist principles of faith and practice. The Fellowship's purpose is to serve Christians and churches as they discover and fulfill their God-given mission. One of the Fellowship's strategic initiatives is engaging in holistic missions and ministries among the most neglected in a world without borders.

2930 Flowers Road South, Ste. 133
Atlanta, GA 30341
Phone: (770) 220-1600
www.thefellowship.info

Evangelical Covenant Church is an effective and efficient humanitarian aid ministry of the Evangelical Covenant Church with a 60 year history. Covenant World Relief collaborates with partners around the world to provide relief, rehabilitation, and transformational community development. These partnerships empower local ministries, increase local involvement, reduce overhead, and facilitate immediate response to disaster and human suffering. Our charge is to love, serve, and work together with the poor, the powerless, and the marginalized.

8303 W Higgins Road
Chicago, IL 60631
Phone: (773) 784-3000
www.covchurch.org/cwr
Blog: blogs.covchurch.org/cwr
Facebook: www.facebook.com/covenantworldrelief

Evangelical Lutheran Church in America World Hunger, the anti-hunger program of the Evangelical Lutheran Church in America, responds to hunger and poverty in the United States and around the world by addressing root causes. Through a comprehensive program of relief, development, education, and advocacy, people are connected to the resources they need to lift themselves out of poverty. The international work of ELCA World Hunger is carried out through ELCA companion relationships as well as through trusted partners like Lutheran World Relief (LWR) and The Lutheran World Federation (LWF). Because of these long-held connections to partners around the world, ELCA World Hunger efforts are efficient and effective. The domestic work of ELCA World Hunger is carried out primarily through the Domestic Hunger Grants Program (relief, development, and community organizing projects).

8765 W. Higgins Road
Chicago, IL 60631-4101
Phone: (800) 638-3522, ext. 2815
www.elca.org

Food and Agriculture Organization (FAO) of the United Nations was founded with a mandate to raise levels of nutrition and standards of living, improve agricultural productivity and better the condition of rural populations. FAO is also a source of knowledge and information, helping developing countries and countries in transition modernize and improve agriculture, forestry, and fisheries practices.

Viale delle Terme di Caracalla
00153 Rome, Italy
Phone: +39 06 57051
www.fao.org

Foods Resource Bank is a Christian response to world hunger. Its goal is for hungry people to know the dignity and hope of feeding themselves by making it possible for them, through sustainable smallholder agricultural programs, to produce food for their families with extra to share, barter or sell. Foods Resource Bank endeavors to build networks with various agricultural communities in "growing projects" in the United States, allowing participants to give a gift only they can give. These volunteers grow crops or raise animals, sell them in the United States and the resulting money is used by implementing members (denominations and their agencies) to establish food security programs abroad.

4479 Central Avenue
Western Springs, IL 60558
Phone: (312) 612-1939
www.FoodsResourceBank.org

Presbyterian Hunger Program

provides a channel for congregations to respond to hunger in the United States and around the world. With a commitment to the ecumenical sharing of human and financial resources, the program provides support for direct food relief efforts, sustainable development and public policy advocacy. The Presbyterian Hunger Program helps thousands of Presbyterian Church (USA) congregations become involved in the study of hunger issues, engage with the communities of need, advocate for just public policies and business practices, and move toward simpler corporate and personal lifestyles.

100 Witherspoon Street
Louisville, KY 40202
Phone: (502) 569-5832
Fax: (502) 569-8963
www.pcusa.org/hunger

United Church of Christ (National)

supports 1.2 million members in congregations and other settings of the United Church of Christ in developing relationships with the greater church community that are global, multiracial and multicultural, open and affirming, and accessible to all. Programs of United Church of Christ National include Volunteer Ministries and National Disaster Ministries, as well as ministries of Refugee

& Immigration, Health & Wholeness Advocacy, and One Great Hour of Sharing and Neighbors In Need special mission offerings.

700 Prospect Ave.
Cleveland, Ohio 44115
Phone: 216-736-2100
www.ucc.org

United Methodist Committee on Relief

is the not-for-profit global humanitarian aid organization of the United Methodist Church. UMCOR is working in more than 80 countries worldwide, including the United States. Its mission, grounded in the teachings of Jesus, is to alleviate human suffering—whether caused by war, conflict or natural disaster, with open hearts and minds to all people. UMCOR responds to natural or civil disasters that are interruptions of such magnitude that they overwhelm a community's ability to recover on its own. UMCOR partners with people to rebuild their communities, livelihoods, health, and homes. In times of acute crisis, UMCOR mobilizes aid to stricken areas–emergency supplies, fresh water, and temporary shelter–and then stays, as long as it takes, to implement long-term recovery and rehabilitation.

475 Riverside Dr., Rm. 1520
New York, NY 10115
Phone: (212) 870-3951
umcor@gbgm-umc.org
www.umcor.org

World Relief

serves the most vulnerable, regardless of religion, race, ethnicity or gender. In 20 countries and 20

locations in the United States, World Relief's innovative ministries focus on economic development, health and social development, and refugee care. World Relief equips churches to minister to people's physical, emotional, and spiritual needs. Since 1944, World Relief has been empowering churches to serve the world's most vulnerable.

7 E. Baltimore Street
Baltimore, MD 21202
Phone: (443) 451-1900
www.WorldRelief.org

World Vision

is a Christian relief and development organization dedicated to providing emergency assistance to children and families affected by natural disasters and civil conflict. It works with communities to develop long-term solutions to alleviate poverty, and advocates for justice on behalf of the poor. World Vision serves more than 100 million people in nearly 100 countries around the world.

34834 Weyerhaeuser Way
South Federal Way, WA 98001 USA
Phone: (888) 511-6593
www.worldvision.org

Friends
(Donations under $5,000)

African Methodist Episcopal Zion Church
www.amez.org

Baptist World Alliance
www.bwanet.org

Bon Secours Health System
www.bshsi.com

Catholic Relief Services
www.crs.org

**Christian Church
(Disciples of Christ)**
www.disciples.org

**Christian Methodist
Episcopal Church**
www.c-m-e.org

**Christian Reformed
Church in North America**
www.crcna.org

**Congressional Hunger
Center**
www.hungercenter.org

Islamic Relief USA
www.islamicreliefusa.org

**Lutheran Church-Missouri
Synod World Relief and
Human Care**
www.lcms.org/worldrelief

Lutheran World Relief
www.lwr.org

**Nazarene Compassionate
Ministries**
www.ncm.org

**Reformed Church
in America**
www.rca.org

**Salvation Army National
Corporation**
www.salvationarmyusa.org

**Willow Creek Community
Church**
www.willowcreek.org/compassion

Index

T

Taiwan   14
Targeting   14, 45, 97, 101
Tariff   30, 43
Tax credits   30, 54, 58
Taxpayers   24, 30, 33, 41, 43
Technology   12, 14, 24, 25, 31, 39, 63, 100, 109, 111, 114
Temporary Assistance for Needy Families (TANF)   77
Temporary legal immigration status   84
Tennessee   35
Texas   31, 44, 81, 84, 102
The Emergency Food Assistance Program (TEFAP)   68, 69, 119
The Grapes of Wrath   73
The Lancet   94, 95, 96
Therapeutic feeding   98
Thompson, Robert L.   29, 32
Thompson-Maier, Linda   51
Thornberry, Sharon   56-57
Thriftway   56
Thune, Sen. John   42
Tobacco   34-35
Tolar, Bryan   83
Tractor   24, 25, 79, 109, 117
Trade   14, 22, 23, 32, 42-44, 60, 97, 108, 109
Trade compliance   43
Trade deficit   22
Trade-distorting   32
Trading partners   9, 14, 17
Trans Atlantic Food Assistance Dialogue (TAFAD)   106
Transport costs (Food aid)   102, 103, 104, 105, 108
Transportation   30, 50, 62, 88
Tufts University   101, 102, 105
Tutwiler, Ann   108

U

U.S. Agency for International Development (USAID)   7, 93, 99, 100, 101, 102, 104, 105, 109, 111, 113
U.S. Agricultural Assistance Act of 1933   22
U.S. Apple Association   77
U.S. Department of Agriculture (USDA)   11, 13, 14, 15, 22, 27, 28, 29, 31, 32, 33, 39, 41, 42, 44, 48, 49, 52, 54, 55, 57, 59, 60, 61, 62, 63, 65, 66, 67, 68, 73, 74, 76, 82, 99, 102, 104, 105, 107, 108, 109, 110, 117, 118, 119
U.S. Department of Labor (DOL)   86, 89

U.S. economy   vii, 5, 10, 11, 14, 22, 40, 47, 49, 59, 87
U.S. Global Change Research Program   26
U.S. Global Hunger and Food Security Initiative   3, 7, 9, 16, 93
   (*see also* Feed the Future)
U.S. government   vii, 3, 4, 5, 7, 9, 10, 11, 13, 14, 15, 16, 21, 22, 23, 24, 26, 27, 28, 31, 33, 34, 35, 36, 37, 38, 39, 40, 41, 42, 43, 44, 45, 47, 48, 54, 58, 59, 60, 63, 66, 68, 69, 73, 86, 91, 93, 99, 104, 106, 114, 117, 118, 119
U.S. Government Accountability Office (GAO)   99, 100, 102, 103, 104, 105, 107, 108
U.S. House of Representatives   vii, 80
U.S. Millennium Challenge Corporation   109
U.S. State Department   79, 104
Uganda   107, 111
Unauthorized immigrants   72, 73, 76, 80, 83, 84
Undernutrition   34, 94, 104
Unemployment   viii, 5, 11, 31, 47, 54, 55, 56, 67, 76, 86, 91
Unhealthy foods   13, 36
UNICEF   95, 98
United Nations   16, 26, 94, 95
United Nations Food and Agriculture Organization (FAO)   26
United Nations High-Level Task Force on Global Food Security   95
United Way   118
University of South Carolina   54
Urban   50, 65, 81, 90, 102
Utilities   62

V

Value chain   108
Value-added   22, 27, 28, 38, 85
Value-added producer grant   28
Vander Meulen, Rebecca J.   96-97
Vegetables   4, 6, 12, 13, 21, 27, 28, 33, 34, 35, 37, 39, 40, 41, 50, 51, 52, 61, 63, 64, 65, 66, 71, 72, 81-83, 85, 106
Vermont   65
Vilsack, Tom   36, 37
Virginia   35, 87
Vitamins and minerals   4, 21, 33, 94, 96, 98, 101
Volatile food prices   15, 17
Volunteer Efforts for Development Concerns (VEDCO)   111

W

Wabwire, Faustine   16
Wages   6, 67, 71, 73, 74, 76, 84, 86, 91
Wall Street   48
Wal-Mart   18, 36, 50
Washington   76, 77, 80, 81, 91
Washington Growers League   77, 80
Washington, DC   37, 80, 95, 117, 118
Wasting   96, 104
Water   10, 26, 27, 28, 78, 80, 97, 99, 103, 109
Water pollution   26
Waiver   59
Weill, Jim   58
Welfare Reform   77
West Africa   110
West Coast   23, 74
Wheat   16, 31
White House   11, 18, 58
Whole food   18
Whole Foods   36
Whole-farm insurance   62
Williams, Rob   87
Winne, Mark   51, 52
Witnesses to Hunger   3, 54, 60
Woodruff County, AR   31
Worker Protection Standards   78
World Bank   95, 106
World Food Program   16, 98, 100, 102-104, 107
World Health Organization   99
World Trade Organization (WTO)   32, 43, 44, 114
World Vision   102
World War II   49, 73, 74

Y

Yale   51, 52, 61

Z

Zambia   25, 107